CBS SERIES FOR CAT

# Analytical Reasoning for

# CAT

COMMON ADMISSION TEST

## PROBLEMS and SOLUTIONS

*Other book in the series by the same author:*

**Mathematics for CAT**

CBS SERIES FOR CAT

# Analytical Reasoning for CAT

COMMON ADMISSION TEST

## PROBLEMS and SOLUTIONS

KAUSHAL KUMAR

CBS

CBS PUBLISHERS & DISTRIBUTORS

New Delhi ⊙ Bangalore

CBS Series for CAT

*Analytical Reasoning for CAT*



ISBN : 81-239-1230-7

First Edition: 2005

Reprint : 2007



*Production Director :* Vinod K. Jain

*Published by :*
Satish Kumar Jain for CBS Publishers & Distributors,
4596/1-A, 11 Darya Ganj, New Delhi - 110 002 (India)
E-mail : cbspubs@vsnl.com
Website : www.cbspd.com

*Branch Office :*
Seema House, 2975, 17th Cross, K.R. Road,
Bansankari 2nd Stage, Bangalore - 560070
Fax : 080-26771680 • E-mail : cbsbng@vsnl.net

*Typeset at CBS P&D Typesetting unit and printed at*
India Binding House, Noida (UP).

# Preface

This book is designed on the pattern of mathematical reasoning problems that are routinely asked in CAT. Every year CAT asks a few innovative questions based on analytical reasoning which are difficult to crack as they cannot be solved through conventional methods and needs ingenuity. The book contains 360 original questions, almost all typical and each problem needs to be dealt uniquely. The author has tried to develop a mathematical approach towards the solutions of these problems which otherwise are very abstract and not amenable to direct solution through any common conventional methods.

The purpose of this book is to expose the readers to numerous forms of abstract questions, each one requiring unique non-conventional method of solving problems which are being progressively employed in all national and international level entrance exams. Although the questions might seem formidable at the first instance, it is urged that the readers go through the problems and solutions, if necessary, so as to develop a mental ability and skill for handling such problems. Some of the problems here may not conform to the time limits set by CAT but they could be highly innovative and conceptual, and modified by the examiners to bring them under desired time limits.

The book, though written exclusively for CAT, will nevertheless serve the purpose of other management entrance exams, various competitive exams and campus interviews which regularly employ the analytically reasoning section to test the mental level of the candidates.

Alternatively, this book can be seen as one on the mathematical puzzles that will definitely tease the brains of puzzle lovers.

The first section of this volume contains the PROBLEMS, at the end of which KEYS have been given for the convenience of the reader. The second section contains SOLUTIONS which have been given in details. The students should first attempt to solve the problem on his/her own, and should proceed to look at the key and the solution only after making a reasonable attempt to workout the problem. This method, if followed earnestly by the reader, will greatly help in honing the sense of analysis, widen the vision of reasoning and give deftness in handling the problems with good technique and competence. I do hope that this publication will set the standards high and be a trailblazer in its category.

I have ensured that the patterns and structures of all the problems set and included in the book are original and exclusive in most respects.

I have attempted my best to weed out all the errors as much as possible, but still a few might have remained undetected or uncorrected. I will be thankful to the readers for pointing out those errors, so that I could rectify them in the next reprint/edition. Kindly send me your critical comments and suggestions at my e-mail address: kaushalkumar00@yahoo.co.in.

**KAUSHAL KUMAR**
e-mail: <kaushalkumar00@yahoo.co.in>

March 15, 2005
New Delhi

# Contents

# Analytical Reasoning for CAT

# Problems

# Analytical Reasoning for CAT

## Problems

1. A circle is divided into $n$ parts and the parts are being over-written with red (R), blue (B) and green (G) colour pencil in the fashion as shown in the adjoining figure. Let the process start at $A_1$ in the clockwise manner. If $A_1 A_n$ is overwritten with red pencil, then $n$ can be equal to

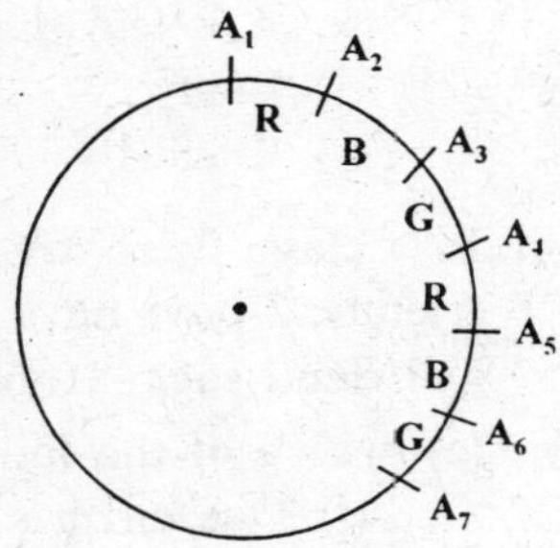


(i) 1257 (ii) 2357 (iii) 1438 (iv) 2876

2. $A_1 \; A_2 \; A_3$ ......................... $A_n$

Shown above is $n$ (> 50) lampposts arranged as given. A boy runs to and from between $A_1$ and $A_n$ counting each post he gets past. If the boy starts running from $A_1$, then

(a) which of the following count will always come on a fixed lamppost for any integral value of $m$?

(i) $2\,mn - m$ (ii) $2\,mn + m$

(iii) $2\,mn - n$ (iv) $2\,mn + n$

(b) the count 100 $n$ will come on the lamppost

(i) $A_{47}$ (ii) $A_{48}$ (iii) $A_{49}$ (iv) $A_{50}$

3. To deal with a situation, let

(a) A be as competent as B and C together and B as competent as C and A together. Which the following inference can be made?

**I. C is fully incompetent to deal with the situation.**

**II. A and B are alone fully competent to deal with the situation.**

**III. A and B are together fully competent to deal with the situation but not alone.**

(i) I only (ii) I and II

(iii) I and III (iv) none of the these

**(b) A be half as competent as B and C together and B be half as competent as C and A together. Then which of the following inference can be made?**

**I. C is less competent than A.**

**II. A is less competent than C.**

**III. C is less than twice as competent as A.**

**IV. A is less than twice as competent as C.**

(i) I only (ii) II only

(iii) II and III (iv) I and IV

**4. In a class, there are 6 boys and 6 girls. 1 boy has 3 girl-friends, 2 boys have 2 girlfriends each and 3 boys have 1 girlfriend each. If every girl has a boyfriend, then**

**(a) which of the following is possible?**

(i) One girl has six boyfriends

(ii) Two girls have three boyfriends each and another girls has two boyfriends

(iii) Four girls have two boyfriends each

(iv) none of these

**(b) which of the following is not possible?**

(i) One girl has five boyfriends

(ii) Two girls can have three boyfriends in common

(iii) Only three girls have two boyfriends each

(iv) none of these

**5. A, B, C and D are four siblings, two males (M) and two females (F). It is known that B is younger to A, D is younger to C and D is female.**

**(a) The sex of A can be determined if the siblings in the decreasing order of their ages are**

(i) MMFF (ii) MFFM

(iii) FMFM (iv) FMMF

**(b) The sex of B cannot be determined if the siblings in the deceasing order of their ages are**

(i) MFMF (ii) MFFM
(iii) FMFM (iv) FMMF

**(c) The sex of C cannot be determined if the siblings in the deceasing order of their ages are**

(i) MFFM (ii) FFMM
(iii) FMFM (iv) FMMF

**6. There are *n* males and *m* (< *n*) females in a room. A few persons start leaving room in the groups of threes until the numbers of males and females are same. If once, during the process, the number of females became more than the number of males, then the least member of**

**(a) males who went out of the room cannot be**

(i) $n - m + 1$ (ii) $n - m + 2$
(iii) $n - m + 3$ (iv) $n - m + 4$

**(b) females who went out of the room cannot be**

(i) 1 (ii) 2 (iii) 3 (iv) 3

**(c) females who went out of the room, given that $n = 40$ and $m = 10$, is**

(i) 1 (ii) 2 (iii) 3 (iv) 3

**7. $A_1$, $A_2$, $A_3$, $A_4$, $A_5$, and $A_6$ are three couples. If $A_1$ is not married to $A_2$ or $A_3$, $A_2$ is not married to $A_3$ or $A_4$, $A_3$ is not married to $A_4$ or $A_5$, then $A_1$ is married to**

(i) $A_4$ (ii) $A_5$
(iii) $A_6$ (iv) cannot be determined

**8. $A_1$, $A_2$, $A_3$, $A_4$, $A_5$, and $A_6$ are three couples. If $A_1$ is not married to $A_2$, $A_2$ is not married to $A_3$ .................., $A_6$ is not married to $A_1$, then**

**(a) all the couples can be known if it is given that following is a couple**

(i) $A_4A_3$ (ii) $A_1A_4$ (iii) $A_2A_5$ (iv) $A_3A_6$

**(b) the probability that other two couples can be known if one of specified is**

(i) $\frac{1}{6}$ (ii) $\frac{1}{3}$ (iii) $\frac{1}{2}$ (iv) $\frac{2}{3}$

**9. 56 apples are being distributed among four persons, A, B, C and D in the batches of 14 apples such that every one gets at least one apple and no two of them get the same numbers of apples in the distribution of any batch. Let, in the distribution of four batches, everyone get two times odd number of apples and two times even number of apples. If the first two batches are distributed as shown below:**

| A | B | C | D | |
|---|---|---|---|---|
| 3 | 2 | 5 | 4 | |
| 4 | 3 | 1 | 6 , | then |

**(a) the subsequent distributions to which of the following two persons can be exactly known?**

(i) A and D (ii) B and D
(iii) C and D (iv) none of these

**(b) the total number of ways in which the third batch can be distributed is**

(i) 2 (ii) 4 (iii) 6 (iv) 8

**10.**

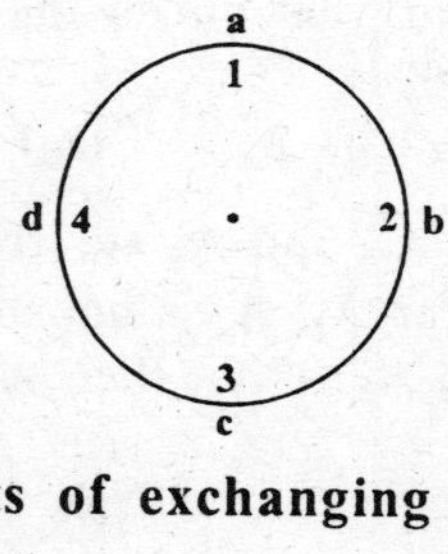


**A process consists of exchanging the letters at the positions**

**(a) (1, 2); (2, 3); (3, 4) and (4, 1) in succession. Which letter will be at the position 3 when the process is executed 100 times successively?**

(i) a (ii) b (iii) c (iv) d

**(b) (1, 2); (2, 4); (3, 4) in succession. Which letter will be at the position 1 when the process is executed 100 times successively?**

(i) a (ii) b (iii) c (iv) d

**(c) (1, 2); (2, 3); (3, 4); (4, 2); (4, 1); (3, 1); (3, 2) and (2, 4) in succession. The whole subprocesses are**

**redundant except the exchange of letters at the positions**

(i) (1, 2) (ii) (1, 3) (iii) (1, 4) (iv) (3, 4)

**11.**

| | | |
|---|---|---|
| a | b | c |
| d | e | f |
| g | h | i |

fig (i)

| | | |
|---|---|---|
| f | h | b |
| c | g | d |
| a | i | e |

fig (ii)

**9 alphabets are placed in 9 blocks as shown in the fig (i). One of the alphabet exchanges its place successively eight times with all the other alphabets once and their positions after the process is shown in the fig (ii).**

**(a) The alphabet which started exchanging its place with other alphabets is**

(i) a (ii) b
(iii) f (iv) cannot be determined

**(b) If the alphabet which exchanged its place exactly after four exchanges took place is e, then the alphabet which exchanged its place exactly after seven exchanges took place is**

(i) c (ii) d
(iii) f (iv) cannot be determined

**12. Consider a $m \times n$ square blocks as shown in the adjoining figure. Two pupils start numbering the blocks one downward and one across, and after they reach the end of the column and row respectively, they start again from the next column and row respectively in the previous fashion.**

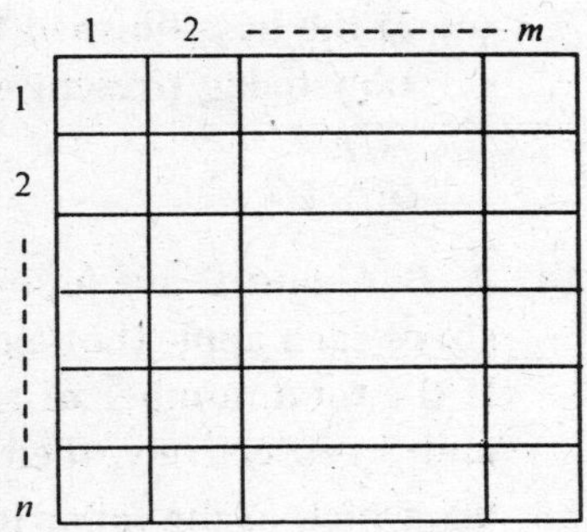


**(a) If $m = 21$ and $n = 41$, then the number of blocks which got the same number by both the pupils is**

(i) 2 (ii) 7 (iii) 13 (iv) 21

**(b) If $m = 20$ and $n = 40$, then the number of blocks which got the same number by both the pupils is**

(i) 2 (ii) 6 (iii) 12 (iv) 20

**(c) Let the first and seventeenth block be same for the two kinds of numbering. If $m = n$, then $m$ can be equal to**

(i) 7, 11 (ii) 7, 15
(iii) 11, 15 (iv) none of these

**13. A boss can do a job in two days if his four secretaries A, B, C and D are all present. His efficiency got reduced to $\frac{1}{6}, \frac{1}{4}, \frac{1}{3}, \frac{1}{2}$ respectively according as A, B, C and D remain absent. In any day only one secretary remains absent. Also the boss finishes his work exactly in integral number of days.**

**(a) Which of following secretary cannot be absent for an odd number of days?**

(i) A (ii) B (iii) C (iv) D

**(b) If each secretary remained absent for at least one day, then in how many days the boss could finished the work?**

(i) 5, 6 or 7 days (ii) 6, 7 or 8 days
(iii) 6, 8 or 9 days (iv) 7, 8 or 9 days

**(c) If the boss finished his work in 6 days with one secretary being present everyday, then the secretary was**

(i) A (ii) B
(iii) C (iv) cannot be determined

**14. A, B, C and D are four brothers who get apples and they share each apple (half and half) with one of their brothers. If the total number of apples eaten by them are 13, 11, 9 and 7 respectively, then**

**(a) which of the following pair of brothers shared exactly equal numbers of apples?**

(i) (A, B) and (C, D) (ii) (A, C) and (B, D)
(iii) (A, D) and (B, C) (iv) none of these

**(b)** the number of apples which B, C and D shared exclusively among themselves is
(i) 9 (ii) 10 (iii) 11 (iv) 12

**15.** $A_1, A_2, A_3, A_4$ are four variables connected by a linear equation. If

| $A_1$ | $A_2$ | $A_3$ | $A_4$ |
|---|---|---|---|
| 0 | 0 | 0 | 0 |
| 1 | 2 | 3 | 4 |
| 4 | 5 | 6 | 8 |

where numbers in column denote values of the corresponding variables and each row denotes the values of variables satisfying the equation.

**(a)** The value of $A_1$, given $A_2 = 5$, $A_3 = 9$ and $A_4 = 12$, is
(i) 1 (ii) 2
(iii) 3 (iv) cannot be determined

**(b)** If $A_1 = A_4 = 0$ , then which of the following necessarily follows?
(i) $A_1 = A_2$ (ii) $A_1 = A_2 = 0$
(iii) $A_1 = 2A_2$ (iv) none of these

**(c)** Let $A_1$, $A_2$ and $A_3$ be given. The value of $A_1$ can be uniquely determined if
(i) $A_3 = 2A_2 - A_1$ (ii) $2A_3 = A_2 - 3A_1$
(iii) $2A_3 = 2A_2 - A_1$ (iv) none of these

**16.** 9 consecutive positive integers are placed in each block of the adjoining figure.

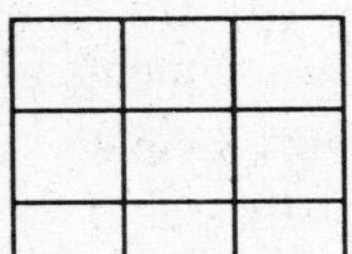

Let S be the total sum of the sum of numbers in the diagonal blocks and the middle (row and column) blocks.

**(a)** If $446 \le S \le 454$, then the least number placed in a block is
(i) 39 (ii) 40 (iii) 41 (iv) 42

**(b)** S cannot be equal to
(i) 154 (ii) 175 (iii) 186 (iv) 199

**17.** $A_1, A_2, A_3, A_4$ are four persons each having few coins of 1 rupee.

**(a)** If $A_1$ retains a rupee coin and can distribute his rest of money among other such that others have equal

**number of coins and $A_2$ retains *m* rupee coins and can distribute his rest of money among others such that others have equal number of coins, then *m* can be equal to**

(i) 2 (ii) 3 (iii) 4 (iv) all of these

**(b) If $A_1$, $A_2$, $A_3$, and $A_4$ retain 0, 3, 6 and 9 coins respectively and can distribute their rest of money among others such that others have equal number of coins, then the least number of coin, they can have together is**

(i) 27 (ii) 30 (iii) 33 (iv) 36

**(c) Let the number of coins with $A_1$, $A_2$, $A_3$, $A_4$ be *a*, *a* + 3, *a* + 6, *a* + 9 respectively. If they respectively retain 0, 3, and 9 coins and can distribute their rest of money among others such that others have equal number of coins, then the least value of *a* is**

(i) 3 (ii) 12 (iii) 15 (iv) 18

**18. Let $S_1$ be the set of sum of variables in each row and $S_2$ be the set of sum of variables in each column. Then which of the following is necessarily true?**

| | | |
|---|---|---|
| x | b | α |
| β | y | c |
| a | γ | z |

(i) If one of the elements of $S_1$ is equal to an element of $S_2$, then the other elements of set are also pairwise equal

(ii) If two of the elements of $S_1$ is equal to two of the elements of $S_2$, then the third elements of both sets must be equal

(iii) Both (iv) None

**19. Six birds, all of a different kinds ($X_1$, $X_2$, $X_3$, $X_4$, $X_5$, $X_6$), are put in pair in 3 cages. ($X_1$, $X_2$), ($X_2$, $X_3$), ($X_3$, $X_4$), ($X_4$, $X_5$), and ($X_5$, $X_6$) cannot be put together in a cage.**

**(a) All the required pair cannot be determined if it is known that $X_1$ is put together with**

(i) $X_3$ (ii) $X_4$ (iii) $X_5$ (iv) $X_6$

**(b) If one of the pair is given, then what is the probability that all the other required pairs can be determined?**

(i) $\frac{4}{10}$ (ii) $\frac{5}{10}$ (iii) $\frac{5}{11}$ (iv) $\frac{6}{11}$

**20.** **$X_1$, $X_2$, $X_3$, $X_4$, $X_5$ and $X_6$ are 6 persons of which only two have the same height. Let all persons of the triplets ($X_1$, $X_2$, $X_3$); ($X_4$, $X_5$, $X_6$); ($X_2$, $X_3$, $X_4$); ($X_5$, $X_6$, $X_1$); ($X_1$, $X_3$, $X_6$) and ($X_4$, $X_2$, $X_5$) are of different heights.**

**(a) The persons with same height are necessarily**

(i) $X_1$ and $X_4$ (ii) $X_2$ and $X_6$
(iii) $X_3$ and $X_5$ (iv) none of these

**(b) How many pairs are possible which can have the same height?**

(i) 1 (ii) 2 (iii) 3 (iv) 4

**21.** **$X_1$, $X_2$, $X_3$, $X_4$ and $X_5$ entered into a race and it was found that had the speeds of $X_1$, $X_2$, $X_3$ been twice in succession, they would've stood third, second and first respectively in the race. Also the speed of each person was less than twice of that of the person just behind him. Which of the following is necessarily correct?**

(i) $X_1$ was just behind $X_2$ (ii) $X_2$ was just behind $X_3$
(iii) BOTH (iv) None

**22.** **$a_1$, $a_2$, $a_3$, .............. $a_6$ are six consecutive integers (not necessarily in orders). If**

**$5a_1 + 6a_2 + 10a_3 = 5a_4 + 6a_5 + 10a_6$**

**and the integers are written in increasing order, then**

**(a) the extreme terms are**

(i) ($a_1$, $a_2$) (ii) ($a_2$, $a_5$)
(iii) ($a_3$, $a_6$) (iv) cannot be determined

**(b) the middle terms are**

(i) ($a_1$, $a_6$) (ii) ($a_1$, $a_4$)
(iii) ($a_3$, $a_4$) (iv) cannot be determined

**23.** **Eight delegates from a guest country handshaked with ten delegates from the host country. If the total handshakes between men and women was 40, then it can be concluded that the**

(i) delegates of one of the country have equal number of males and females
(ii) delegates of both the countries have equal number of males and femaies
(iii) total number of male delegates (both countries) is nine
(iv) none of these

**24. A, B and C are three persons sitting on a bench. They exchange their places such that each of them is not sitting on their previous positions. If now two of them exchange their places again, then**

(i) two of them will be at their original positions
(ii) one of them will be at their original positions
(iii) none of them will be at his original positions
(iv) cannot be determined

**25. A, B, C and D are four children playing a game by passing a ball to one another, the child receiving the ball just not passing it immediately to one from whom he gets it. Let during the game A, B and C held the ball 3, 5 and 7 times respectively. If C started the game and first/last holding of the ball also counts, then**

**(a) the minimum number of times D held the ball would have been**

(i) 1 (ii) 2 (iii) 3 (iv) 4

**(b) the minimum number of times D held the ball, given that he held the ball in the last, would have been**

(i) 3 (ii) 4 (iii) 5 (iv) 6

**(c) the maximum number of times D held the ball would have been**

(i) 6 (ii) 7 (iii) 8 (iv) 9

**26. A man divided his property among his 4 sons A, B, C and D who get 10%, 20%, 30%, and 40% of the property respectively. The sons divided their properties equally among other three brothers and hence their share of properties got changed. If this process is continued for**

**(a) 5 times, then the share of A will be about**

(i) 26% (ii) 27% (iii) 28% (iv) 29%

**(b) large number of times, then the share of D will be nearly**

(i) 25% (ii) 28% (iii) 31% (iv) 33%

**27. A boy spends $x_1$, $x_2$, $x_3$ ........... $x_{30}$ per cent of his money he is left with *n*th day after he has received his pocket money on the first day of a month. If the boy spends same**

amount of money everyday, then which of the following can be the element of the set $\{x_1, x_2, x_3 \ldots\ldots\ldots\ldots x_{30}\}$?

(i) 4 (ii) 8 (iii) 16 (iv) any of these

28. **A man can buy three of the articles A, B or C. With all the money he has , he can buy as many articles of A as one of its article cost. He could as well buy as many articles of B as one of its article cost with Rs 57 being left; as many articles of C as one of its article cost with Rs 10*x* being left where *x* is a single digit integer. Then**

**(a) $x =$**

(i) 3 (ii) 4 (iii) 7 (iv) 9

**(b) what is the difference between the cost of an article of B and C?**

(i) Rs 1 (ii) Rs 3 (iii) Rs 4 (iv) Rs 5

29. **$F_1$, $F_2$, $F_3$, $F_4$, $F_5$, $F_6$ and $F_7$ are seven different food products, each deficient in exactly one of vitamins A, B, C and D and each vitamin is deficient in at least one of the food products. If it is known that at best one of the combination of food products**
**$(F_1, F_2)$; $(F_3, F_4)$; $(F_5, F_6)$ is deficient in vitamin A,**
**$(F_2, F_3)$; $(F_7, F_5)$; $(F_1, F_6)$ is deficient in vitamin B and**
**$(F_1, F_7)$; $(F_3, F_5)$; $(F_2, F_4)$ is deficient in vitamin C, then**

**(a) $F_1$ is deficient in vitamin**

(i) A (ii) B (iii) C (iv) D

**(b) $F_2$ is deficient in vitamin**

(i) A (ii) B (iii) C (iv) D

**(c) which of the following is deficient in vitamin D?**

(i) $F_1$ (ii) $F_4$ (iii) $F_6$ (iv) $F_7$

30. **A, B and C are three different food products of calories 200, 300 and 400 kcal respectively. If one wants to buy foods of total calorie 1000 kcal out of the three food products, one need to spend either Rs 29 or Rs 32 or Rs 38 or Rs 41 where one does not buy only of the food products. Given that the cost of each food products are integer,**

**(a) what can be the price of A?**

(i) Rs 8 (ii) Rs 9 (iii) Rs 10 (iv) Rs 11

**(b) which will be the costliest?**

(i) A (ii) B

(iii) C (iv) cannot be determined

**31. A, B and C are three persons having Rs 90, Rs 100 and Rs 120 (not in order). They together bought three articles P, Q and R, the shares of A, B and C in them being 1:1:2, 2:3:1, 2:1:2 respectively. Assuming that all the money the persons had was spent,**

**(a) how much money A initially had?**

(i) Rs 90 (ii) Rs 100

(iii) Rs 120 (iv) cannot be determined

**(b) how much money C initially had?**

(i) Rs 90 (ii) Rs 100

(iii) Rs 120 (iv) cannot be determined

**(c) the cost of Q is**

(i) Rs 72 (ii) Rs 94

(iii) Rs 96 (iv) cannot be determined

**(d) which is the cheapest article?**

(i) P (ii) Q

(iii) R (iv) cannot be determined

**(e) which is the costliest article?**

(i) P (ii) Q

(iii) R (iv) cannot be determined

**32. P, Q, R and S are four persons with one of then having Rs 150, Rs 100, Rs 50 more than the other three. A, B, C and D are four articles with one of them having its price Rs 30, Rs 20, Rs 10 more than the other three. It is found that with all their money, P can buy one article each of A, B, C and D; Q can buy an article each of C and D; R can buy 3 articles of B and an article of D; S can buy 3 articles of C and an article of A.**

**(a) What is the price of D?**

(i) Rs 40 (ii) Rs 50

(iii) Rs 60 (iv) cannot be determined

**(b) The price of which article can be only either the least the or most?**

(i) A (ii) B (iii) C (iv) B or C

**(c) If Q has Rs 120, then the price of the least expensive article is**

(i) Rs 30 (ii) Rs 40 (iii) Rs 50 (iv) Rs 55

**(d) If B the is most expensive article, then its price is**

(i) Rs 60 (ii) Rs 65 (iii) Rs 70 (iv) Rs 75

**(e) The difference between the initial money of Q and that of which other person is constant for all possible cases?**

(i) P (ii) R

(iii) S (iv) none of these

**33. A, B, C and D are four towns all interconnected by roads of same length equal to 1 mile. A car is going from one town to another without just returning back by the same road.**

**(a) If the car starts from A and after covering 100 miles, it is again at A, then the least number of times the car would have passed through D is**

(i) 0 (ii) 1 (iii) 2 (iv) 3

**(b) If the car starts from A and after covering 101 miles, it is again at A, then the least number of times the car would have passed through D is**

(i) 0 (ii) 1 (iii) 2 (iv) 3

**(c) If the car starts from A and after covering (30 + $i$) ($i$ = 1 or 2) miles, it is at B, then the least number of time it would have passed through D is**

(i) 0 (ii) $i - 1$ (iii) $i$ (iv) none of these

**34. A, B, C, D and E are five students who appeared in a test of total marks 100. Study the following observations:**

**(i) If E had got 30 marks more, he would have got the number equal to the topper.**

**(ii) If D had got 20 marks more, he would have got the number equal to the second topper.**

**(iii) If C had got 20 marks less, he would have got the number equal to the student getting the least number.**

**(iv) If A had got 30 marks less, he would have got the number equal to the student getting the least number.**

**Now answer the following questions:**

**(a) The topper**

(i) must be A (ii) must be B

(iii) must be A or C (iv) must be A, B or C

**(b) The student who got the least number**

(i) must be E (ii) must be D

(iii) must be E or D (iv) can be E, D or A

**(c) The second topper**

(i) must be B (ii) must be C

(iii) must be B or C (iv) can be B, C or A

**(d) The student who got the fourth rank**

(i) must be D (ii) must be E

(iii) must be D or E (iv) can be D, E or C

**35. A, B, C, D, E, F, G and H are four couples, they are said to arrange themselves in pairs of one man and one woman. Let four ways of their arrangement be as shown by the rows shown below.**

**A.**

| Rows | Arrangement in Pairs | | | |
|---|---|---|---|---|
| I | AD | BG | CE | FH |
| II | AE | BH | CD | FG |
| III | AG | BD | CH | FE |
| IV | AH | BE | CG | FD |

**(a) Which of the following must be true?**

(i) There must be a couple in each row

(ii) There must be a couple in each column

(iii) Both (iv) None

**(b) If A is married to D, B is not married to G, C is not married to E, then F can be married to**

(i) E or G (ii) G or H

(iii) E or H (iv) E, G or H

**B.**

| Rows | Arrangement in Pairs | | | |
|---|---|---|---|---|
| I | AE | BH | CD | FG |
| II | AG | BE | CD | FH |
| III | AD | BH | CG | FE |
| IV | AH | BD | CE | FG |

**If each row and each column has exactly one couple, then**

**(a) A is married to**
(i) D (ii) E (iii) G (iv) H

**(b) B is married to**
(i) D (ii) E (iii) G (iv) H

**(c) C is married to**
(i) D (ii) E (iii) G (iv) H

C.

| **Rows** | **Arrangement in Pairs** | | | |
|---|---|---|---|---|
| **I** | **AD** | **BG** | **CE** | **FH** |
| **II** | **AE** | **BH** | **CD** | **FG** |
| **III** | **AG** | **BD** | **CH** | **FE** |
| **IV** | **AH** | **BE** | **CG** | **FD** |

**If each row has exactly one couple,**

**(a) then B cannot be married to**
(i) D (ii) E (iii) G (iv) H

**(b) and A is married to D, then C is married to**
(i) E (ii) G
(iii) H (iv) cannot be determined

**(c) and if A is married to E, then G is married to**
(i) B (ii) C
(iii) F (iv) cannot be determined

**36. A, B, C, D, E and F are grouped into 3 pairs, viz. (A, D), (B, F) and (C, E). The pair is splited and then again combined to form 3 pairs all distinct from previous ones. Again the pairs is splited and then combined to from another set of 3 pairs, viz. (A, B), (C, D) and (E, F) all distinct from the previous pairs. Then all the pairs of the intermediate steps**

**(a) can be known if it is known that following is a pair:**
(i) A, F (ii) B, C
(iii) D, F (iv) none of these

**(b) cannot be known if it is known that following is a pair:**
(i) A, C (ii) A, E
(iii) A, F (iv) none of these

**(c) could have exhibited themselves in *n* different ways where *n* =**
(i) 3 (ii) 4 (iii) 5 (iv) 6

**37. A, B, C, D, E are five persons who are asked to pick one of 5 coins of Rs 1, 2, 3, 4 and 5.**

**A. A process consists of exchanging coin of Rs 1 with that of Rs 2, then Rs 2 with that of Rs 3 and so on until the coin of Rs 5 has been exchanged.**

**(a) This process is executed twice and after that A has the coin of Rs 1. Then originally A has the coin of Rs**

(i) 2 (ii) 3
(iii) 4 (iv) cannot be determined

**(b) The least number of execution of the process after which all the persons will have the same coins as originally picked by them is**

(i) 5 (ii) 20 (iii) 60 (iv) 120

**(c) Let after the execution of this process a few times, the sequence in which they have the coin of Rs 1 to 5 be BDAEC. If originally A had the coin of Rs 1, then the sequence in which they had the coins of Rs 1 to 5 was**

(i) AECBD (ii) ADBCE
(iii) ADEBC (iv) AEDCB

**B. A process consist of exchanging coins of Rs 1 with that of Rs 2, Rs 2 with that of Rs 3, Rs 3 with that of Rs 4, Rs 4 with that of Rs 5, and Rs 5 with that of Rs 1 in sequence as given. For three consecutive exchanges, the difference between holding of two particular persons is**

**(a) Rs 1. After fourth consecutive exchange, the difference in their holdings will be**

(i) Rs 1 (ii) Rs 2 (iii) Rs 3 (iv) Rs 4

**(b) Rs 2. After fourth consecutive exchange, the difference in their holdings will be**

(i) Rs 1 (ii) Rs 2 (iii) Rs 3 (iv) Rs 4

**38. Five persons A, B, C, D and E are asked to pick one of coins of Rs 1, 2, 3, 4 and 5. Let the coins be denoted by *v*, *w*, *x*, *y* and *z*. A process consist of exchanging *v* with *w*; *w* with *x*; *x* with *y*; *y* with *z* in sequence as given. Consider the following data.**

| Coins | A | B | C | D | E |
|---|---|---|---|---|---|
| Originally | 1 | 2 | 3 | 4 | 5 |
| After the process is executed ones | 2 | 3 | 4 | 5 | 1 |
| After the process is executed twice | $k_1$ | $k_2$ | $k_3$ | $k_4$ | $k_5$ |

**Then**

**(a)** $k_5$ =
(i) 2 (ii) 3
(iii) 4 (iv) cannot be determined

**(b)** $x$, **given** $v = 3$, **is**
(i) 1 (ii) 2 (iii) 4 (iv) 5

**(c)** $w$, **given** $y = 4$, **is**
(i) 1 (ii) 2 (iii) 3 (iv) 5

**39.** ***n* persons each having a coin or Rs 1, 2, and 3 distribute them among 3 donation boxes A, B and C, no person putting two coins in the same box. The collection of boxes A, B and C are respectively Rs 20, Rs 30 and Rs 40 respectively.**

**(a) Which of the following box must got the equal number of coins of Rs 1 and Rs 3?**
(i) A (ii) B
(iii) C (iv) none of these

**(b) The number of coins of Rs 1 in box A cannot be**
(i) 9 (ii) 10 (iii) 11 (iv) 12

**(c)** $n$ =
(i) 9 (ii) 12 (iii) 15 (iv) 18

**40.** **$A_1$, $A_2$, $A_3$ and $A_4$ are four friends who went to a restaurant, three at a time. Each one went to the restaurant three times and each one paid the bill once. The bill paid by $A_1$, $A_2$, $A_3$ and $A_4$ was Rs 300, 400, 500 and 600 respectively while they ate the food costing Rs 500, 300, 600 and 400 respectively. At a time, each one ate the food costing either Rs 100 cr 200.**

**(a) When $A_1$, $A_2$, $A_3$ went together, then the bill was paid by**

(i) $A_1$ (ii) $A_2$
(iii) $A_3$ (iv) cannot be determined

**(b) When $A_1$, $A_2$, $A_4$ went together, then the bill was paid by**

(i) $A_1$ (ii) $A_2$
(iii) $A_4$ (iv) cannot be determined

**(c) When $A_2$, $A_3$, $A_4$ went together, then the bill was paid by**

(i) $A_2$ (ii) $A_3$
(iii) $A_4$ (iv) cannot be determined

**41. A, B, C are three containers of capacity $2(n + 1)$, $n + 2$ and $n$ litres respectively. A process consists of pouring water from one containers to another. Let, initially, A is empty while B and C are full with water. The least number of process after which**

**(a) C will hold 2 litres of water is**

(i) 3 (ii) 4 (iii) 5 (iv) 6

**(b) C will hold 4 litres of water is**

(i) 5 (ii) 6 (iii) 7 (iv) 8

**(c) A and B both will hold $(n + 1)$ litres of water, given $n$ is odd is**

(i) $2n - 1$ (ii) $2n$ (iii) $2n + 1$ (iv) $2n + 2$

**42. Consider the matrix given below:**

$$\begin{vmatrix} 0 & a & a \\ a & 0 & a \\ a & a & 0 \end{vmatrix}$$

**Let $C_{ij}$ denote the cofactor of the element in $i$th row and $j$th column. The cofactor $C_{ij}$ is calculated by writing down the four elements which are not in $i$th row or in $j$th column as such and then calculating the difference between the product of the diagonal elements (upper left × down right – down left × upper right) and then this difference multiplied with $(-1)^{i+j}$. For example, in the matrix**

$$\begin{vmatrix} a_1 & a_2 & a_3 \\ b_1 & b_2 & b_3 \\ c_1 & c_2 & c_3 \end{vmatrix},$$

$$C_{11} = (-1)^{1+1}\begin{vmatrix} b_2 & b_3 \\ c_2 & c_3 \end{vmatrix} = (b_2c_3 - c_2b_3),$$

$$C_{22} = (-1)^{2+2}\begin{vmatrix} a_1 & a_3 \\ c_1 & c_3 \end{vmatrix} = (a_1c_3 - c_1a_3) \text{ and}$$

$$C_{12} = (-1)^{1+2}\begin{vmatrix} b_1 & b_3 \\ c_1 & c_3 \end{vmatrix} = -(b_1c_3 - c_1b_3)$$

**A process consists of forming matrix of cofactors of its preceding matrix i.e.**

$$\begin{vmatrix} C_{11} & C_{12} & C_{13} \\ C_{21} & C_{22} & C_{23} \\ C_{31} & C_{32} & C_{33} \end{vmatrix}$$

**Let after the execution of the process a few number of times, the given matrix is modified to**

$$\begin{vmatrix} 0 & b & b \\ b & 0 & b \\ b & b & 0 \end{vmatrix}$$

**(a) If $a = 1$ and $b = 2$, then the number of execution of process is**

(i) 1 (ii) 2

(iii) 4 (iv) none of these

**(b) If $a = 1$, then $b$ can be equal to**

(i) 4 (ii) 8

(iii) 16 (iv) none of these

**(c) If $a = 1$ and the process has been executed $2n$ times, then $b =$**

(i) $2^{\frac{4^n-1}{3}}$ (ii) $2^{\frac{4^{n+1}-1}{3}}$

(iii) $2^{\frac{4^{n+1}-5}{3}}$ (iv) none of these

**(d) If $a = 2$ and the process has been executed $2n$ times, then $b =$**

(i) $2^{\frac{4^n-1}{3}}$ (ii) $2^{\frac{4^{n+1}-1}{3}}$

(iii) $2^{\frac{4^{n+1}-5}{3}}$ (iv) none of these

**43. There are three persons, each of them, either speaks truth or lies. They are asked in pairs, the questions:**

**I. "DO YOU BOTH SPEAK THE TRUTH?"**

**and the responses (Yes or No) are recorded pairwise in a set $S_1$.**

**II. "DO YOU BOTH LIE?"**

**and the responses (Yes or No) are recorded pairwise in a set $S_1$ in the same sequence as they have been done in set $S_1$.**

**(a) $S_1$ cannot have**

(i) 6 Yes (ii) 4 Yes, 2 No

(iii) 2 Yes, 4 No (iv) All are possible

**(b) If a pair is in agreement for both questions asked, then the third persons can give responses for the four question asked (note that each person is asked above questions twice) as**

(i) 4 Yes or 4 No (ii) 2 Yes, 2 No

(iii) Both (iv) None

**(c) Which of the following is necessarily correct?**

(i) If a pair have same responses in both sets, then the third person is speaking truth

(ii) For part (i), the third person is speaking lie

(iii) If a pair have opposite responses in set $S_2$ from that in $S_1$, then the third person is speaking truth

(iv) none of these

**44. A, B, C, D, E are five person; each person speaks truth to only two other persons and lie to other two persons. Let A speaks truth to one of (B, C) and one of (D, E); B speaks truth to one of (C, D) and one of (A, E); C speaks truth to one of (A, B) and one of (D, E).**

**Also any two persons speak either only truth or only lies to each other. If A speaks truth to**

**(a) B, then E must speak truth to**

(i) A (ii) C
(iii) D (iv) cannot be determined

**(b) C, then both the persons to whom a person speak truth can be known if the person is**

(i) B (ii) D
(iii) E (iv) none of these

**(c) D, then E must speak truth to**

(i) B (ii) C
(iii) D (iv) cannot be determined

**(d) E, then D must speak truth to**

(i) B (ii) C
(iii) E (iv) cannot be determined

**45. A, B, C and D have certain sums of money each. When A divided his money among B,C, D according to the ratio of money they already had, their total amounts are found to be Rs 45, Rs 60 and Rs 75 respectively. If at least one of (B, C, D) can also split his money likewise on the condition that others get only integral number of rupees, then**

**(a) the money possessed by A initially was**

(i) Rs 36 (ii) Rs 72
(iii) Rs 108 (iv) cannot be determined

**(b) who will be able to split his money likewise?**

(i) B (ii) C (iii) D (iv) B or C

**46. Each of four boys A, B, C, D have a pair of marbles of different colour from four distinct colours, no two persons having marbles of same set of two colours. A round consist of exchanging of a marble between two persons who have no marbles of same colour. Let in first round, (A, C) and (B, D) exchanged a marble. In the second round, (A, B) and (C, D) exchanged a marble. In the third round, (A, D) and (B, D) exchanged a marble.**

**(a) After second round, which of the following is correct?**

(i) (A, C) and (B, D) have marbles of same set of colours
(ii) (A, C) and (B, D) have marble of exactly one colour in common

(iii) A, B have marbles of same set of colours as initially possessed by C, D respectively
(iv) none of these

**(b) If after second round, A has the marbles of same set of colours as he initially had, then who else has also the marbles of same set of colours as he initially had?**

(i) B (ii) C
(iii) D (iv) none of these

**(c) If in part (b), had B been there instead of A, then the marbles with C would have been of same set of colours as initially possessed by**

(i) A (ii) C
(iii) D (iv) none of these

**(d) After second round , the colours of set of marbles possessed by the person can be of same set of colours as initially possessed by**

(i) A and C (ii) B and D
(iii) Either of these only (iv) May be none of these

**47. A, B, C, D respectively have Rs 20, Rs 22, Rs 24 and Rs 26. Each of them bought exactly four fruits from mango, apple, orange and peach. The price of a mango is Rs 1, Rs 2, and Rs 3 more then that of an apple, an orange and a peach respectively. Assuming that all persons spent their whole money on fruits and four fruits of each kind are purchased, then**

**(a) the cost of a peach is**

(i) Rs 4 (ii) Rs 4.25
(iii) Rs 4.50 (iv) Rs 4.75

**(b) assuming that B did not buy any orange, he bought**

(i) one apple and two peaches
(ii) two apples and one peach
(iii) two apples and two peaches
(iv) cannot be determined

**(c) assuming that C did not buy any mango, he bought**

(i) two apples (ii) two oranges
(iii) three apples (iv) three oranges

**(d) who could have bought each of four fruits?**

(i) B (ii) C (iii) Both (iv) None

**48. Nine blocks shown below are to be filled by letters A to I. It is given that**

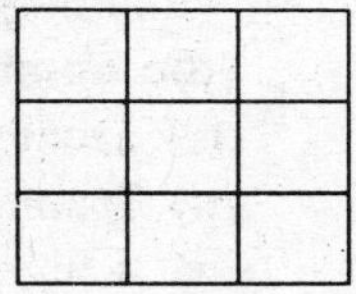

**(1) A is just above B.**

**(2) B is just right to C.**

**(3) D is just left to E.**

**(4) F is just below I.**

**(5) G is just right to H.**

**(a) Which letter is in the centre?**

(i) A (ii) B
(iii) C (iv) cannot be determined

**(b) Which letter is in the bottom left hand corner?**

(i) F (ii) D
(iii) H (iv) cannot be determined

**(c) Elements of which of the following can be fully determined?**

(i) Middle row (ii) Middle column
(iii) Left column (iv) Right column

**49. Nine blocks shown alongside are filled by 3 A's, 3 B's and 3 C's. A sequence consists of the elements in either row (from left to right) or column (from top to bottom)**

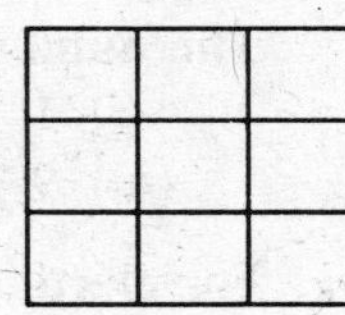

**A. Let there be 3 pairs of unique sequences.**

**(a) If the corresponding elements of the rows of two columns are interchanged, then the number of unique sequences will be**

(i) 3 (ii) 4 (iii) 5 (iv) 6

**(b) If the corresponding elements of the rows of two columns are interchanged, then there will be 3 unique pairs of another sequence where the sequence consists of the elements in either**

(i) row (form left to right) or column (from bottom to top)
(ii) row (form right to left) or column (from top to bottom)
(iii) row (form right to left) or column (from bottom to top)
(iv) none of these

**B. Let the blocks be filled in such a way that the interchanging of any two rows or columns does not alter the number of unique sequences. Then there are**

(i) 2 unique sequences, three of each
(ii) 3 unique sequences, a pair of each
(iii) 4 unique sequences, one of them being triple
(i) none of these

**50. Consider a 3 × 3 arrangement as shown below:**

| | | |
|---|---|---|
| **1** | **2** | **3** |
| **4** | **5** | **6** |
| **7** | **8** | **9** |

**When four pairs of number exchanged their mutual place and the ninth number exchanges its place with one of them, then the arrangement got modified as shown below:**

| | | |
|---|---|---|
| **5** | **4** | **8** |
| **2** | **9** | **7** |
| **6** | **9** | **1** |

**The number which exchanged its place twice is**

(i) 1 (ii) 5
(iii) 9 (iv) cannot be determined

**51. For electing the president of the board of a company out of three candidates, five members of the board are asked to give their choice of president as first, second and third choice for the three candidates. The weightage given to the first choice is twice of that given to the second choice and thrice of that given to the third choice. No members of the board gave the identical choices. The ratio of weightage given to winner to that of the candidate least preferred is**

(i) 3 : 2 (ii) 4 : 3 (iii) 5 : 4 (iv) 6 : 5

**52. A, B, C, P, Q, R, X, Y and Z are nine person who are related as: A is B's only sister; C and P are brothers; Z is son of A; C is unmarried brother-in-law of B; X is sister-in-law of Y; and R is father-in-law of P. If there are three couples and every couple is accounted for, then**

**(a) who is the mother of A?**

(i) Y (ii) X
(iii) Q (iv) cannot be determined

**(b) which of the following is not married?**

(i) X (ii) Y
(iii) Q (iv) all of these are married

**53. A triangular cricket tournament was played in January among three teams A, B and C. There were nine league matches, each country playing three matches with the other. The league matches were divided into three bouts, each bout consisting of three matches played on consecutive days, one match among each of two countries. The bouts were separated by one day for rest and no two teams played in same sequence in any two league matches. Each win was assigned a point. The two teams scoring higher points played three matches on alternate days with each other, the first of these matches started after a day the last of league match was played. The team winning more matches in the last three final matches won the tournament. There were no draws in any of the matches. Now it is known that**

**I. the teams A and C played on Jan 15 in which C won.**
**II. the teams B and C played on Jan 17 in which B won.**
**III. the teams A and B played on Jan 22 in which A won.**
**IV. it was not yet clear on Jan 20 which teams would go to final.**
**V. the teams winning the first of the league matches lost the tournament although it had the highest points in the leaguematches.**
**VI. the teams winning the last of the league matches also won the tournament.**

**(a) Who won the tournament?**

(i) A (ii) B
(iii) C (iv) cannot be determined

**(b) On which date the last match of the tournament was played?**

(i) 28th Jan (ii) 29th Jan
(iii) 30th Jan (iv) 31th Jan

**(c) Which team could not have won two league matches successively?**

(i) A (ii) B
(iii) C (iv) cannot be determined

**(d) Which team won the first of the league matches?**

(i) A (ii) B
(iii) C (iv) cannot be determined

**(e) If the team winning on 18th Jan won the tournament, then which team won match played on 14th Jan?**

(i) A (ii) B
(iii) C (iv) cannot be determined

**54. Shown alongside is a network of road. To go from A to B, a man walks either towards east or towards north only (In the figure, towards right or towards up)**

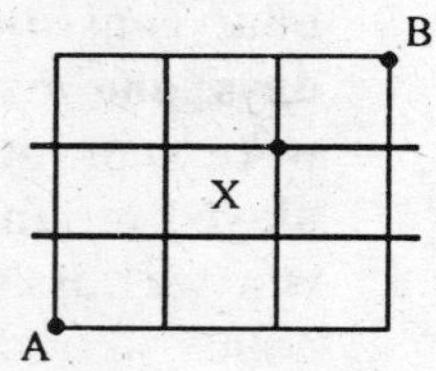


**In how many different ways can the man go from**

**(a) A to B?**

(i) 16 (ii) 18 (iii) 20 (iv) 21

**(b) A to B without crossing the junction X?**

(i) 7 (ii) 8 (iii) 9 (iv) 10

**55. Shown alongside is a signal processing circuit in which each nodes are maintained at two states, viz. 0 or 1. The signal can pass through a branch only if the states at its end nodes are different. Also it does not pass through the same node twice. The number of different ways in which the signal could have passed through A to B for the figure shown below**

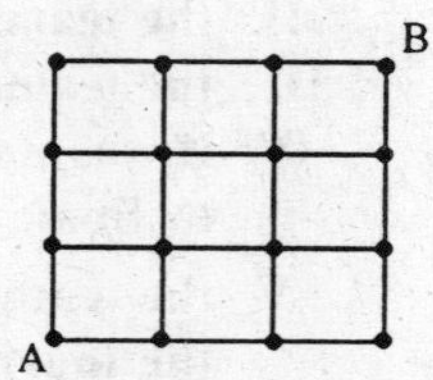


**(a)**

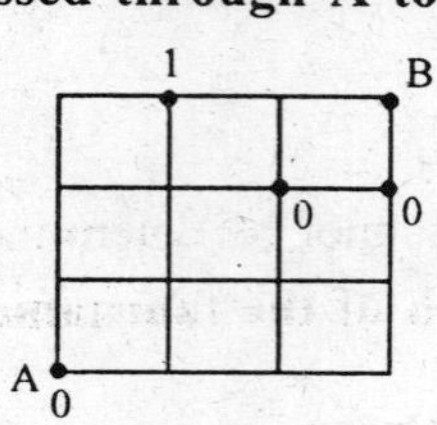


**is ( the digits 0, 1 show the states of nodes near which they are given)**

(i) 16 (ii) 18 (iii) 20 (iv) 21

**(b)** 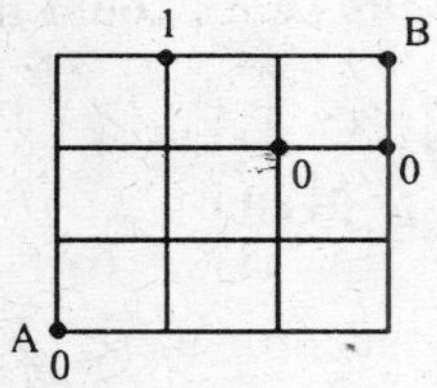

**is**

(i) 21 (ii) 24
(iii) 28 (iv) none of these

**56. Shown alongside is a network of road with each branch of 1 km. A man walks from A to C never going along branches in the same direction successively or along the same branch again. If he walks for as much time as possible,**

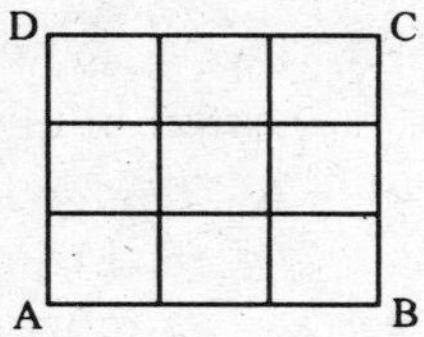


**(a) then how many kilometers does he walk?**

(i) 15 (ii) 16 (iii) 17 (iv) 18

**(b) but without passing through either B or D, then how many kilometers does he walk?**

(i) 10 (ii) 12 (iii) 14 (iv) 15

**57. There are four pairs of similar black shoes but are of different sizes. Four persons A, B, C and D whose foot sizes are different can wear one of the given pairs of the shoes. The shoes are arranged in a line. No person knows which pair of shoes can fit him beforehand (but knows that there is a pair of shoes for each of them). Each person starts trying from left to right to find the positions of the pair of the shoes fitting him. The persons can recognise whether a shoe is for left foot or right foot. Let A, B, C and D found the positions of both the shoes fitting them after 4th, 4th, 5th and 5th trial respectively. Let the positions of left shoes of A and C be earlier than that of their respective right shoes while the case for B and D are vice versa (note that person having one of his pair of shoes at last of the shoes of the same foot can well recognise it by trying the third shoes of the same foot). If the first shoe is the left shoe of A, then**

**(a) in how many distinct way, the shoes could have been arranged?**
(i) 3 (ii) 6 (iii) 12 (iv) 18

**(b) the position of which shoe is fixed?**
(i) left shoe of C (ii) right shoe of B
(iii) right shoe of C (iv) none of these

**(c) which of the following position has a fixed shoe?**
(i) Second (ii) Third
(iii) Fourth (iv) none of these

**58. Two men, two women, two boys and two girls are to be seated in eight seats numbered 1 to 8 in a row.**

**A. The girls can be seated in seat number (2, 5); (3, 4); (6, 8) or (1, 7) only. The boys can be seated in seat number (1, 8); (2, 3); (4, 6) or (5, 7) only. The women can be seated in seat numbers (1, 4); (2, 8); (3, 7) or (5, 6) only. The men can be seated in seat numbers (1, 6); (2, 7); (3, 5) or (4, 8) only.**

**(a) The seats occupied by the girls are**
(i) (1, 7) (ii) (2, 5) (iii) (3, 4) (iv) (6, 8)

**(b) The seats occupied by the boys are**
(i) (1, 8) (ii) (4, 6)
(iii) (5, 7) (iv) cannot be determined

**(c) The men are separated by**
(i) 1 seat (ii) 3 seats
(iii) 4 seats (iv) cannot be determined

**B. If the girls can be seated in seat numbers 2, 5 or 8 only; the boys can be seated in seat numbers 3, 6 or 8 only, the men can be seated only in seat numbers 2, 4 or 7 only; and the women can be seated only in seat numbers 1, 5 or 7 only, then the seat number of which of the following can be definitely known?**
(i) Girls (ii) Boys
(iii) Men (iv) Women

**59. 6 men and 3 women (A1, A2, ........... $A_9$) are to be seated in a row such that no two women sit together. Let three of the possible arrangements be $A_1A_2A_3A_4A_5A_6A_7A_8A_9$; $A_5A_3A_8A_1A_6A_2A_4A_7A_9$ and $A_4A_9A_2A_8A_5A_1A_7A_3A_6$.**

**(a) How many distinct possible triplets of females can exists?**

(i) Two (ii) Three (iii) Four (iv) Five

**(b) Which of the following cannot be found in any of the possible triplets of female?**

(i) $A_4$ (ii) $A_7$ (iii) $A_8$

(iv) all will be found in at least one of the triplets

**(c) If $A_9$ is a female, then which of the following must be a female?**

(i) $A_1$ (ii) $A_5$

(iii) $A_6$ (iv) none of these

**(d) Which of the following is correct?**

(i) If $A_4$ is a female, then $A_1$ is also a female

(ii) If $A_5$ is a female, then $A_9$ is also a female

(iii) If $A_9$ is a female, then $A_3$ is also a female

(iv) none of these

**60. A, B, C, D, E, F are six persons (three male and three females) seated in a line such that no males are together and two females are together.**

**(a) Let E be flanked by B and C while F be flanked by A and D. Sex of every person can be known if it is given that**

(i) E is a female (ii) F is a female

(iii) B is a female (iv) none of these

**(b) Let A is adjacent to B and C is adjacent to D. Which of the following is necessarily true?**

(i) If E is not adjacent to F, then both are males

(ii) If E is not adjacent to F, then both are of opposite sex

(iii) If E is adjacent to F, then both are of opposite sex

(iv) none of these

**61. Consider a parent and their three children: two males and one female, out of which one male and one female are married. Let the persons described above be A, B, C, D, E, F, G (not in order) which are arranged in a line as A B C D E F G. Now it is known that the only couple together is parent, the unmarried brother is adjacent to his married brother and brother-in-law, and C is a female.**

**(a) The unmarried brother can be known if it is known that**

(i) B is a male (ii) D is a male
(iii) G is a male (iv) none of these

**(b) If D is not a parent, then it is necessarily married to**

(i) A (ii) B
(iii) G (iv) none of these

**(c) If G is married to A, then which of the following is necessarily acouple?**

(i) BE (ii) CF (iii) BD (iv) DF

**(d) Which of the following must be true?**

(i) A must be a female
(ii) E cannot be married to G
(iii) D and F are siblings
(iv) none of these

**62. On any clock, there are 12 marks indicating hours. Two dices A and B move from one mark to another, they move alternately as many marks ahead as the number thrown by them. Let the number thrown by the dices A and B in six throws be**

| **Throw** | **First** | **Second** | **Third** | **Fourth** | **Fifth** | **Sixth** |
|---|---|---|---|---|---|---|
| **A** | **3** | **2** | **5** | **4** | **6** | **1** |
| **B** | **2** | **3** | **4** | **6** | **1** | **5** |

**Initially A is at mark indicating 12 'O' clock and moves first and the position of B is not given.**

**A. Let A and B both move clockwise.**

**(a) What is the maximum number of times for which both dices will be at the same position?**

(i) One (ii) Two (iii) Three (iv) Four

**(b) If after third toss, they are at the same position, then after which toss they were/will be at the same position?**

(i) First (ii) Fourth
(iii) Fifth (iv) none of these

**(c) If after fourth toss, they are at the diagonally opposite positions, then they were/will be closest to each other after**

(i) first toss (ii) second toss
(iii) third toss (iv) fifth toss

**(d) If after two intermediate consecutive tosses, the difference in their positions increased by two marks, then by how many marks will the difference between their positions increase/decrease after the next toss?**

(i) Increase by 4 (ii) Increase by 5
(iii) Decrease by 4 (iv) Decrease by 5

**B. Let A moves clockwise while B moves anti-clockwise.**

**(a) What is the maximum number of times for which both the dices will be at the same position?**

(i) One (ii) Two (iii) Three (iv) Four

**(b) Let the dices be at the same position after a few tosses (not initially). After how many tosses will they be again at the same position?**

(i) One (ii) Two
(iii) Three (iv) none of these

**63. In the adjoining figure, X is a child who moves two blocks in one direction and then one block in another direction at one go to halt temporarily. He also does not halt in the same block again. It is given that the child only moves right, left, up or down and starts moving from a corner which is to be regarded as the first halt.**

| | | | |
|---|---|---|---|
| | | | |
| | | | |
| | | | |
| X | | | |

**(a) How many maximum halts can he make?**

(i) 12 (ii) 13 (iii) 14 (iv) 15

**(b) After how many minimum halts he would not be left with any block to move in?**

(i) 7 (ii) 8 (iii) 9 (iv) 10

**(c) Suppose another child Y, moving in a similar manner as X, starts moving from a block at corner (not diagonally opposite to the block at the corner from which X starts moving). If both X, Y move alternately (X moving first), then after how many minimum moves of X, both will be in the same block?**

(i) 3 (ii) 4 (iii) 5 (iv) 6

**64.**

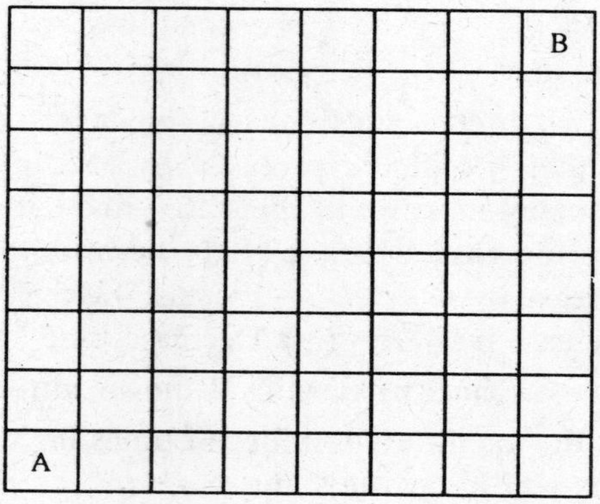


**Consider the arrangement of 8 × 8 square blocks as shown in the above figure. Two players (A and B) initially on the opposite corner blocks move alternately and they can move one block up, down left or right but not diagonally.**

**(a) If they move so as to meet each other in minimum number of moves, then the number of different possible blocks in which they can meet will be**

(i) 2 (ii) 4 (iii) 8 (iv) 12

**(b) Suppose they meet after each of them made exactly 9 moves. If none of them move in the same block twice, then the number of different possible blocks in which they can meet will be**

(i) 12 (ii) 20 (iii) 22 (iv) 34

**65. A, B, C, D, E, F, G, H, I fills the nine blocks shown alongside and their positions are then taken fixed. Now four pairs are chosen and their places are exchanged with the ninth letter retaining its original position. If three of such modified blocks can be**

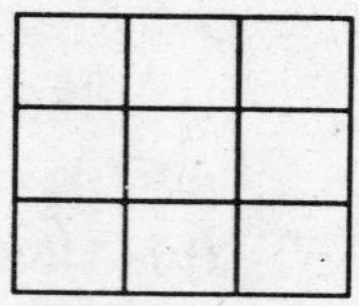

| | | |
|---|---|---|
| A | D | H |
| F | E | C |
| B | I | G |

**Fig: 1**

| | | |
|---|---|---|
| F | H | I |
| G | C | B |
| E | D | A |

**Fig: 2**

| | | |
|---|---|---|
| I | F | G |
| B | H | A |
| D | C | E |

**Fig: 3**

,

then

(a) in Fig. 1, the letters which retained its original position is

(i) A (ii) B (iii) C (iv) D

(b) the letter at the centre of the original block is

(i) D (ii) F (iii) G (iv) I

(c) the letter at the right upper corner of the original block is

(i) B (ii) C (iii) D (iv) E

**66.** **There are 16 square blocks with two players occupying a block as shown in the alongside figure. They can move a block up, down, left or right but cannot move diagonally. Also none of them move in the same block twice or move in the block initially occupied by them.**

| | | | |
|---|---|---|---|
| | | | |
| | | | B |
| | | | |
| A | | | |

**(a) Suppose A moved in a block in exactly 10 moves. He could as well move in that block in exactly**

(i) 9 moves (ii) 11 moves

(iii) 12 moves (iv) all of these

**(b) Let S be the set of numbers of moves A can possibly make before he has any block left to move in. Then the number of unequal elements of S will be equal to**

(i) 6 (ii) 7 (iii) 8 (iv) 9

**(c) Suppose A and B meet in a block, making moves alternatively after they move exactly equal number of times, say *n*. Then how many distinct values of *n* are possible?**

(i) Zero (ii) One (iii) Two (iv) Four

**67.** **Study carefully the pattern of filling 25 numbers $x_1$, $x_2$, $x_3$, .............. $x_{25}$ in 5 × 5 blocks as shown alongside. The pattern has unique property that the sum of subscripts of any row, column or diagonal are same.**

| | | | | |
|---|---|---|---|---|
| $x_{17}$ | $x_{24}$ | $x_1$ | $x_8$ | $x_{15}$ |
| $x_{23}$ | $x_5$ | $x_2$ | $x_{14}$ | $x_{16}$ |
| $x_4$ | $x_6$ | $x_{13}$ | $x_{20}$ | $x_{22}$ |
| $x_{10}$ | $x_{12}$ | $x_{19}$ | $x_{21}$ | $x_3$ |
| $x_{11}$ | $x_{18}$ | $x_{25}$ | $x_2$ | $x_9$ |

**A. If another such pattern filled from $x_1$ to $x_{25}$ in a similar way is**

| | | | | |
|---|---|---|---|---|
| | | | | |
| | | | | |
| | | | | |
| | | | $a$ | |
| | $x_1$ | | | |

,

**then $a$ =**

(i) $x_7$ (ii) $x_{12}$

(iii) $x_{22}$ (iv) none of these

**(b) Suppose the pattern is not filled in similar way but it has the same property. If few of the elements of the pattern are**

| | | | | |
|---|---|---|---|---|
| | $x_{22}$ | | | |
| | | | $x_{11}$ | |
| | | $x_1$ | | |
| | | | | $x_5$ |
| $a$ | | | | |

,

**then $a$ =**

(i) $x_8$ (ii) $x_{14}$ (iii) $x_{16}$ (iv) $x_{20}$

**B. By using the similar pattern, it is possible to fill 7 × 7 blocks with numbers 1-49 such that the sum of numbers in any row, column or diagonal are same. Consider one such pattern as:**

| | | | | | | |
|---|---|---|---|---|---|---|
| | | | | | | |
| | | $x$ | | | | |
| | | | | | | 2 |
| 1 | | | | | | |
| | | | | | | |
| | | | | | $z$ | |
| $y$ | | | | | | |

**(a) The sum of numbers in any row is equal to**
(i) 168 (ii) 175 (iii) 182 (iv) 189

**(b)** $x =$
(i) 26 (ii) 32 (iii) 35 (iv) 44

**(c)** $y =$
(i) 22 (ii) 20 (iii) 28 (iv) 30

**(d)** $z =$
(i) 23 (ii) 27
(iii) 47 (iv) none of these

**68. Consider a 10 × 10 square blocks similar to that of a chessboard. The blocks are numbered 1-100 rowwise starting from top left corner. Out of two players A and B who can occupy one block at a time, A can move a block up, down, right or left only while B can move a block diagonally only. Each player makes one move alternately. Also they do not move in the block they already occupied once. Suppose initially A and B occupy the block numbered *m* and *n* respectively. If A makes a first move, then in how many minimum number of their moves (sum of moves of both players) they can meet if**

**(a)** $m = 1$ **and** $n = 60$**?**
(i) 10 (ii) 11 (iii) 12 (iv) 13

**(b)** $m = 4$ **and** $n = 95$ **?**
(i) 11 (ii) 12 (iii) 13 (iv) 14

**69.** 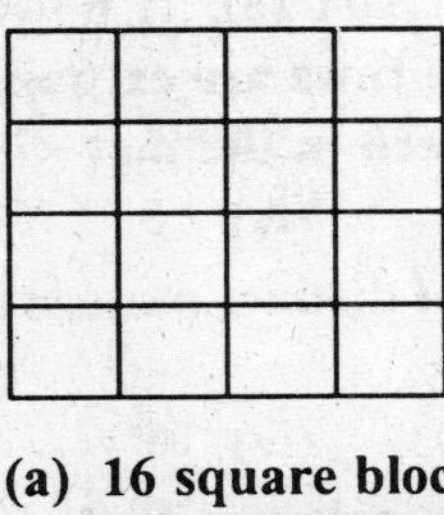

**(a) 16 square blocks are filled with letters A to P, a letter in each block. Squares of four adjacent blocks are then chosen and written as such (without any rotation). If four such squares are**

| | |
|---|---|
| O | I |
| H | D |

,

| | |
|---|---|
| B | M |
| L | F |

,

| | |
|---|---|
| E | J |
| I | B |

and

| | |
|---|---|
| N | P |
| J | K |

,

then in the original 4 × 4 blocks, the letter in the third row of last column is

(i) F (ii) K (iii) M (iv) P

(b) Suppose in part (a), one out of four such squares chosen is rotated. If the four squares are

| | |
|---|---|
| G | L |
| I | B |

,

| | |
|---|---|
| N | G |
| J | D |

,

| | |
|---|---|
| E | H |
| B | K |

and

| | |
|---|---|
| I | O |
| C | M |

,

then the letter in the last row and third column is

(i) B (ii) C (iii) I (iv) J

70. A mat having 16 squares as shown above are to be filled by four different colours such that each column and each row has colours of all types. Pattern is defined as the sequence of four colours in any row (forward or backward) or any column (up or down).

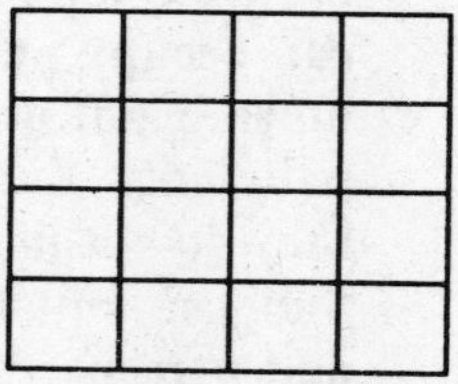

A. (a) What is the minimum number of distinct pattern that can be there in the mat?

(i) 8 (ii) 10 (iii) 12 (iv) 14

(b) Consider a way of filling the squares with colours corresponding to the condition of part (a). If now the sequence of colours in two of the rows are exchanged, then the number of distinct pattern in the mat will be

(i) 10 (ii) 12 (iii) 14 (iv) 16

(c) What is the maximum number of distinct pattern that can be there in the mat?

(i) 10 (ii) 12 (iii) 14 (iv) 16

B. Let the mat be filled with four colours: Red, Blue, Green and Yellow: and no two patterns in the mat be same. Also let the first row has the forward pattern as: Yellow, Red, Blue, Green. Then the forward pattern in the

**(a) third row will be**
(i) Blue, Green, Yellow, Red
(ii) Red, Blue, Green, Yellow
(iii) Green, Yellow, Red, Blue
(iv) cannot be determined

**(b) fourth row will be**
(i) Blue, Green, Yellow, Red
(ii) Red, Blue, Green, Yellow
(iii) Green, Yellow, Red, Blue
(iv) cannot be determined

**71. There are four couples among nine persons: A, B, C, D, E, F, G, H and I.**

| | | |
|---|---|---|
| E | A | F |
| B | I | C |
| D | G | H |

**Fig (i)**

| | | |
|---|---|---|
| I | B | E |
| C | A | D |
| G | H | F |

**Fig (ii)**

**In fig (i), all couples are adjacent to each other (i.e. in these blocks having one of their sides common) while in Fig (ii) no couples are in adjacent blocks.**

**(a) Which of the following must be a couple?**
(i) A, E (ii) F, A (iii) C, H (iv) G, I

**(b) Which of the following cannot be a bachelor?**
(i) D (ii) E (iii) F (iv) H

**(c) Which of the following must be a couple?**
(i) B, D (ii) C, H (iii) F, A (iv) F, C

**(d) A can be married to**
(i) E only (ii) E or F only
(iii) E or I only (iv) E, F or I only

**72. Consider 9 persons: A, B, C, D, E, F, G, H, and I, a few males and a few females. In 3 × 3 square blocks shown alongside, females always occupy fixed blocks and males occupy remaining blocks. The two ways in which they can occupy the blocks are as:**

| | | |
|---|---|---|
| | | |
| | | |
| | | |

| | | |
|---|---|---|
| B | A | E |
| D | C | H |
| G | F | I |

and

| | | |
|---|---|---|
| G | D | H |
| F | B | C |
| E | I | A |

**Given that the number of females is less than that of males,**

**(a) the number of females is**

(i) 1 (ii) 2 (iii) 3 (iv) 4

**(b) which of the following are males?**

(i) A, F (ii) A, H (iii) B, F (iv) B, H

**73. A, B, C, D, E, F, G, H, I are 9 elements to be filled in 3 × 3 blocks as shown below (with their numbers):**

| | | |
|---|---|---|
| 1 | 2 | 3 |
| 4 | 5 | 6 |
| 7 | 8 | 9 |

**Let none of the element as shown in the figure below**

| | | |
|---|---|---|
| A | B | C |
| D | E | F |
| G | H | I |

**actually fills the row or column, they are shown to occupy. Also in actual filling of blocks, A, C, G occupy the block numbers 6, 7, 2 respectively.**

**(a) The position of which of the following can be definitely known?**

(i) E (ii) H

(iii) I (iv) none of these

**(b) If F is in block number 1, then the position of which of the following can be definitely known?**

(i) D only (ii) D and B

(iii) D and E (iv) D and H

**(c) If D is in block number 3, then the position of which of the following can be definitely known?**

(i) F only (ii) F and B
(iii) F and E (iv) F and H

**74. Nine blocks as shown alongside are filled by nine different elements A, B, C, D, E, F, G, H and I. It is observed that there is a common element in row/column occupied by (G, H) and (C, F); (A,C) and (E, H); (E, F) and (A, G). Also A, C lie in the first row with A in the first column.**

| | | |
|---|---|---|
| | | |
| | | |
| | | |

**(a) Who occupies the block in the centre?**

(i) E (ii) F
(iii) H (iv) cannot be determined

**(b) Which of the following is necessarily true?**

(i) G occupies second row
(ii) H occupies third row
(iii) E occupies second column
(iv) F occupies second column

**(c) The occupants of which of the following blocks can be only B, D or I?**

(i) First row, second column
(ii) Second row, first column
(iii) Third row, second column
(iv) Third row, third column

**75. Nine elements A, B, C, D, E, F, G, H and I are to be filled in nine numbered cells as shown alongside. The cells are filled in a particular cyclic sequence (for example if the sequence is 1457863921, then the elements will be filled successively starting with any numbered cell and then going around the sequence). Similarly the elements are themselves also in a cyclic sequence which fill the cells with each successive element filling a cell just after its preceding element in the sequence fills a cell. Let two of the possible arrangements be**

| | | |
|---|---|---|
| 1 | 2 | 3 |
| 4 | 5 | 6 |
| 7 | 8 | 9 |

| | | |
|---|---|---|
| A | C | F |
| H | D | B |
| E | G | I |

and

| | | |
|---|---|---|
| G | I | C |
| E | A | H |
| B | D | F |

**(a) A and G in their cyclic sequences must be separated by**
(i) no or seven elements
(ii) one or six elements
(iii) two or five elements
(iv) three or four elements

**(b) The cells numbered 2 and 3 in their cyclic sequences must be separated by**
(i) no or seven cells
(ii) one or six cells
(iii) two or five cells
(iv) three or four cells

**(c) If, in an arrangement, C and F are in cells numbered 4 and 6 respectively, then I will be in the cell numbered**
(i) 3 (ii) 7
(iii) 8 (iv) cannot be determined

**(d) If the sequences are**
**A B C __ E __ D X __ A and**
**1 2 4 5 __ 9 __ Y __ 1 , then**
(i) X is determinable while Y is not
(ii) Y is determinable while X is not
(iii) X and Y are both determinable
(iv) none of X, Y are determinable

**76. The nine cells shown alongside are numbered 1-9 hapazardly. Three letters A, B, C are placed in three different cells. The arrangement is now to be changed such that no letters occupy any other cells in the row or column in which they are presently placed (although they can retain their previous positions). If for new arrangement,**

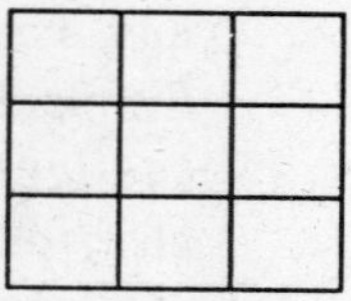

**I A cannot occupy the cells numbered (1, 5) in a column and (3, 6) in a row.**

**II B cannot occupy the cells numbered (6, 7) in a column and (2, 5) in a row.**

**III C cannot occupy the cells numbered (3, 9) in a column and (4, 5) in a row, then**

**(a) A occupies the cell numbered**

(i) 2 (ii) 4
(iii) 8 (iv) cannot be determined

**(b) B occupies the cell numbered**

(i) 1 (ii) 4
(iii) 8 (iv) cannot be determined

**(c) C occupies the cell numbered**

(i) 2 (ii) 6
(iii) 8 (iv) cannot be determined

**77. Consider a 3 × 3 blocks as shown alongside. A counter can move along the first row (left to right), then second row (left to right) and then third row (left to right) after which it again repeats the earlier path in similar fashion. The counter when placed in any cell will move as many block ahead along the path as number written in that cell after which it temporarily stops and then again move in the similar fashion. The counter stops permanently when it again stops in the cell from which it has started or the cell it has already temporarily stopped once.**

| | | |
|---|---|---|
| 1 | 2 | 3 |
| 4 | 5 | 6 |
| 7 | 8 | 9 |

**(a) During a move, which of the following can be the total number of temporary stops it can have (barring the cell in which it is initially placed)?**

(i) 0, 1 and 5 only
(ii) 0, 1, 4 and 5 only
(iii) 0, 1, 3, 4 and 5 only
(iv) 0, 1, 2, 3, 4 and 5 only

**(b) Had the places of 8, 9 been switched in the given figure, then from which cell the counter must start so as to have maximum temporary stops?**

(i) 1 (ii) 5
(iii) 7 (iv) none of these

**(c) Which of the following two numbers in the given figure must be switched so that the counter can have six temporary stops (barring the cell in which it is initially placed)?**
(i) 4, 8 (ii) 8, 7
(iii) 7, 5 (iv) all of these

**78. In the above figure A, B, ............ I are nine persons. Let there be four couples who are adjacent to each other.**

| | | |
|---|---|---|
| A | B | C |
| D | E | F |
| G | H | I |

**(a) How many different possibilities for the four set of couples exist?**
(i) 14 (ii) 15 (iii) 18 (iv) 20

**(b) How many different possibilities for the unmarried persons exist?**
(i) 4 (ii) 5 (iii) 8 (iv) 9

**79. Nine cells shown alongside are to be filled by nine letters A, B, C, D, E, F, G, H, I (in that order). Each successive letter must be filled adjacent (two cells sharing a side) to its predecessor. Also there can be only one letter in any cell. The process of filling the cells terminates if there is no cell left for any letter to go into according to the above stated condition.**

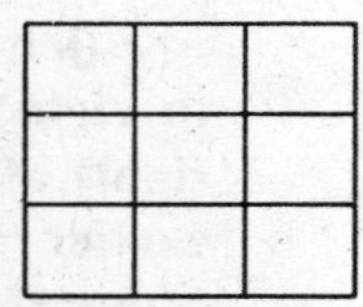

**(a) Let, in a process, one cell remains empty with H on the right top corner. The process could have well been complete in the middle with the filling of cells by letters up to F only. In the former case, the block which is left empty is**
(i) left top corner
(ii) left bottom corner
(iii) right bottom corner
(iv) cannot be determined

**(b) Let, in a process, two cells remain empty. Which of the following can never be together?**
(i) B, G (ii) C, F
(iii) D, G (iv) all of these can be together

(c) Let $m$ be the number of different initial positions of A for which no cell can remain empty and $n$ be the number of different initial positions of A for which at least one cell must remain empty. Which of the following is true?

(i) $m = 1, n = 4$ (ii) $m = 5, n = 4$
(iii) $m = 5, n = 1$ (iv) $m = 4, n = 4$

**80.**

| | | |
|---|---|---|
| 1 | 2 | 3 |
| 4 | 5 | 6 |
| 7 | 8 | 9 |

**Fig: (i)**

| | | |
|---|---|---|
| 3 | 2 | 1 |
| 4 | 5 | 6 |
| 9 | 8 | 7 |

**Fig: (ii)**

A, B, C, D, E, F, G, H, I are filled (in that sequence) in the cells of the above two figures which are themselves to be filled in the cyclic sequence 1, 2, 3, 4, 5, 6, 7, 8, 9, 1 (for example if A is filled in cell number 3, then B should be filled in cell number 4 and so on). Let the position of A (the row and the column) in both the figure shown above be same.

(a) For how many different positions of A, there will be four more letter which corresponding position in both the figures will be same?
(i) 2 (ii) 3 (iii) 4 (iv) 5

(b) For how many different positions of A in the second figure, there will be at least one letter having same relative position in both the figures?
(i) 5 (ii) 6 (iii) 7 (iv) 9

(c) For how many different positions of A, D will also have the same position in both the figures?
(i) 2 (ii) 4 (iii) 5 (iv) 6

(d) For how many different positions of A, G will also have the same position in both the figures?
(i) 2 (ii) 3 (iii) 4 (iv) 5

**81.** Letters A to I are filled in nine cells, as shown alongside, starting from cell number 1 to cell number 9 (in the

| | | |
|---|---|---|
| 1 | 2 | 3 |
| 4 | 5 | 6 |
| 7 | 8 | 9 |

**increasing order of 1-9). The letters to be filled are in cyclic sequences ADEFCBGIHA and AFGHBIDCEA. If a letter of any sequence is filled in any cell, then the next cell to be filled must be filled by the letter following the previous letter in the given sequence.**

**(a) Suppose in filling of cells by both the sequences, two of the letters have same position for the two fillings. How many such pairs of letters exist?**

(i) 1 (ii) 2 (iii) 3 (iv) 4

**(b) Which of the following letters is not in any of such pairs mentioned in part (a)?**

(i) D (ii) F (iii) G (iv) H

**(c) Suppose in filling of cells by both the sequences, the positions of two particular letters are switched in the two fillings. How many such pairs of letters exist?**

(i) 1 (ii) 2 (iii) 3 (iv) 4

**(d) Which of the following letters is not in any of such pairs mentioned in part (c)?**

(i) A (ii) B (iii) C (iv) D

**82.**

| | | |
|---|---|---|
| | | |
| | | |
| | | |

**A counter is at rest in one of the nine cells shown above. Let this cell be numbered 1. In one move, the counter moves across five different cells (any two successive cells in a move being adjacent) to stop in the fifth cell. The stop of *n*th move is numbered ($n + 1$). Let after the seven moves the number of cells be as**

| | | |
|---|---|---|
| 5 | *b* | 7 |
| *a* | *c* | 8 |
| 1 | *d* | *e* |

**where *a*, *b*, *c*, *d*, *e* represent the cells they are written in.**

**(a) Which of the following cell will be numbered 3?**

(i) *b* (ii) *c*

(iii) e (iv) cannot be determined

**(b) Which of the following cell will be numbered 4?**

(i) *a* (ii) *b*

(iii) *d* (iv) cannot be determined

**83. A counter can move in the cells shown alongside, first along the first row (left to right), then second row (left to right), then third row (left to right) and then again repeat the earlier path. The counter, initially at left hand top corner,**

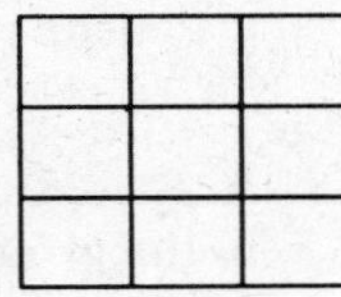

**move as many cells along the path as number thrown up by a dice after which it comes to rest until the dice is thrown again. The dice is thrown five times throwing 4 in the third throw while in other four throws, it threw each 2, 3, 5, and 6 once. If the counter did not rest in any block twice, then the number thrown in**

**(a) first toss is**

(i) 2 (ii) 3

(iii) 5 (iv) the given case is not possible

**(b) fourth toss is**

(i) 2 (ii) 3

(iii) 6 (iv) the given case is not possible

**(c) fifth toss is**

(i) 3 (ii) 5

(iii) 6 (iv) the given case is not possible

**84. (a) Consider a set of 70 natural number arranged in 10 rows and 7 columns. Let the number be arranged rowwise and columnwise as shown in the figure given below:**

| | | | | | | | | | | | | | | | | |
|---|---|---|---|---|---|---|---|---|---|---|---|---|---|---|---|---|
| **1** | **2** | **3** | . | . | . | **7** | | **1** | **11** | . | . | . | . | . | . | |
| **8** | **9** | **10** | . | . | . | . | | **2** | **12** | . | . | . | . | . | . | |
| . | . | . | . | . | . | . | | **3** | . | . | . | . | . | . | . | |
| . | . | . | . | . | . | . | **and** | . | . | . | . | . | . | . | . | |
| . | . | . | . | . | . | . | | . | . | . | . | . | . | . | **69** | |
| . | . | . | . | . | **69** | **70** | | **10** | . | . | . | . | . | . | **70** | |

**The numbers which retained its position in both the arrangements barring 1 and 70 are**

(i) 24, 47 (ii) 27, 49
(iii) 31, 53 (iv) none of these

**(b) Had there been 25 rows and 37 columns in part (a) instead of 10 and 7, other things remaining unchanged, then the total number of such numbers which would have retained there position in both the arrangement would have been**

(i) 11 (ii) 12 (iii) 13 (iv) 14

**85. A, B, C, D, and E are five persons, there being two couples in the group. Let (A, B); (B, C) and (C, D) are of opposite sex but they are not couples.**

**(a) Which of the following will necessarily be a couple?**

(i) B, E (ii) C, E (iii) A, E (iv) A, D

**(b) If D, E are of opposite sex, then which of the following will be a bachelor in the group?**

(i) A (ii) B
(iii) C (iv) cannot be determined

**86. In a parliament of 100 members, a bill was stuck (50 for it and 50 against it) due to cross voting on either side, viz. the government and the opposition. If every member voted and the cross voting were integral percent (< 25) of the votes of their groups, then**

**(a) how many members does the government has?**

(i) 60 (ii) 72 (iii) 75 (iv) 80

**(b) the percent crossvoting occurred on the government side is**

(i) 5 (ii) 10 (iii) 15 (iv) 20

**(c) the percent crossvoting occurred on the opposition side is**

(i) 5 (ii) 10 (iii) 15 (iv) 20

**87. Let** $x_1 + x_2 + x_3 = 1$

$$x_2 + x_3 + x_4 = 1/2$$

$$x_3 + x_4 + x_5 = 1/4 \quad \text{and so on,}$$

**where each successive term is less than its preceding term and decreases progressively to zero.**

**(a) Then** $x_1 =$

(i) 2/3 (ii) 4/7
(iii) 8/15 (iv) none of these

**(b) Then $x_2 =$**

(i) 1/3 (ii) 2/7
(iii) 4/15 (iv) none of these

**(c) Had $x_1 + \frac{x_2}{2} + \frac{x_3}{4} = 1$, $x_2 + \frac{x_3}{2} + \frac{x_4}{4} = 1$, $x_3 + \frac{x_4}{2} + \frac{x_5}{4} = 1$ and so on, where each successive term is less than its preceding term and decreases progressively to zero, then $x_1 =$**

(i) 2/3 (ii) 4/7
(iii) 8/15 (iv) none of these

**88. $M_1, M_2, M_3, M_4, M_5$ are five students who are asked three questions of Yes/No type. Their responses are as follow:**

| | $M_1$ | $M_2$ | $M_3$ | $M_4$ | $M_5$ |
|---|---|---|---|---|---|
| 1. | Y | Y | Y | N | N |
| 2. | N | N | Y | Y | Y |
| 3. | Y | N | N | N | Y |

**If it is known that one of them always gave the answers correctly, one of them always gave the answers wrongly and the total number of correct responses of all three questions is less than that of incorrect responses, then**

**(a) the student who always gave correct answers is**

(i) $M_1$ (ii) $M_2$ (iii) $M_3$ (iv) $M_4$

**(b) the student who always gave incorrect answers is**

(i) $M_1$ (ii) $M_3$ (iii) $M_4$ (iv) $M_5$

**(c) $M_3$ gave**

(i) no answer correctly
(ii) one answer correctly
(iii) two answers correctly
(iv) all answers correctly

**89. $M_1$, $M_2$, $M_3$ and $M_4$ bought a computer and decided to share the time of each day according to the money they**

**contributed. The price of the computer in rupees as well as the hours of the day, the computer is used (> 10), are integers. If $M_1$ contributed Rs 5000, $M_2$ contributed 25% of the total money, $M_3$ uses 20% of the time of the computers and $M_4$ uses it for 2 hours, then**

**(a) $M_1$ uses the computer for**

(i) 6 hrs. (ii) 6 hrs 15 minutes
(iii) 6 hrs. 30 minutes (iv) 6 hrs 45 minutes

**(b) $M_4$ contributed**

(i) Rs 1500 (ii) Rs 1600
(iii) Rs 1800 (iv) Rs 2000

**(c) If another person $M_4$ wanted to use the remaining free hours at the computer each day by paying them a rent of Rs 100 for certain number of days and after which he could have it free because he would have contributed by then the money had he contributed the same money at the purchase of it for his share of time of computer, then he would have paid the rent for**

(i) 42 days (ii) 45 days
(iii) 48 days (iv) 54 days

**90. Four persons bet on two horses A and B. Each ticket for A and B are sold at Rs 10 and Rs 20 respectively and better gets double if the horses he bets on wins (and loses the money of his ticket if it loses). All of them bought at least one ticket of each horse and invested equal amount of money. Tickets of both horses sold are found to be equal. First better bets such that he cannot lose while no betters bought the same number of tickets of a horse.**

**(a) The minimum number of tickets of a horse sold can be**

(i) 12 (ii) 16 (iii) 20 (iv) 24

**(b) The amount invested by each person corresponding to part (a) is**

(i) Rs 120 (ii) Rs 150
(iii) Rs 180 (iv) Rs 200

(c) **The maximum number of tickets of a horse B bought by any better corresponding to part (a) will be**
(i) 6 (ii) 7 (iii) 8 (iv) 9

**91. A, B, C, D, E, E are five persons who spent equal amount of money on buying apples and oranges. Each bought at least one of each fruits and none of them bought the same number of any fruits. A bought 5 apples and 2 oranges; B bought same number of apples and oranges; C bought 2 apples and twice the number of oranges as B bought; D bought less number of fruits together than that bought by E.**

(a) **The number of oranges bought by D is**
(i) 2 (ii) 4 (iii) 6 (iv) 8

(b) **The total number of oranges bought is**
(i) 24 (ii) 28 (iii) 30 (iv) 32

(c) **The total number of apple bought is**
(i) 15 (ii) 16 (iii) 17 (iv) 18

**92. A, B, C and D bought (9 apples, 25 oranges); (11 apples, 22 oranges); (15 apples, 16 oranges) and (21 apples, 8 oranges) respectively. It is known that three of them spent the equal amount of money.**

(a) **Who did not spend the same amount of money as others did?**
(i) A (ii) B (iii) C (iv) D

(b) **The fourth person would have spend the same amount of money as others spent had he bought**
(i) one apple more (ii) one orange more
(iii) one apple less (iv) one orange less

**93. A tank has three inlet pipes and three outlet pipes. When one inlet pipe and one outlet pipe are opened together, the tank is found to be filled in $x, \frac{6}{5}, \frac{4}{3}, \frac{8}{3}$, 3, 4, $\frac{24}{5}$, 6 and 12 hours for various combination of the pipes where $x$ is the least value in the above series.**

(a) **$x$ can be equal to**

(i) $\frac{24}{20}$ (ii) $\frac{24}{21}$ (iii) $\frac{24}{22}$ (iv) $\frac{24}{23}$

**(b) When all pipes are opened together, then the time in which tank will get filled for the corresponding value of *x* in part (a) is**

(i) $\frac{24}{30}$ hrs (ii) $\frac{24}{31}$ hrs

(iii) $\frac{24}{32}$ hrs (iv) $\frac{24}{33}$ hrs

**(c) *x* can be equal to**

(i) $\frac{24}{24}$ (ii) $\frac{24}{25}$

(iii) $\frac{24}{26}$ (iv) $\frac{24}{27}$

**(d) When all pipes are opened together, then the time in which tank will get filled for the corresponding value of *x* in part (c) is**

(i) $\frac{24}{30}$ hrs (ii) $\frac{24}{31}$ hrs

(iii) $\frac{24}{32}$ hrs (iv) $\frac{24}{33}$ hrs

**94. A shopkeeper gives one article free for every three articles purchased together and two articles free for every five articles purchased together. He sold 100 articles.**

**(a) Had he not given discount, which of the following can be the number of articles sold?**

(i) 68 (ii) 70

(iii) 72 (iv) all of these

**(b) Let the shopkeeper made 10% profit. Had he not given discount,he could have made *x*% profit. Then *x* can be equal to**

(i) 20 (ii) 25 (iii) 40 (iv) 50

**95. X bought four articles, viz. A, B, C, D for Rs 100. He used article A and sold the remaining articles to Y for**

**Rs 100. Y used article B and sold the remaining article to Z for Rs 100. Z used article C and sold article D for Rs 100. Let the profit percents of X, Y and Z be 20%, 25% and 50% respectively.**

**(a) Which is the cheapest article?**

(i) A (ii) B (iii) C (iv) D

**(b) Which is the costliest article?**

(i) A (ii) B (iii) C (iv) D

**(c) What is the cost of article D?**

(i) Rs 10 (ii) Rs 20 (iii) Rs 30 (iv) Rs 40

**96. A. Let A, B, C, D and E be the vertices of a regular pentagon and O be a point inside it such that OA > OB > OC > OD > OE. Which of the following is correct?**

(i) A and B are adjacent vertices
(ii) B and C are adjacent vertices
(iii) C and D are adjacent vertices
(iv) all of these

**B. Let A, B, C, D, E and F be the vertices of a regular hexagon and O be a point inside it such that OA > OB > OC > OD > OE > OF.**

**(a) Which of the following is necessarily true?**

(i) A lies between the adjacent vertices B and C
(ii) B lies between the adjacent vertices A and C
(iii) C lies between the adjacent vertices B and D
(iv) none of these

**(b) Which of the following is necessarily wrong?**

(i) D lies between the adjacent vertices B and F
(ii) E lies between the adjacent vertices D and F
(iii) F lies between the adjacent vertices D and E
(iv) all of these are necessarily true

**(c) The perpendicular dropped from O on which of the following lines will be longest in length?**

(i) AF (ii) BE
(iii) CD (iv) cannot be determined

**97. ABCD is a quadrilateral and O is a point inside it such that OA < OB < OC < OD. The point O can lie anywhere inside the triangle PQR but not outside it.**

**(a) How many sides of PQR will be necessarily perpendicular to a side of ABCD?**
(i) Zero (ii) One (iii) Two (iv) Three

**(b) Which of the sides of the quadrilateral ABCD is not bisected when the sides of triangle PQR are produced (considering that the triangle PQR lies inside the quadrilateral ABCD)?**
(i) AB (ii) BC (iii) CD (iv) DA

**(c) Which of the following segment of lines will have its perpendicular bisector split the triangle PQR?**
(i) AD (ii) AC (iii) BD (iv) DA

**98. ABC is a triangle with BC > CA > AB. Let D, E, F be the midpoints of the sides.**

**(a) If AD > BE > CF, then on which of the sides will D lie?**
(i) AB (ii) BC
(iii) CA (iv) the case is not possible

**(b) If BD > CE > AF, then on which of the sides will D lie?**
(i) AB (ii) BC
(iii) CA (iv) cannot be determined

**99. Four rows and four columns are to be filled by 16 elements, viz. $A_i$, $B_i$, $C_i$, $D_i$ ($i$ = 1, 2, 3, 4). Rows 1-4 are filled by $A_i$, $B_i$, $C_i$ and $D_i$ respectively. No columns contains any two elements of same subscript. Let $C_1$, $B_2$, $A_4$ and $D_3$ be in first, second, third and fourth column respectively.**

**(a) How many different kind of arrangements are possible?**
(i) 1 (ii) 2 (iii) 3 (iv) 4

**(b) When $B_1$ is just below $A_4$, then**
(i) $C_2$ is just below $B_4$
(ii) $C_3$ is just above $D_4$
(iii) $B_1$ is just above $C_4$
(iv) none of these

**(c) Which of the following cannot be correct?**

(i) $B_1$ is above $C_3$ (ii) $A_2$ is above $B_3$

(iii) $C_2$ is above $D_4$ (iv) $D_1$ is below $C_4$

**(d) Which of the following cannot be correct?**

(i) $D_2$ is below $C_4$ (ii) $C_4$ is below $B_3$

(iii) $A_1$ is above $B_3$ (iv) none of these

**100. A, B, C, and D are four persons having Rs 8 each. Each of them bet once with others and they give half of their money to the opponent if they lose and get half of the money of one's opponent if one wins.**

**(a) If D wins all his bets, then his final amount will be Rs**

(i) 16 (ii) 18

(iii) 20 (iv) cannot be determined

**(b) If D wins all his bets, and A losses all his bets, then the difference in amount of B and C will be Rs**

(i) 1 (ii) 2

(iii) 5 (iv) cannot be determined

**101. Five points are arranged around a circle on five fixed positions and each of the position is assigned a number through 1 to 5. The points shifted their positions clockwise as many in numbers as that is assigned to their positions. It is found that none of them shared the same position after the movement.**

**(a) How many distinct numbering of positions are possible?**

(i) 1 (ii) 2 (iii) 3 (iv) 4

**(b) For an arrangement, the maximum number of times the points can successively shift according to the aforementioned rule is**

(i) 1 (ii) 2 (iii) 3 (iv) 4

**(c) Had the points moved anti-clockwise instead of clockwise, they would've still not shared the same position for**

(i) one type of arrangement

(ii) two distinct types of arrangements

(iii) three distinct types of arrangements

(iv) four distinct types of arrangements

**102. 100 coins are to be distributed among 6 children A, B, C, D, E and F such that the numbers of coins given to children increases in that order with no children getting less than twice or more than thrice the number of coins the child just preceding him in order gets.**

**(a) The maximum number of coins F can get is**

(i) 63 (ii) 64 (iii) 65 (iv) 69

**(b) The minimum number of coins F will get is**

(i) 51 (ii) 52 (iii) 53 (iv) 54

**(c) If D gets 13 coins, then how many coins F gets?**

(i) 52 (ii) 53

(iii) 54 (iv) cannot be determined

**103. In class tests of four subjects: Maths, Physics, Chemistry and Biology four students A, B, C and D scored relatively as A > B > C > D; B > D > C > A; C > A > D > B and D > B > A > C respectively. The total marks of a test was 10 and no student got marks in decimal or less than 4 or same marks in two subjects. If the average marks obtained by students in the subjects were 7, 8, 6 and 8 respectively, then total marks obtained by**

**(a) A was**

(i) 28 (ii) 29 (iii) 30 (iv) 31

**(b) B was**

(i) 28 (ii) 29 (iii) 30 (iv) 31

**(c) A was**

(i) 28 (ii) 29 (iii) 30 (iv) 31

**104. A, B, C, D, E, F and G are seven children who have few marbles with them, the number of marbles with them form a series of consecutive integers. Let S be the set of three children, one of the children having sum of number of marbles possessed by other two children. Let all possible kind of set S be**

**A. {A, B, C}; {E, F, G}; {B, D, F}; {C, E, G}; {A, F, G}; {A, B, G}; {C, D, F}; {B, E, F} and {A, D, E}**

**(a) Which of the following has the least number of marbles?**

(i) A (ii) E (iii) F (iv) G

**(b) Which of the following has the maximum number of marbles?**

(i) B (ii) C (iii) D (iv) E

**(c) Which of the following has the number of marbles which is equal to average number of marbles possessed by all of them?**

(i) A (ii) 8 (iii) G (iv) E

**(d) Which of them has 5 marbles?**

(i) B (ii) F (iii) G (iv) D

**(e) How many marbles does D have?**

(i) 5 (ii) 6 (iii) 7 (iv) 8

**B. {A, C, D}; {B, D, E}; {D, F, G} and {A, B, F}**

**(a) Which of the following has the maximum number of marbles?**

(i) C (ii) E
(iii) F (iv) cannot be determined

**(b) How may marbles G has?**

(i) 5 (ii) 6 (iii) 7 (iv) 8

**(c) Who has got the least number of marbles?**

(i) A (ii) B
(iii) G (iv) cannot be determined

**105. Two identical circular pieces of papers have written (A, B, C, D) and (P, Q, R, S) on the ends of their two perpendicular diameters, not necessarily in that order. Also
when P is over A, Q is not over B;
when Q is over B, R is not over C;
when R is over C, S is not over D;
and when S is over D, P is not over A.**

**(a) When P is against Q, then A is against**

(i) B (ii) C
(iii) D (iv) cannot be determined

**(b) When P is against R, then A is against**

(i) B (ii) C
(iii) D (iv) cannot be determined

**(c) When P is against S, then A is against**

(i) B (ii) C
(iii) D (iv) cannot be determined

**(d) When S is over C (S, R being against each other, then P is over**

(i) A (ii) C
(iii) D (iv) cannot be determined

**(e) When S is over B (S, P being against each other), then R is over**

(i) A (ii) C
(iii) D (iv) cannot be determined

**106. Two identical circular pieces of papers have written (A, B, C, D, E, F) and (P, Q, R, S, T, U) on the vertices of regular hexagons (vertices being on the edge). They are kept one over the other. It is observed that**

**I. when P is between A and F (adjacent vertices), then D is between Q and T (adjacent vertices).**

**II. when R is between B and E (adjacent vertices), then F is between S and V (adjacent vertices).**

**III. when Q is between C and D (adjacent vertices), then A is between P and S (adjacent vertices).**

**(a) S must be against**

(i) Q (ii) R
(iii) T (iv) cannot be determined

**(b) If Q is against P, then R is against**

(i) S (ii) T
(iii) U (iv) cannot be determined

**(c) If A is against B, then F is against**

(i) C (ii) D
(iii) E (iv) cannot be determined

**(d) If A is against C, then F is against**

(i) B (ii) D
(iii) E (iv) cannot be determined

**(e) If Q is against U, then C is against**

(i) A (ii) F
(iii) B (iv) cannot be determined

**(f) If R is against U, then A is against**

(i) B (ii) C (iii) D (iv) E

**107. A game is being played by three players A, B and C with a dice. Each round of games consist of throwing of the dice once by each player. Each player is accorded two**

**numbers, turning up of one of them gives one point while the turning up of another deducts a point from the score of the player. A player can get a point or lose a point regardless of who threw up his corresponding numbers. They played three rounds. In round one, A, B, C threw up 5, 4, 6 respectively and their scores were –1, 1, 1 (may not be in order). In round two, A, B, C threw up 2, 3, 4 respectively and their scores were –1, 1, 1 (may not be in order). In round three A, B, C gets 1, –1, 1 respectively while they threw different numbers from what they had thrown in earlier rounds. Also A, B, C got/lost points on the numbers thrown up by C, A, B respectively.**

**(a) B gets –1 when the number turned up is**

(i) 1 (ii) 2
(iii) 4 (iv) cannot be determined

**(b) Who gets/loses point when the number turned up is 4?**

(i) A (ii) B
(iii) C (iv) cannot be determined

**(c) If A gets + 1 in first round, then C gets + 1 in turning up of**

(i) 1 (ii) 2 (iii) 3 (iv) 4

**(d) If A gets + 1 in first round, then which of the following is correct?**

(i) A gets –1 when 5 turns up
(ii) A gets –1 when 6 turns up
(iii) A gets +1 when 3 turns up
(iv) none of these

**108. Mrs. X gave birth to six children A, B, C, D, E and F in the span of eight years, no two children being born within 18 months. Let the date of births of A, B, C, D, E and F be 5th Jan, 3rd Feb, 6th Apr, 7th Jun, 8th Sep and 9th Nov respectively.**

**(a) Who is the first child to be born?**

(i) B (ii) C
(iii) E (iv) cannot be determined

**(b) Who is the second child to be born?**

(i) D (ii) E
(iii) F (iv) cannot be determined

**(c) Who is the third child to be born?**

(i) A (ii) C
(iii) F (iv) cannot be determined

**(d) Who is the fourth child to be born?**

(i) B (ii) D
(iii) F (iv) cannot be determined

**(e) Who is the sixth child to be born?**

(i) A (ii) B
(iii) D (iv) cannot be determined

**109. In a class test of four subjects: Maths, Physics chemistry and Biology, four students Rose, Monica, Lily and Tina got one of the grades: A, B, C in each of the four subjects. The weightage given to A is twice that of B and thrice that of C. Let in the subjects mentioned above, the grades given are (2A, B, C); (A, 2B, C); (2A, 2B) and (A, B, 2C) respectively. Let Rose got grades A and C in Maths and Biology respectively; Monica got grades C and B in Physics and Chemistry respectively; Lily got grades C and A in Maths and Chemistry respectively; and Tina got same grade B in Physics and Biology. Also no two students got the same rank and each of them got grades A and B in at least one of the subjects.**

**(a) Who is ranked first?**

(i) Rose (ii) Monica
(iii) Lily (iv) Tina

**(b) Who is ranked fourth?**

(i) Rose (ii) Monica
(iii) Lily (iv) Tina

**(c) The grades of Lily are**

(i) 2A, B, C (ii) A, 2B, C
(iii) A, B, 2C (iv) cannot be determined

**(d) The rank of Monica is**

(i) FIRST (ii) SECOND
(iii) THIRD (iv) FOURTH

**110. A, B, C, D are four students who took exams in four subjects, viz. Maths, Physics, Chemistry and Biology. They respectively got (8, 9, 10, 11); (7, 8, 9, 12); (7, 8, 10, 11);**

**and (8, 9, 10, 12) while marks obtained in Maths, Physics, Chemistry and Biology by four students are (8, 9, 10, 11); (7, 8, 10, 11); (7, 8, 9, 12) and (8, 9, 10, 12) respectively. All of them got different marks in different subjects and no two students got same mark in any subject.**

**(a) Let C get 11 marks in the subject in which A got 8. Then who got the least marks in Chemistry and Biology?**
- (i) B and C respectively
- (ii) C and D respectively
- (iii) B and D respectively
- (iv) C for both subjects

**(b) For part (a), B get 8 marks in**
- (i) Maths and Chemistry
- (ii) Maths and Physics
- (iii) Physics and Biology
- (iv) Chemistry and Biology

**(c) For part (a), which of the following can be determined?**
- (i) Marks of B in Chemistry
- (ii) Marks of B in Biology
- (iii) Marks of D in Maths
- (iv) Marks of D in Physics

**(d) Let C got 11 marks in the subject in which A got 9. Then C got the least marks in**
- (i) Maths and Chemistry
- (ii) Physics and Chemistry
- (iii) Physics and Biology
- (iv) Chemistry and Biology

**(e) For part (d), marks obtained by students can be definitely known for which of the following subjects?**
- (i) Maths and Physics
- (ii) Maths and Chemistry
- (iii) Physics and Biology
- (iv) Chemistry and Biology

**(f) For part (d), D got 8 marks in**
- (i) Maths
- (ii) Physics
- (iii) Chemistry
- (iv) Biology

**111. In a class test of four subjects: Maths, Physics, Chemistry and Biology, four students P, Q, R, S got one of the grades A, B, C in each of the four subjects. Let the grades given to P, Q, R, S be (A, A, B, C); (A, B, C, C); (A, B, C, C) and (A, B, B, C) respectively while the grades given in Maths, Physics, Chemistry and Biology be (A, A, B, C); (A, B, B, C); (A, B, C, C) and (A, B, C, C) respectively.**

**(a) Who will definitely get A in Maths?**

(i) P (ii) Q
(iii) R (iv) cannot be determined

**(b) Who will definitely get B in Physics?**

(i) Q (ii) R
(iii) S (iv) cannot be determined

**ADDITIONAL INFORMATIONS FOR (C, D, E):**
**Let P gets A in Maths and one of the other subjects, say X and B, C in remaining two subjects, say Y, Z respectively. Also let one of the other students, say L gets B in Maths while remaining two students, say M, N gets A, C respectively (in Maths)**

**(c) How many grades of L, M, N in subjects (X, Y, Z) can be definetly known?**

(i) 3 (ii) 4 (iii) 5 (iv) 6

**(d) If M gets B in X, then which of the following will be correct?**

(i) L gets A in Y (ii) N gets A in Z
(iii) L gets C in X (iv) N gets B in Z

**(e) In which of the following pair (subject/student) only one of the grades remains to be determined?**

(i) (L, X) (ii) (M, Y)
(iii) (N, Z) (iv) none of these

**112. In an exam, three grades are given, viz. A, B and C. Grades A, B and C denote that one gets (8 or 9); (6 or 7) and (4 or 5) marks out of 10. Four students P, Q, R and S took exams in four subjects: Maths, Physics, Chemistry and Biology. The grades obtained by the students in exams are tabulated as below:**

| Students | Maths | Physics | Chemistry | Biology |
|---|---|---|---|---|
| P | A | B | C | B |
| Q | C | B | B | A |
| R | B | C | A | C |
| S | C | A | B | B |

**Let each of them gets different marks in different subjects and no two of them gets same marks in same subject. Also the total marks obtained by each of them is different and that obtained in each of the subject is also different. Also R gets 7 marks in Maths.**

**(a) The total marks obtained in Maths is**
(i) 23 (ii) 24
(iii) 25 (iv) cannot be determined

**(b) In which of the following subjects, the marks obtained cannot be maximum?**
(i) Physics (ii) Chemistry
(iii) Biology (iv) cannot be determined

**(c) The total marks obtained by which of the following students cannot be maximum?**
(i) P (ii) Q
(iii) S (iv) cannot be determined

**(d) If Q got 8 marks in Biology, then the total marks obtained by P is**
(i) 25 (ii) 26
(iii) 27 (iv) cannot be determined

**(e) If S got 9 marks in Physics, then the total marks obtained in biology will be**
(i) 25 (ii) 26
(iii) 27 (iv) cannot be determined

**113. Six apples and six oranges (cheaper than apples) are distributed among four children A, B, C and D. The children who got fruits worth lesser amounts are compensated with cash so that net worth of cash plus fruits is equal for all of them. Let B, C and D received Rs 1, Rs 8 and Rs 9 respectively while A received no cash.**

**(a) The cost of an apple cannot be**
(i) Rs 3 (ii) Rs 4 (iii) Rs 6 (iv) Rs 8

(b) **The cost of an orange cannot be**
(i) Rs 1 (ii) Rs 2 (iii) Rs 3 (iv) Rs 4

(c) **If A got 2 oranges, then which of the following will be definitely correct?**
(i) B got 1 orange (ii) C got 2 oranges
(iii) D got 1 orange (iv) none of these

(d) **Which of the following is incorrect?**
(i) A could get 1, 2 or 3 oranges
(ii) B could get 1, 2 or 3 oranges
(iii) C could get 0, 1 or 2 oranges
(iv) D could get 0, 1 or 2 oranges

**114. 8 marbles: 3 green, 3 red and 2 blue are distributed among four persons A, B, C and D, each of whom get a pair of marbles (no two of them getting the same pair). The price of marbles of each colour are different. Let after the distribution, the worth of marbles C and D have be the least and the most respectively. Also the worth of marbles A has is more than that of B. Also A and B have at least one marble of red and green colour respectively.**

(a) **Who will definitely have both the marbles of same colour?**
(i) C (ii) D
(iii) Both (iv) None

(b) **When A has a red and a green marble, then which of the following is correct?**
(i) R is the most expensive and G is the least
(ii) R is the most expensive and B is the least
(iii) B is the most expensive and G is the least
(iv) cannot be determined

(c) **In how many certain ways, the marbles would have been distributed?**
(i) 5 (ii) 6 (iii) 7 (iv) 8

(d) **For part (c), in how many ways, blue marble would be least expensive?**
(i) 0 (ii) 1 (iii) 2 (iv) 3

**115. 20 marbles are distributed among four persons A, B, C, D (each getting at least one marble) such that A, B got even number of marbles while C got an odd number of marble.**

**(a) If C got the average of what A, B got and D got $x$ (> 0) marbles more than C, then $x$ =**
(i) 2 (ii) 4 (iii) 6 (iv) 8

**(b) If D got 8 marbles more than one of them and least number of marble anyone got is 2, then how many marbles D got?**
(i) 10 (ii) 11
(iii) 13 (iv) cannot be determined

**116. A can of capacity of $n$ litres ($n$ being a two-digit multiple of 10) is full with diluted milk. Half of this milk is given to P, after which a litre of water is added to it. Again half of the milk in the can is given to Q, after which again a litre of water is added to it. Similarly R and S (in that sequence) is also given milk. Water is not added to it after the milk is given to S. On analysis of remaining milk in the can, it is found that it contains 90 % water as against 80% water found naturally in the pure milk. Assuming that each of the persons had integral number of litres of diluted milk given to them, the percent dilution of amount of milk with**

**(a) P is**
(i) 30% (ii) 33% (iii) 36% (iv) 38%

**(b) Q is**
(i) 37% (ii) 38% (iii) 40% (iv) 42%

**(c) R is**
(i) 40% (ii) 43% (iii) 45% (iv) 47%

**(d) S is**
(i) 44% (ii) 46% (iii) 48% (iv) 50%

**117. Let A, B, C, D, E, F, G, H, I, J, K, L be four persons, each person having two nicknames. Let each of the groups (A, C, D, E); (C, I, K, L); (D, F, H, J); (A, G, H, L) and (B, G, J, K) have all the four persons. Then**

**(a) the nickname of B can be**
(i) A (ii) C (iii) F (iv) E

**(b) the nickname of I can be**
(i) B (ii) D (iii) E (iv) H

**(c) the nickname of E can be**

(i) B (ii) G (iii) I (iv) H

**(d) the nickname of F can be**

(i) E (ii) I (iii) G (iv) L

**118. Four students A, B, C, D took exam in four subjects: Maths, Physics, Chemistry and Biology. Between any two students, the marks obtained in two subjects by one of them is greater than other one while that in other two subjects, they are less.**

**(a) How many of them must get all the possible ranks in four subjects?**

(i) One (ii) Two (iii) Three (iv) All Four

**(b) Let the least number of students who must get ranks 1, 2 and 3 be *m*, *n* and *p* respectively. Which of the following will be correct?**

(i) $m = m = p$ (ii) $m = n + 1$

(iii) $n = p + 1$ (iv) $p = m + 1$

**(c) If A gets highest marks in Maths and Physics, B gets highest and second highest marks in Chemistry and Physics respectively and C got highest marks in Biology and second highest marks in Maths, then which of the following will be correct?**

(i) D gets lowest marks in Maths

(ii) D gets lowest marks in Physics

(iii) D gets second lowest marks in Maths

(iv) D gets second lowest marks in Chemistry

**(d) Let A get second highest marks in three of the subjects and B get lowest marks in Maths and Physics. If C gets lowest marks in chemistry, then D must get second lowest marks in**

(i) Maths (ii) Physics

(iii) Chemistry (iv) Biology

**(e) Let A get second highest marks in two subjects, viz. Physics and Maths and B get lowest marks in two subjects, viz. Chemistry and Biology. Which of the following can be correct?**

(i) C gets second lowest marks in Chemistry

(ii) D get highest marks in Maths
(iii) D gets second lowest marks in Biology
(iv) none of these

**119. A, B, C, D are four students who took exams in four subjects. Maths, Physics, Chemistry and Biology. In any subject, the students get one of the ranks 1, 2, 3 or 4. Let**

**A get rank 1 in Maths and rank 4 in Chemistry;**
**B get rank 1 Physics and rank 3 in Maths;**
**C get rank 3 in Chemistry and rank 2 in Biology;**
**D get rank 2 in Physics and rank 4 in Biology;**

**(a) How many distinct possibilities of rankings of students in all subjects are possible?**
(i) 8 (ii) 12 (iii) 16 (iv) 20

**(b) How many distinct possibilities of rankings of students in all subjects are possible if the sums of ranks obtained by A and D in four subjects are same?**
(i) 1 (ii) 2 (iii) 3 (iv) 4

**(c) The sum of ranks (consider their face values) for which of the following student will be least?**
(i) B (ii) C
(iii) D (iv) cannot be determined

**120. In an exam, instead of marks, grades A, B, C and D are given. Two systems of evaluation can be employed:**

**SYSTEM I. The weightage of A is twice that of B, thrice that of C and four times that of D.**

**SYSTEM II. The weightage of D is half that of B, one-third that of C and one-fourth that of A.**

**P, Q, R and S are four students who took exam in three subjects. By evaluation of system I, they got ranks 2, 4, 1, 3 respectively while by evaluation of system II, they got ranks 3, 2, 2, 1 respectively. [Note that the rank 1 is highest and rank 4, the lowest]. Also P got grade C in one of the subjects.**

**(a) The grades obtained by which of the following students cannot be uniquely determined?**
(i) P (ii) Q (iii) R (iv) S

(b) At least how many students must have got grade A?
(i) Zero (ii) One
(iii) Two (iv) Three

(c) Which of the following students must have got grade C in at least one of the subjects?
(i) Q (ii) R (iii) S (iv) R and S

(d) Which of the following students cannot get grade B in any of the subjects?
(i) P (ii) Q (iii) R (iv) S

(e) The total number of which of the following grades obtained by the students can be uniquely determined?
(i) A (ii) B (iii) C (iv) D

**121. A, B, C and D are four children playing a game by passing a ball to one another, the child receiving the ball not just passing it back to one from he got it. Let during the game, A, B, C and D held the ball for 5, 3, 4 and 4 times respectively (The holding of ball by a person at the start of the game is also counted). Also let initially a held the ball and passed it to C and finally D passed the ball to A. The number of times the ball is passed**

**A. successively twice among**

**(a) A, B and C only (in any order) is**
(i) 3 (ii) 4
(iii) 5 (iv) cannot be determined

**(b) A, C, and D only (in any order) is**
(i) 3 (ii) 4
(iii) 5 (iv) cannot be determined

**B.**

**(a) among A, B or C only is**
(i) 6 (ii) 7
(iii) 8 (iv) cannot be determined

**(b) among A, C or D only is**
(i) 7 (ii) 8
(iii) 9 (iv) cannot be determined

**122. A, B, C, D, E, F, G and H are eight books to be kept on three shelves: lowest, middle or top. The books are of four subjects: Mathematics, Physics, Chemistry and Biology,**

**two books of each subjects. No two books of same subject are kept on one shelf. Also**

**I. A is above D; G is below B; E is below F and H is below C.**

**II. top shelf has no chemistry book; middle shelf has no math book and lowest shelf has no physics book.**

**III. E and biology book are not together; H and physics book are not together; F and math book are not together and B and chemistry book are not together.**

**(a) Which of the following books will always be together?**

(i) H, E (ii) D, H (iii) D, G (iv) F, G

**(b) Which of the following will not be on the top shelf?**

(i) A (ii) B
(iii) C (iv) all will be on the top shelf

**(c) If E, G are books of same subject, then their subject is**

(i) Maths (ii) Physics
(iii) Chemistry (iv) cannot be determined

**(d) The book of which of the following subject cannot be on the shelf having two books?**

(i) Maths (ii) Physics
(iii) Chemistry (iv) Biology

**123. A man has certain amount of money with which he can buy three kinds of articles A, B or C. With his money, he can buy at most 5 articles of A and 1 articles of B; or 4 articles of B and 2 articles of C; or 3 articles each of A and C, with the money left in each case being not enough to buy any other article.**

**(a) The cheapest article is**

(i) A (ii) B
(iii) C (iv) cannot be determined

**(b) The costliest article is**

(i) A (ii) B
(iii) C (iv) cannot be determined

**124. A, B, C are three kind of articles for sale. Study the table below:**

| Article Type | A | B | C | Total Articles Purchased |
|---|---|---|---|---|
| | $x$ | $y$ | $z$ | 28 |
| | $x$ | $z$ | $y$ | 29 |
| Money Spent | $y$ | $z$ | $x$ | 31 |
| | $y$ | $x$ | $z$ | $k$ (< 32) |
| | $z$ | $x$ | $y$ | 31 |
| | $z$ | $y$ | $x$ | $k'$ |

**(a)** $k =$

(i) 28 (ii) 29 (iii) 30 (iv) 31

**(b)** $k' =$

(i) 30 (ii) 31 (iii) 32 (iv) 33

**(c) Let $p$, $q$, $r$ be the number of articles bought by A, B and C with Rs $x$. Then which of the following is correct?**

(i) $p + q = 2r$ (ii) $p + r = 2q$
(iii) $2p + r = 3q$ (iv) $p + 2r = 3q$

**(d) Which of the following is correct?**

(i) $x + z = 2y$ (ii) $x + 2z = 3y$
(iii) $2x + z = 3y$ (iv) $x + y = 2z$

**125. A, B, C are three types of articles for sale with the price of a being highest and that of C being lowest. With certain amount it is found that one can buy 3, 4, 5, 6 or 7 articles.**

**(a) When the seven articles bought are 7C, then the three articles bought with the same amount will be**

(i) 2A, B (ii) 2B, A
(iii) 2 C, A (iv) cannot be determined

**(b) When the seven articles bought are A and 6C, then the three articles bought with the same amount will be**

(i) 2 A, B (ii) 2 B, A
(iii) 2 C, A (iv) cannot be determined

**(c) When the seven articles bought are B and 6C, then the three articles bought with the same amount will be**

(i) 2 A, B (ii) 2 B, A
(iii) 2 A, C (iv) cannot be determined

**(d) In how many different ways three articles could be bought?**
(i) 3 (ii) 4 (iii) 5 (iv) 6

**(e) In how many different ways seven articles could be bought?**
(i) 3 (ii) 4 (iii) 5 (iv) 6

**126. Three kind of articles A, B, C are for sale, the prices of all articles being different. With Rs 240, one can buy four articles of A and an article of B ; or two articles of one kind and two articles of another kind, or one article of one kind, one article of another kind and three articles of third kind.**

**(a) The costliest article is**
(i) A (ii) B
(iii) C (iv) cannot be determined

**(b) The cheapest article is**
(i) A (ii) B
(iii) C (iv) cannot be determined

**(c) With Rs 240, when two articles of one kind and two articles of another kind are bought, then which of the following article is not purchased?**
(i) A (ii) B
(iii) C (iv) cannot be determined

**(d) With Rs 240, when one article of one kind, one article of another kind and three articles of third kind are bought, then this third kind is**
(i) A (ii) B
(iii) C (iv) cannot be determined

**127. Three kind of articles are for sale while P, Q, R are three buyers having Rs 160, Rs 180 and Rs 210 respectively. The buyers do not buy until they can use all of their money. It is found that total number of articles bought by P, Q, R can be 4 or 5 only; 4, 5 or 6 only; 5, 6 or 7 only respectively.**

**(a) In how many different ways P can buy the articles using all his money?**
(i) 2 (ii) 3 (iii) 4 (iv) 5

**(b) In how many different ways Q can buy the articles using all his money?**
(i) 3 (ii) 4 (iii) 5 (iv) 6

**(c) In how many different ways R can buy the articles using all his money?**
(i) 3 (ii) 4 (iii) 5 (iv) 6

**(d) What is the price of least expensive article?**
(i) Rs 25 (ii) Rs 30 (iii) Rs 35 (iv) Rs 40

**(e) What is the price of most expensive article?**
(i) Rs 45 (ii) Rs 50 (iii) Rs 55 (iv) Rs 60

**128. (a) $P > Q > R > S > T > U$ are six numbers. The minimum number of distinct elements of set containing the sum of them taken three at a time will be**
(i) 10 (ii) 12 (iii) 15 (iv) 17

**(b) In part (a), assume that there exists three distinct triplets from the given numbers such that the sums of elements of triplets are equal. How many possibilities of such distinct pair of triplets exist?**
(i) 1 (ii) 2 (iii) 3 (iv) 4

**129. A, B, C, D, E, F are six teachers who teach two of the subjects from Maths, Physics, Chemistry and Biology, no two teachers teaching the same pair of subjects. Now**
**(A, C) do not teach Physics;**
**(B, D) do not teach Chemistry;**
**(E, F) do not teach Maths;**
**only one of (B, E) teaches Biology and**
**only one of (C, D) teaches Biology.**

**(a) If C, D teach exclusive pair of subjects, then which of the following pair will also necessarily teach exclusive pair of subjects?**
(i) A, F (ii) B, E (iii) Both (iv) None

**(b) All the pair of subjects taught by each teacher can be known if it is known that**
(i) A teaches Maths and Chemistry
(ii) B teaches Maths and Physics
(iii) F teaches Physics and Chemistry
(iv) none of these

**(c) If D teaches Biology, then both the subjects taught by how many teachers can be known?**
(i) 1 (ii) 2 (iii) 3 (iv) 4

**(d) If C teaches Biology, then both the subjects taught by which of the following teacher can be known?**
(i) B (ii) C (iii) E (iv) F

**(e) Which of the following pair cannot teach biology together?**
(i) B, C (ii) C, E (iii) D, E (iv) B, F

**130. In a company, there are few supervisors, few managers and a director, viz. A, B, C, D, E, F, G, H, I and J (not in order). Each supervisor reports to few manager or director. All managers report to the director. Now**
**E reports to A and B only;**
**F reports to two persons only, not C;**
**G reports to two persons only, not A;**
**H reports to two persons only, not B;**
**I reports to two persons only, C and D;**
**J reports to two persons only, not D.**
**Also A, B, D each gets reports from four persons.**

**(a) From how many persons does C gets report from?**
(i) 2 (ii) 3
(iii) 4 (iv) cannot be determined

**(b) If there are three supervisors who report to same pair of managers, then the director is**
(i) A (ii) B (iii) C (iv) D

**(c) If there are two pairs of supervisors, each pair reporting to same exclusive pair of managers, then one of the pair of managers must be**
(i) A and B (ii) C and D
(iii) A and D (iv) B and D

**131. A, B, C, D, E, F G and H are eight books; two each of subjects: Maths, Physics, Chemistry and Biology.**
**Let the subject of**
**one of (A, B) be Physics ; one of (D, F) be Biology;**
**one of (C, G) be Maths ; one of (E, H) be Chemistry;**
**one of (E, F) be Maths ; one of (C, D) be Physics;**
**one of (A, G) be Chemistry; one of (B, H) be Biology.**

**(a) If A is a Physics book, then the subject of F is**
(i) Maths (ii) Physics
(iii) Chemistry (iv) Biology

**(b) If D is a biology book, then the subject of G will be**
(i) Maths (ii) Physics
(iii) Chemistry (iv) Biology

**(c) If the subjects of (G, H) are same, then the subjects of which of the following pairs of books will also be same?**
(i) (B, F) and (A, E) (ii) (B, C) and (A, D)
(iii) (C, E) and (B, F) (iv) none of these

**(d) Which of the following can have the same subjects?**
(i) (A, C) (ii) (B, D)
(iii) (F, H) (iv) none of these

**132. $X_1$, $X_2$, $X_3$, $X_4$ and $X_5$ are five persons taking part in three different events for gold, silver and bronze medals. The following are the outcome of three events:**

**I. No medal is shared by any two or more persons.**
**II. $X_1$ got a bronze and two medals of same kind.**
**III. $X_2$ got two medals, one gold and one silver.**
**IV. $X_3$ got two medals.**
**V. $X_4$ got one silver medal only.**
**VI. $X_5$ got one bronze medal only.**

**Now answer the following question:**

**(a) In an event, when $X_1$ got a bronze, then which of the following statement must be true?**
(i) $X_2$ got gold (ii) $X_2$ got silver
(iii) $X_3$ got silver (iv) $X_4$ got silver

**(b) Which of the following will be correct?**
(i) When $X_4$ got silver, then $X_1$ got gold
(ii) When $X_4$ got silver, then $X_2$ got gold
(iii) When $X_5$ got bronze, then $X_1$ got gold
(iv) When $X_5$ got bronze, then $X_2$ got silver

**(c) Which of the following cannot be possible?**
(i) When $X_4$ got silver, then $X_3$ got bronze
(ii) When $X_4$ got silver, then $X_5$ got bronze
(iii) When $X_5$ got bronze, then $X_3$ got silver
(iv) all of the above are possible

**133. A, B, C, D are four persons who need to take 1600, 1800, 2200 and 2400 kilocalorie respectively per day for being healthy. They can choose from four different packets P, Q, R, S which give respectively 400, 450, 500 and 650 kcal. One day they together bought 4 packets of each food and distributed it among themselves according to their calorie needs. While distribution, B preferred to have only three packets.**

**(a) D must have a packet**

(i) P (ii) Q (iii) R (iv) S

**(b) In how many different ways the packets can be distributed?**

(i) 3 (ii) 4 (iii) 5 (iv) 6

**(c) Which of the following is not a feasible combination of packets for C?**

(i) 2 Q and 2 S (ii) 3 P and 2 R
(iii) P, R, and 2 S (iv) 2 P, 2 Q, and R

**(d) Which of the following is not a feasible combination of packets for D?**

(i) 2 Q and 3 R (ii) P, 3 Q and S
(iii) 2 P, Q, R and S (iv) all of these are possible

**134. Three kind of articles are for sale. With Rs 23, 24, 25 or 26, one can buy four articles if at least two kinds of articles are to be purchased with no money being left. Given that cost of each articles are integral number of rupees,**

**(a) the cost of the least expensive article is**

(i) Rs 4 (ii) Rs 5
(iii) Rs 6 (iv) cannot be determined

**(b) The cost of the most expensive article is**

(i) Rs 6 (ii) Rs 7
(iii) Rs 8 (iv) cannot be determined

**(c) The cost of third article is**

(i) Rs 5 (ii) Rs 6
(iii) Rs 7 (iv) cannot be determined

**135. Each articles of A, B, C, D cost Rs 80, Rs 90, Rs 100 and Rs 120 respectively. With all the money P, Q, R, S have,**

**they can buy 2 or 3 articles only; 3 or 4 articles only; 4 or 5 articles only; 5 or 6 articles only respectively.**

**(a) What is the minimum sum of money that can be possessed by all the persons together?**

(i) Rs 1360 (ii) Rs 1420
(iii) Rs 1440 (iv) Rs 1460

**(b) What is the maximum sum of money possessed by all the persons together?**

(i) Rs 1590 (ii) Rs 1610
(iii) Rs 1630 (iv) Rs 1640

**(c) What is the maximum number of article B that R can buy?**

(i) 4 (ii) 5 (iii) 6 (iv) 7

**(d) What is the minimum number of article C that S can buy?**

(i) 4 (ii) 5 (iii) 6 (iv) 7

**(e) Which of the following is incorrect?**

(i) P cannot buy article B
(ii) Q cannot buy article C
(iii) R cannot buy two items of article B
(iv) S cannot buy three items of article C

**136. P. Q, R are three persons having some initial amounts. There are four different kind of articles for sale, viz. A, B, C and D, all of different prices (integral number of Rupees). It is observed that with all the money they have,**

**I. P can buy either two articles of A or C and D;**
**II. Q can buy either three articles of C or two articles of B and D;**
**III. the minimum and maximum number of articles R can buy are three and five respectively;**
**IV. B is the cheapest article sold at Rs 30 and R has Rs 150.**

**(a) Which is the costliest item?**

(i) A (ii) B
(iii) D (iv) cannot be determined

**(b) The cost of A is**

(i) Rs 48 (ii) Rs 50
(iii) Rs 54 (iv) cannot be determined

**(c) The difference in cost of C and A can not be Rs**
(i) 10 (ii) 12 (iii) 15 (iv) 20

**(d) Which of the following will have definitely the most money?**
(i) P (ii) Q (iii) R (iv) Q or R

**(e) If R can buy four articles, then he cannot buy**
(i) C (ii) A
(iii) D (iv) all items could be bought

**137. A, B, C, D, E are five persons holding certain amount of money each (all different).**

**When B, C, D, E exchanged their amounts among themselves so that no one have their original amount, it is observed that**

**I. B possesses the highest amount among all persons.**
**II. D possesses the lowest amount among all persons which is Rs 20 less than what A has.**
**III. E and C possess Rs 50 and Rs 70 respectively.**

**When A, C, D, E exchanged their initial amounts among themselves so that no one have their original amount, it is observed that**

**I. A has the highest amount among all persons which is Rs 40 more than what B has.**
**II. C has Rs 30 less than what A has.**
**III. E has Rs 10 less than what D has.**

**(a) The initial amount possessed by A was**
(i) Rs 40 (ii) Rs 60
(iii) Rs 80 (iv) cannot be determined

**(b) The initial amount possessed by B was**
(i) Rs 40 (ii) Rs 50
(iii) Rs 60 (iv) cannot be determined

**(c) The initial amount possessed by C was**
(i) Rs 50 (ii) Rs 70
(iii) Rs 80 (iv) cannot be determined

**(d) The initial amount possessed by D was**
(i) Rs 50 (ii) Rs 60
(iii) Rs 80 (iv) cannot be determined

**(e) The initial amount possessed by E was**

(i) Rs 60 (ii) Rs 70
(iii) Rs 80 (iv) cannot be determined

**138. A, B, C, D have certain amounts: Rs 100, 200, 300 and 400 respectively. Six exclusive pairs are chosen once and successively. After each selection, the pair interchanged their money. Let after third and sixth selection, the respective amounts with A, B, C, D be Rs (200, 300, 400, 100) and Rs (100, 200, 300, 400) respectively.**

**(a) If the first pair selected is (A, B), then the last pair selected can be**

(i) (A, D) or (B, C) (ii) (A, C) or (B, D)
(iii) (A, D) or (C, D) (iv) (B,C) or (C, D)

**(b) If the first pair selected is (A, C), then the last pair selected will be**

(i) (A, B) (ii) (B,C)
(iii) (B, D) (iv) (C, D)

**(c) If the first pair selected is (A, D), then the last pair selected can be**

(i) (A, B) or (C, D) (ii) (A, C) or (B, D)
(iii) (A, C) or (B, C) (iv) (B, C) or (C, D)

**(d) If the first pair selected is (B, C), then the last pair selected can be**

(i) (A, B) or (C, D) (ii) (A, C) or (B, D)
(iii) (A, D) or (C, D) (iv) (B, D) or (C, D)

**(e) If the first pair selected is (B, D), then the last pair selected will be**

(i) (A, B) (ii) (A, C)
(iii) (B, C) (iv) (C, D)

**(f) If the first pair selected is (C, D), then the last pair selected can be**

(i) (A, B) or (B, C) (ii) (A, C) or (B, D)
(iii) (A, D) or (B, C) (iv) (A, B) or (B, D)

**139. A, B, C, D are four persons having same initial amounts (all different). Two of them are selected and they divided their money equally between each other. Every possible pair is chosen once and in succession. Let after third**

**and sixth selection, A, B, C, D have Rs (36, 42, 42, 40) and Rs (39, 41, 40, 40) respectively.**

**(a) What is the initial amount B had?**
(i) Rs 32 (ii) Rs 38 (iii) Rs 42 (iv) Rs 48

**(b) What is the initial amount C had?**
(i) Rs 32 (ii) Rs 38 (iii) Rs 42 (iv) Rs 48

**(c) What is the initial amount A had?**
(i) Rs 38 (ii) Rs 42
(iii) Rs 48 (iv) cannot be determined

**(d) Which of the following is first pair to be chosen?**
(i) (A, B) (ii) (A, C) (iii) (A, D) (iv) (B, D)

**(e) Which of the following is correct?**
(i) After fifth selection, C has Rs 41
(ii) The pair chosen for fourth selection is B, D
(iii) After fourth selection, D has Rs 40
(iv) none of these

**140. A, B, C, D are four persons each having some amount of money (all integers) who can buy mango, orange or apple (cost of one fruit of any kind being integer). Let with the money,**
**A and C have together, they can buy 35 mangoes;**
**B and D have together, they can buy 45 mangoes;**
**A and B have together, they can buy 52 oranges;**
**C and D have together, they can buy 76 oranges;**
**A and D have together, they can buy 85 apples;**
**B and C have together, they can buy 35 *n* apples where *n* is an integer between 50 and 100. Given that the money A, B, C and D have together is a multiple of Rs 10 and less than Rs 4000, then**

**(a) $n$ =**
(i) 60 (ii) 75
(iii) 80 (iv) cannot be determined

**(b) the amount possessed by which of the following is least?**
(i) A (ii) B
(iii) C (iv) cannot be determined

**(c) the number of apples that can be bought by A, B and D together will be**
(i) 100 (ii) 108 (iii) 120 (iv) 128

**(d) the number of oranges that can be bought by B, C and D together will be**

(i) 100 (ii) 104 (iii) 108 (iv) 112

**141. A, B, C, D are four articles for sale, their cost and weights being different. Let the cost of (B, C); (A, D) and (B, D) be 130, Rs 140 and Rs 150 respectively while the weights of (A, C), (B, D) and (C, D) be Rs 4, 6 and 7 kg respectively. Also the weight of the article which price is Rs 80 is 3 kg.**

**(a) The weight of B is**

(i) 2 (ii) 3
(iii) 4 (iv) cannot be determined

**(b) The cost of A is**

(i) Rs 30 (ii) Rs 40
(iii) Rs 50 (iv) cannot be determined

**(c) Which article is costliest per kg weight?**

(i) A (ii) B (iii) C (iv) D

**142. Three kinds of fruits: orange, apple and mango are for sale. Let the cost of**
**1 dozen orange be equal to that of 1.5 kg of mango;**
**1 dozen apple be equal to Rs 2 more than that of 1 kg of orange;**

**Also 1 dozen of any kind of fruit weigh only 1, 2 or 3 kg (each one weigh differently). Given that the cost of any fruit per kg is an integer (in rupees) less than 30,**

**(a) the cost of 1 kg of orange is**

(i) Rs 15 (ii) Rs 18
(iii) Rs 21 (iv) cannot be determined

**(b) the cost of 1 kg of apple is**

(i) Rs 15 (ii) Rs 18
(iii) Rs 21 (iv) cannot be determined

**(c) the cost of 1 kg of mango is**

(i) Rs 18 (ii) Rs 21
(iii) Rs 24 (iv) cannot be determined

**143. A, B, C, D are four persons who can buy three fruits: apple, mango and orange. With the money A, B, C, D**

**have, they can respectively buy at most 11, 12, 10, 14 apples; 10, 11, 9, 12 mangoes; 13, 15, 12, 16 oranges. Let the cost of an apple, a mango or an orange be an integer.**

**(a) The least value of cost of an apple will be**
(i) 5 (ii) 6 (iii) 7 (iv) 8

**(b) The least value of cost of a mango will be**
(i) 5 (ii) 6 (iii) 7 (iv) 8

**(c) The least value of cost of an orange will be**
(i) 5 (ii) 6 (iii) 7 (iv) 8

**(d) For the values obtained in above parts, the amount with A, if it is a multiple of 5, will be**
(i) Rs 70 (ii) Rs 75 (iii) Rs 80 (iv) Rs 85

**144. X, Y, Z are three articles and A, B, C, D, E, F are six persons, each having some amount of money. It is observed that**
**X can be bought by (A, B, C) or (D, E, F) only;**
**Y can be bought by (A, C, D) or (B, D, F) only and**
**Z can be bought by (A, C, F) only [all the amounts with persons in triplets have are used]. Given that A, B, C, D, E, F have Rs (400, 450, 500, 600, 700, 750) (not in order),**

**(a) the cost of X is**
(i) Rs 1700 (ii) Rs 1800
(iii) Rs 1900 (iv) cannot be determined

**(b) the cost of Y is**
(i) Rs 1700 (ii) Rs 1800
(iii) Rs 1900 (iv) cannot be determined

**(c) the cost of Z is**
(i) Rs 1700 (ii) Rs 1800
(iii) Rs 1900 (iv) cannot be determined

**(d) the amount with F is**
(i) Rs 600 (ii) Rs 700
(iii) Rs 750 (iv) cannot be determined

**145. Consider five kind of fruits: apple, peach, orange, mango and guava. Let**
**1 kg of apple has same number of fruits as 0.5 kg of guava and 1 kg of orange;**

**2 kg of mango has same number of fruits as 0.5 kg of guava and 0.8 kg of orange;**
**1 kg of guava has 2 fruits less than 1 kg of peach and 1 kg of mango;**
**2 kg of peach has 3 fruits more than 1 kg of apple.**
**If the total number of fruits in a kg of any kind of fruits given is less than 25, then the number of fruits in 1 kg of**

**(a) apple is**
(i) 7 (ii) 8
(iii) 9 (iv) cannot be determined

**(b) peach is**
(i) 5 (ii) 6
(iii) 7 (iv) cannot be determined

**(c) mango is**
(i) 3 (ii) 4
(iii) 5 (iv) cannot be determined

**146. Four persons A, B, C and D start running simultaneously from a point on a circle around it, each with constant speed in clockwise direction. A met B after A made 2 revolutions; B met C after B made 3 revolutions and C met D after C made 4 revolutions.**

**(a) If the speed of A is greater than that of C, then A met C after A made**
(i) 3/2 or 2 revolution (ii) 3/2 or 3 revolution
(iii) 4/3 or 2 revolution (iv) 4/3 or 3 revolution

**(b) If the speed of A is less than that of C, then C met A after C made**
(i) 3/2 revolution (ii) 4/3 revolution
(iii) 2 revolution (iv) 3 revolution

**(c) If the speed of B is less than that of D, then D met B after D made**
(i) 3/2 revolution (ii) 2 revolution
(iii) 5/2 revolution (iv) 3 revolution

**(d) The ratio of speeds of A and D cannot be**
(i) 2 : 1 (ii) 4 : 3 (iii) 3 : 4 (iv) 2 : 5

**147. Four persons A, B, C, D are asked about three qualities of a stick, viz. its length, shape and weight.**

**(a) They may or may not tell the truth about all the three qualities. Let the description of stick by**

**A be as long, thin and light;**
**B be as short, thin and light;**
**C be as long, thick and heavy;**
**D be as short, thick and heavy;**

**Which of the following must be true?**

(i) One of them is speaking truth about all qualities
(ii) One of them is speaking lie about all qualities
(iii) Both
(iv) None

**(b) One of them speaks only truth while other three speak at least one lie and one truth about the qualities. Let the description of stick by**

**A be as short, thin and heavy;**
**B be as short, thick and light;**
**C be as long, thin and light;**
**D be as long, thick and heavy;**

**D cannot speak truth about**

(i) just one quality (ii) just two qualities
(iii) any quality (iv) all qualities

**148. A, B, C, D, E are five persons, each person speaks truth to two persons and lie to other two persons Let**
**A speaks truth to exactly one of B, C;**
**B speaks truth to exactly one of C, E;**
**C speaks truth to exactly one of B, D;**
**D speaks truth to exactly one of A, E;**
**E speaks truth to exactly one of A, D;**
**Also each person is told truth by exactly two persons and lie by exactly two persons.**

**(a) If B, E speak truth of A, then B and C speak truth to**

(i) C and B respectively
(ii) C and D respectively
(iii) E and B respectively
(iv) E and D respectively

**(b) If C, D speak truth of A, then B and C speak truth to**

(i) C and B respectively

(ii) C and D respectively
(iii) E and B respectively
(iv) E and D respectively

**(c) If A, B speak truth of E, then B and C speak truth to**
(i) A and B respectively
(ii) A and D respectively
(iii) D and B respectively
(iv) C and D respectively

**149. A, B, C, D, E are five persons living in a five storey building, each one on a separate floor. Now one of each of the following pairs of information is incorrect:**

**A lives on the first floor, B lives on the second floor;**
**B lives on the third floor, D lives on the ground floor;**
**C lives on the third floor, E lives on the top floor;**

**(a) Who cannot be on the second floor?**
(i) A (ii) B (iii) D (iv) E

**(b) Who cannot be on the top floor?**
(i) A (ii) B (iii) C (iv) E

**150. In a triangular cricket series for Pepsi Cup among Australia, India and Pakistan, the bookies offer to double, triple or quadruple the amount invested on the teams (in the order as given) regarding their winning of the cup. A, B, C are three betters who invested money on these teams. If**

**Australia wins, then A, B, C will respectively lose Rs 700, Rs 500 and Rs 700;**
**India wins, then they will respectively lose Rs 400, lose Rs 400 and gain Rs 200;**
**Pakistan wins, then they will respectively gain Rs 1300, Rs 1100 and Rs 700;**
**They money invested by three betters on**

**(a) Australia is**
(i) Rs 1200 (ii) Rs 1300
(iii) Rs 1400 (iv) Rs 1500

**(b) India is**
(i) Rs 1300 (ii) Rs 1400
(iii) Rs 1500 (iv) Rs 1600

**(c) Pakistan is**

(i) Rs 1600 (ii) Rs 1700

(iii) Rs 1800 (iv) Rs 1900

**151. A, B, C, D, E, F are six siblings (no twins). It is given that one of the following pairs of informations is incorrect:**

**A is elder to C and B is younger than D;**

**C is elder to F and E is younger than D;**

**E is elder to A and B is younger than F;**

**Also the incorrect informations are ones such that the relative ages of all the siblings can be known.**

**(a) If D is the youngest sibling, then the eldest sibling is**

(i) A (ii) B (iii) E (iv) F

**(b) If C is the youngest sibling, then the eldest sibling is**

(i) A (ii) B (iii) E (iv) F

**(c) If E is the youngest sibling, then the eldest sibling is**

(i) A (ii) B (iii) C (iv) D

**(d) If F is the youngest sibling, then the eldest sibling is**

(i) A (ii) B (iii) C (iv) D

**(e) Which of the following can be second eldest or second youngest sibling?**

(i) A or B only (ii) A, B, C or D only

(iii) A, B, E or F only (iv) A, B, C, D, E or F

**152. A, B, C, D are professor, artist, lawyer and doctor (not in order) who live in blue, green, red and yellow (not in order) house. It is given that only one of the information in the following statements is correct:**

**A is professor and lives in blue house;**

**B is artist and lives in green house;**

**C is lawyer and lives in red house;**

**D is doctor and lives in yellow house;**

**Professor lives in red house and artist lives in yellow house;**

**Lawyer lives in blue house and doctor lives in green house.**

**(a) If A is not a professor, then he can be**

(i) artist or lawyer

(ii) lawyer or doctor

(iii) doctor or artist

(iv) artist, lawyer or doctor

**(b) If B is not an artist, then he can be**

(i) professor or lawyer
(ii) doctor or lawyer
(iii) doctor or professor
(iv) professor, lawyer or doctor

**(c) C cannot be**

(i) professor (ii) artist
(iii) lawyer (iii) doctor

**(d) If D is not a doctor, then he can be**

(i) professor (ii) artist
(iii) lawyer (iv) doctor

**153. Let A, B, C, D, E, F be professor, doctor, lawyer, chemist, actor and accountant (not in order). It is given that two of the informations in the following statements are wrong:**

**I. A is professor, B is doctor, C is lawyer, E is accountant;**

**II. B is chemist, D is lawyer, E is professor, F is accountant;**

**III. A is actor, C is doctor, D is professor, E is accountant;**

**IV. B is chemist, C is lawyer, E is doctor, F is actor.**

**(a) A is**

(i) professor (ii) actor (iii) doctor (iv) lawyer

**(b) Who is the accountant?**

(i) C (ii) D (iii) E (iv) F

**(c) Who is the chemist?**

(i) B (ii) D (iii) E (iv) F

**(b) Who is the doctor?**

(i) A (ii) B (iii) C (iv) E

**154. A, B, C, D, E are four males and one female, the female being the youngest. It is given that one of the information in each of the following statements is wrong:**

**A is male, B is younger to C;**
**B is female, E is younger to A;**
**C is male, A is younger to D;**
**D is female, C is younger to E;**
**E is female, D is younger to B;**

**(a) Who is female?**

(i) B (ii) D
(iii) E (iv) none of these

**(b) Who is the eldest?**

(i) A (ii) B
(iii) E (iv) cannot be determined

**(c) Who is the youngest?**

(i) B (ii) C
(iii) D (iv) cannot be determined

**155. A, B, C, D, E, F, G and H are eight persons (male or female). It is given that one of the information in the following statements is incorrect:**

**A is male and B is male;**
**C is male and D is female;**
**E is female and F is male;**
**G is female and H is female;**
**B is female and F is male;**
**C is female and G is male;**

**(a) If there are six females in the group, then which of the following is male?**

(i) C (ii) D (iii) G (iv) H

**(b) If there are six males in the group, then which of the following is female?**

(i) A (ii) B (iii) E (iv) F

**(c) If there are four males and four females in the group, and if A is male, then which of the following is female?**

(i) C (ii) D (iii) G (iv) H

**156. A, B, C, D, E are five persons who like one of the four colours: red, blue, green, black and yellow (no two persons like the same colour). It is given that one of the information in the following statements is wrong:**

**A likes green and B likes blue;**
**B likes yellow and C likes red;**
**D likes red and E likes black;**

**(a) If D likes red, then B likes**

(i) green (ii) blue (iii) yellow (iv) black

**(b) If E likes blue, then A likes**

(i) green (ii) red (iii) yellow (iv) black

**(c) How many distinct possibilities of solution are there?**
(i) 1 (ii) 2 (iii) 3 (iv) 4

**157. A, B, C, D are four persons (two males and two females) who like one of four colours: red, blue, green and yellow (no two persons like the same colour). It is given that one of the information in the following statements is wrong:**
**A is male and D likes blue;**
**B is female and C likes green;**
**C is male and A likes yellow;**
**D is female and B likes red;**
**Also it is given that A, C are of opposite sex.**

**(a) Which of the following colours will be liked by males only?**
(i) blue (ii) green (iii) yellow (iv) red

**(b) Which of the following colours will be liked by females only?**
(i) blue (ii) green (iii) yellow (iv) red

**(c) If a male likes green colour, then he can be**
(i) A or B (ii) A or D (iii) B or C (iv) C or D

**(d) If a female likes green colour, then she can be**
(i) A or C (ii) A or D (iii) B or C (iv) B or D

**158. A, B, C, D, E, F, G, H are four couples. It is given that only one of the following informations is incorrect:**
**(A, G), (B, D) and (D, E) are couples;**
**(A, H), (B, E) and (C, G) are couples;**
**(A, F), (C, H) and (D, G) are couples;**
**(B, H), (C, E) and (D, F) are couples;**

**(a) Which of the following can be a couple?**
(i) A, H (ii) B, D (iii) C, E (iv) D, F

**(b) Which of the following cannot be a couple?**
(i) A, F (ii) B, E (iii) C, H (iv) D, G

**159. A, B, C, D, E, F, G, H are four couples:**
**C, D; F, H; G, E; and A, B are of same sex. It is given that one of the information of the following statements is incorrect:**
**A, F is a couple and C, D are male;**
**D, E is a couple and F, H are male;**

**C, H is a couple and G, E are male;**
**B, G is a couple and A, B are female;**

**(a) Which of the following are males?**
(i) A, B (ii) G, E
(iii) F, H (iv) cannot be determined

**(b) Which of the following must be a couple?**
(i) A, F (ii) D, E (iii) C, H (iv) B, G

**(c) Which of the following must not be a couple?**
(i) B, F (ii) C, G (iii) D, H (iv) D, G

**160. Consider three males and three females who are given ranks from 1 to 6. The ranks given to males are 1, 3 and 4. Let the persons be A, B, C, D, E and F. It is given that one of the information in each of the following statements is incorrect:**
**A is male and the rank of E is 4;**
**D is male and the rank of A is 3;**
**E is male and the rank of B is 2;**
**The rank of F is 5 and the rank of C is 1.**

**(a) Which of the following is of sex different from that of others?**
(i) A (ii) B (iii) D (iv) E

**(b) Which of the following is of sex different from that of others?**
(i) A (ii) B (iii) C (iv) F

**(c) If the rank of F is 5, then which of the following is correct?**
(i) The rank of A is 3 (ii) The rank of B is 2
(iii) The rank of D is (iv) The rank of E is 4

**(d) If the rank of C is 1, then which of the following is correct?**
(i) The rank of A, B are 3, 2 respectively
(ii) The rank of A, F are 3, 4 respectively
(iii) The rank of B, F are 2, 4 respectively
(iv) all of these

**161. A, B, C, D, E, F are six persons who are given ranks from 1 to 6. It is given that one of the information in each of the following statement is incorrect:**

**I. The rank of A is 2 and that of C is higher than that of D.**

**II. The rank of B is 1 and that of A is higher than that of E.**

**III. The rank of C is 4 and that of F is higher than that of E.**

**IV. The rank of D is 5 and that of A is higher than that of B.**

**V. The rank of E is 3 and that of F is higher than that of C.**

**VI. The rank of F is 6 and that of D is higher than that of B.**

**Also three of first part of statements and three of second parts of statements are correct.**

**(a) The rank of A is**

(i) 1 (ii) 3
(iii) 5 (iv) cannot be determined

**(b) The rank of B is**

(i) 1 (ii) 4
(iii) 6 (iv) cannot be determined

**(c) The rank of C is**

(i) 2 (ii) 3
(iii) 4 (iv) cannot be determined

**(d) The rank of E is**

(i) 2 (ii) 3
(iii) 5 (iv) cannot be determined

**162. A, B, C, D, E, F are six persons seated in a row. It is given that one of the information in each of the following statements is incorrect?**

**A is adjacent to B and E is adjacent to F;**
**C is adjacent to A and D is adjacent to E;**
**B is adjacent to E and F is adjacent to A;**
**C is adjacent to F and A is adjacent to D.**

**(a) If A is at one end, then which of the following cannot be at the other end?**

(i) C (ii) D (iii) E (iv) F

**(b) If A is adjacent to E, then E is**
(i) adjacent to B or D (ii) adjacent to D or F
(iii) adjacent to B or F (iv) the case is not possible

**(c) If E is at one end, then which of the following will be at the other end?**
(i) B or D (ii) C or D (iii) B or F (iv) D or F

**(d) If F is at one end, then which of the following cannot be at the other end?**
(i) A (ii) B (iii) C (iv) D

**(e) If X is at one end, and adjacent to A, then X cannot be**
(i) B (ii) C (iii) D (iv) F

**163. A, B, C, D, E, F are six persons seated in a row. Now it is known that either**
**A is between C and D or E is between B and F;**
**D is between C and A or B is between F and E;**
**C is between A and E or F is between B and D;**
**D is between A and F or B is between C and E.**

**(a) Which of the following are sitting at ends?**
(i) C and E (ii) D and F
(iii) A and F (iv) C and B

**(b) Which of the following are sitting in the middle?**
(i) C and E (ii) D and F
(iii) A and F (iv) C and B

**164. A, B, C, D, E, F are six persons sitting in a row. It is given that two of the following statements are wrong:**
**I. A is between D and B**
**II. B is between C and F**
**III. C is between F and E**
**IV. D is between C and E**
**V. E is between A and B**
**VI. F is between D and A**

**For which of the following cases, the relative positions of all persons will not be unique (treat the similar arrangements rightwise or leftwise as same)?**

**(a)** (i) I and IV are wrong
(ii) I and V are wrong
(iii) I and VI are wrong
(iv) none of these

**(b)** (i) II and IV are wrong
(ii) II and V are wrong
(iii) II and VI are wrong
(iv) none of these

**(c)** (i) III and IV are wrong
(ii) III and V are wrong
(iii) III and VI are wrong
(iv) none of these

**165. A, B, C, D, E, F, G are seven persons: a man, his two sons and four grandsons, each sons having two sons of their own. It is given that one of the information in the following statements is wrong:**
**A is son of E and B is son of D;**
**G is son of D and C is son of F;**
**A is brother of F and B is brother of G;**
**D is brother of E and C is brother of A;**

**(a) Which of the following pairs are necessarily brothers?**
(i) A, F (ii) B, G (iii) D, E (iv) C, A

**(b) Which of the following will necessarily be a father?**
(i) A (ii) B (iii) C (iv) D

**(c) Which of the following may not necessarily be a grandson?**
(i) B (ii) C (iii) F (iv) G

**(d) When B, G are brothers, then who is the grandfather?**
(i) A (ii) C
(iii) F (iv) cannot be determined

**(e) When A, F are brothers, then who is the grandfather?**
(i) B (ii) E
(iii) G (iv) cannot be determined

**166. A, B, C . . . . . . . H are eight persons who live in house of different colours, viz. red, blue, green, yellow, white, black, pink, and orange. Consider five statements:**
**I. A lives in green house and B in black house.**
**II. F lives in yellow house and H in green house.**
**III. E lives in black house and G in white house.**
**IV. B lives in pink house and D in blue house.**
**V. A lives in red house and C in orange house.**
**VI. F lives in orange house and G in blue house.**

**It is given that three of the statements (both parts) are correct and other three (both parts) incorrect.**

**(a) C can live in house of colour**

(i) red (ii) yellow

(iii) pink (iv) none of these

**(b) D can live in house of colour**

(i) blue (ii) white

(iii) orange (iv) none of these

**(c) Who can live in black house?**

(i) B, E (ii) A, G (iii) A, B (iv) E, G

**167. A, B, C, D, E, F, G, H are four couples. Consider the four statements given below:**

**I. (A, F) and (B, D) are couples.**

**II. (A, G) and (C, E) are couples.**

**III. (C, G) and (B, H) are couples.**

**IV. (D, E) and (F, H) are couples.**

**Now it is given that one of the statements is fully correct, two totally incorrect and one is half correct.**

**(a) A cannot be married to**

(i) B (ii) E (iii) F (iv) G

**(b) C cannot be married to**

(i) B (ii) D (iii) E (iv) G

**(c) G cannot be married to**

(i) A (ii) C (iii) D (iv) H

**(d) H cannot be married to**

(i) B (ii) E (iii) F (iv) G

**168. Let $a$, $b$, $c$, $d$ be four distinct positive integers. It is given that one of the information of the following statements is incorrect:**

**A.** $a + b = 5$ and $c + d = 10$;

$a + c = 4$ and $b + d = 9$;

$a + d = 7$ and $b + c = 8$;

$b - a = 1$ and $d - c = 2$.

**(a)** $a =$

(i) 1 (ii) 2

(iii) 3 (iv) cannot be determined

**(b)** $b =$

(i) 2 (ii) 3
(iii) 4 (iv) cannot be determined

**(c)** $c =$

(i) 3 (ii) 4
(iii) 5 (iv) cannot be determined

**(d)** $d =$

(i) 4 (ii) 5
(iii) 6 (iv) cannot be determined

**169. A, B, C, D are four numbers. It is given that one of the information in the following statements is wrong:**
**A < B or C > D;**
**A > C or B < D;**
**A > D or B > D;**

**(a) If C is the least number, then the greatest number is**

(i) A (ii) B
(iii) D (iv) cannot be determined

**(b) If A is not the extreme number, then the extreme number are**

(i) B, C (ii) C, D
(iii) B, D (iv) cannot be determined

**170. A, B, C, D, E, F are six consecutive numbers. It is given that one of the information of each of the following statements is incorrect:**

**I. A + B = 2F and B + C = 2D;**
**II. C + D = 2E and E + F = 2B;**
**II. A + F = 2C and E + C = 2A.**

**(a) The difference between A and B is**

(i) 2 (ii) 3
(iii) 4 (iv) cannot be determined

**(b) The difference between C and D is**

(i) 2 (ii) 3
(iii) 4 (iv) cannot be determined

**(c) The difference between E and F is**

(i) 1 (ii) 2
(iii) 3 (iv) cannot be determined

**(d) The difference between A and D is**

(i) 2 (ii) 3

(iii) 5 (iv) cannot be determined

**(e) The difference between B and E is**

(i) 1 (ii) 2

(iii) 5 (iv) cannot be determined

**171. Let $y = ax^2 + bx + c$ where $a, b, c$ are the constants to be determined. Let at $x = -1, 0, 1$ and 2, the corresponding values of $y$ is one of (0, –1); (–2, –1); (–2, 1) and (0, 1) respectively. Then**

**(a) $a =$**

(i) –1 (ii) 0

(iii) 1 (iv) cannot be determined

**(b) $b =$**

(i) –1 (ii) 0

(iii) 1 (iv) cannot be determined

**(c) The value of the expression at $x = -1, 1$ and 2 are**

(i) 0, –2, 0 respectively

(ii) 0, 1, 1 respectively

(iii) –1, –2, 1 respectively

(iv) cannot be determined

**172. (a) Let three of the values of $(x, y)$, viz. (1, 2); (–3, 1); (2, –1) and (4, 3) satisfy the relation.**

**$a\,x + b\,y + c = 0$ where $a, b, c$, are non zero real numbers.**

**The value of $(x, y)$ not satisfying the given relation is**

(i) (1, 2) (ii) (–3, 1)

(iii) (2, –1) (iv) (4, 3)

**(b) Let three of the values of $(x, y)$, viz. (–3, –1); (1, –1); (0, 2) and (1, 3) satisfy the relation**

**$(x - a)^2 + (y - b)^2 = c^2$**

**where $a, b, c$ are real numbers.**

**The chosen three values must include the value of $(x, y)$ as**

(i) (–3, –1) (ii) (1, –1)

(iii) (0, 2) (iv) (1, 3)

**173.** ***A*, *B*, *C*, *D*, *E*, *F* are single digit positive integers. Let one of (*A*, *B*, *C*) be 1; (*B*, *C*, *D*) be 2; (*C*, *D*, *E*) be 3; (*D*, *E*, *F*) be 4; (*E*, *F*, *A*) is 5 and (*F*, *A*, *B*) be 6.**

**(a) How many distinct possibilities for the values of letters exist?**

(i) 12 (ii) 15 (iii) 18 (iv) 24

**(b) Let $A = 1$ and $E = 3$. Then which of the following holds true?**

(i) $B = 2$ and $F = 6$ (ii) $B = 2$ and $D = 4$
(iii) $B = 6$ and $F = 4$ (iv) $B = 6$ and $D = 4$

**(c) Let $A = 1$ and the values of *C*, *D* are given so that values of all the letters can be uniquely known. Then**

(i) only *C* has unique value
(ii) only *D* has unique value
(iii) both *C*, *D* have unique values
(iv) none of these

**174.** ***A*, *B*, *C*, *D* are four numbers such that $|A - 2B| = 1$, $|B - 2C| = 2$, $|C - 2D| = 4$ and $|D = 2A| = 3$.**
**If *A* is an integer, then**

**(a) $B =$**

(i) –4 or 4 (ii) –2 or 2
(iii) –2 or 4 (iv) –4, –2, 2 or 4

**(b) $D =$**

(i) –1 or 1 (ii) –3 or 3
(iii) –3 or 1 (iv) –3, –1, 1 or 3

**175. Four students A, B, C and D were asked a few questions (each having four options, one of which is correct and other wrong. In succession in that cyclic order. A student giving the correct answer when asked first a question gets 4 marks but if he gives a wrong answer, then the student next in succession is to choose correct the answer from the remaining three options. If he chooses the correct answer, he gets three marks, but if he gives a wrong answer, then the student next in succession is to choose the correct answer from remaining two options. If he chooses the correct answer, he gets two marks, but if he gives the wrong answer, then the student next in succession gets one**

**mark if he gives the correct answer, otherwise no mark. Let the marks obtained by the students be 10, 8, 11 and 10 respectively.**

**(a) The minimum number of questions asked would be**
(i) 12 (ii) 13 (iii) 14 (iv) 15

**(b) For the case mentioned in subquestion (a), one of the question asked to whom remained unanswered?**
(i) A (ii) B (iii) C (iv) D

**(c) For the case mentioned in subquestion (a), who could not have answered any questions asked first to him?**
(i) A (ii) B (iii) C (iv) D

**176. First 100 natural numbers are written in 10 rows and 10 columns in two different ways. In first method, first row is filled by 1-10 left to right and the second row by 11-20 right to left, third row by 21-30 left to right and so on. In second method, first column is filled by 1-10 top to bottom, second column with 11-20 bottom to top, third column with 21-30 top to bottom and so on.**

**(a) How many blocks will by first numbering be the same as by second numbering?**
(i) 9 (ii) 10 (iii) 11 (iv) 19

**(b) How many blocks will by first numbering be 9 more than by second numbering?**
(i) 0 (ii) 1 (iii) 2 (iv) 3

**(c) How many blocks will by first numbering be 18 more than by second numbering?**
(i) 4 (ii) 6 (iii) 8 (iv) 10

**177. A man starts his journey from point A in the eastward direction and turns at every corner at a right angle which are sequentially denoted by $A_i$ ($i$ = 1, 2, ... 9) as he passes them to return to $A_0$. Let**
**$A_0A_1 + A_2A_3 = A_4A_5 + A_6A_7 + A_8A_9$ and**
**$A_1A_2 + A_5A_6 + A_9A_0 = A_3A_4 + A_7A_8$.**
**Also there are two exclusive pairs of roads which intersect each other.**

**(a) Which of the following pair of roads intersect each other?**

(i) $A_0A_1$ and $A_3A_4$ (ii) $A_0A_1$ and $A_5A_6$
(iii) $A_2A_3$ and $A_5A_6$ (iv) $A_2A_3$ and $A_7A_8$

**(b) Which of the following pair of roads intersect each other?**

(i) $A_0A_1$ and $A_7A_8$ (ii) $A_2A_3$ and $A_9A_0$
(iii) $A_1A_2$ and $A_6A_7$ (iv) $A_5A_6$ and $A_8A_9$

**(c) Which of the following is correct?**

I. The man moved eastward twice and westward thrice.
II. The man moved westward twice and eastward thrice.
III. The man moved northward twice and southward thrice.
IV. The man moved northward thrice and southward twice.

(i) I only (ii) II only
(iii) I and III (iv) II and IV

**178. Three rows and five columns are to be filled by fifteen elements $A_i$, $B_i$, $C_i$ ($i$ = 1, 2, 3, 4, 5) such that first, second and third rows are filled by $A_i$, $B_i$ and $C_i$ respectively and no two elements of a column has the same subscript. Let the positions of a few elements of an arrangement be as shown above.**

| | | | | |
|---|---|---|---|---|
| | $A_1$ | | $A_2$ | |
| | | $B_2$ | | $B_3$ |
| $C_4$ | | | $C_5$ | |

**(a) How many distinct arrangements of all elements are possible?**

(i) 7 (ii) 9 (iii) 12 (iv) 18

**(b) In which of the columns there are maximum different ways to fill it?**

(i) First (ii) Second (iii) Third (iv) Fifth

**(c) If by filling two more additional elements, all other elements can be filled in a unique way, then the two additional elements will be**

(i) 1 A's and 1 B's (ii) 1 A's and 1 C's
(iii) 1 B's and 1 C's (iv) 2 A's

**179. A, B, C, D, E, F, G, H, I, J, K, L are names and nicknames of six persons (each person having a nickname). Now**

**I. A is F's father-in-law.**
**II. E is husband of L.**
**III. B is brother of H.**

**IV. D is brother-in-law of G.**
**V. C is sister-in-law of J.**
**VI. K is son-in-law of I.**
**Assuming that no one is married to one's sibling's spouse's siblings, who is**

**(a) B?**
(i) D (ii) G
(iii) K (iv) cannot be determined

**(b) C?**
(i) L (ii) H
(iii) K (iv) cannot be determined

**(c) F?**
(i) G (ii) J
(iii) K (iv) cannot be determined

**180. A, B, C, D, E, F and G are the vertices of a regular heptagon. Let $AB > DG$, $DF > BE$, $CG > BF$ and $DE > AC$.**

**(a) How many distinct possibilities for the naming of vertices exist?**
(i) 7 (ii) 8 (iii) 9 (iv) 10

**(b) In how many of the above possibilities, D, G are adjacent vertices?**
(i) 4 (ii) 5 (iii) 6 (iv) 7

**(c) In how many of the above possibilities [part (a)] B, E are adjacent vertices?**
(i) 4 (ii) 5 (iii) 6 (iv) 7

**(d) In how many of the above possibilities [part (a)] B, F are adjacent vertices?**
(i) 5 (ii) 6 (iii) 7 (iv) 8

**(e) In how many of the above possibilities [part (a)] A, C are adjacent vertices?**
(i) 4 (ii) 5 (iii) 6 (iv) 7

**181. 16 blocks are to be filled by 8 alphabets A, B, C, D, P, Q, R, S such that the alphabets of group (A, B, C, D) and (P, Q, R, S) are in different rows and columns. Also in each row and column two blocks are empty of which four are shown by cross (×) in the adjoining figure.**

| | Q | S | R | P |
|---|---|---|---|---|
| B | × | | | |
| C | | × | | |
| D | | | | × |
| A | | | × | |

**Let B, C, D, A be in first, second, third and fourth columns respectively. If A is not in the same column or row as S and B is not in the same column or row as R, then**

**(a) how many distinct arrangements are possible?**

(i) one (ii) two (iii) three (iv) four

**(b) which of the following must be a blank?**

(i) third row, first column
(ii) second row, fourth column
(iii) Both
(iv) None

**(c) which of the following must be adjacent?**

(i) S and D (ii) R and D
(iii) C and R (iv) none of these

**(d) When C is in first column, then**

(i) D is in third column and S is in third row
(ii) D is in second column and S is in first row
(iii) D is in third column and S is in first row
(iv) none of these

**(e) When Q is in second row, then**

(i) D is in second column and P is in first row
(ii) D is in second column and P is in fourth row
(iii) D is in third column and P is in first row
(iv) D is in third column and P is in fourth row

**182. A, B, C and D are four students, one of whom was told by his teacher a sequence of five letters which is passed to other students by turns, each giving it to the student next in turn and the last student tells it to the teacher. Each student got confused in two letters at consecutive places (none of them getting confused at the same consecutive place), and the sequence told by A, B, C, D are respectively Q R P T S, Q P R T S, Q R T P S and Q P R S T.**

**(a) If A told the sequence to B, then C got confused in letters at**

(i) first and second places
(ii) second and third places
(iii) third and fourth places
(iv) fourth and fifth places

(b) **Which of the following pair could not have interacted directly?**

(i) A and C (ii) B and D
(iii) C and D (iv) none of these

(c) **If B told the sequence to A, then the sequence told by the teacher was**

(i) P Q R S T (ii) Q P R S T
(iii) Q R P T S (iv) none of these

**183. A, B, C, D, E are five numbers of a sequence $a_n$ ($1 \le n \le 5$) in which each number of the sequence is a fixed quadratic expression of its preceding terms given as**

$$a_{n+1} = k_1 a_n^2 + k_2 a_n + k_3 \quad (n = 1, 2, 3, 4)$$

**Let the value of A, B, C, D and E be respectively 0, 0, 1, 2 and 2.**

(a) **Which term of the sequence is C?**

(i) First (ii) Third
(iii) Fifth (iv) cannot be determined

(b) $k_3 =$

(i) 0 (ii) 1
(iii) 2 (iv) cannot be determined

(c) **If A be the last term of the series, then $k_2 =$**

(i) –2 (ii) –1 (iii) 1 (iv) 2

(d) **If E be the last term of the series, then $k_1 =$**

(i) –2 (ii) –1 (iii) 1 (iv) 2

**184. Five letters, A, B, C, D and E are written in a sequence; a process consists in breaking it at a place and then reversing the sequences of left and right parts.**

(a) **If the initial sequence is A B C D E, then which of the following sequence can be derived by using the process (any number of times)?**

(i) A C D B E (ii) C D B A E
(iii) D E A B C (iv) all of these

(b) **What is the least number of times the process should be used so as to change the sequence A B C D E to E A B C D?**

(i) 1 (ii) 2 (iii) 3 (iv) 4

(c) **What is the least number of times the process should be used so as to again get the initial sequence, given that no two successive processes involve breaking of**

**the sequence at the same place (i.e., after the same number of letters) is**

(i) 3 (ii) 4 (iii) 5 (iv) 6

**185. $A_1$, $A_2$, $A_3$, $A_4$, $A_5$, $A_6$, $A_7$ and $A_8$ are divided into two groups $G_1$ and $G_2$ of four elements each. Now four pairs are to be formed, one from each group, by taking an element from $G_1$ and $G_2$ such that an element having the average of the subscripts of the elements of the pair is found in $G_1$ and this element forms an element of the next pair. Let $A_1$ be found in $G_1$ and be the element of the first pair formed.**

**(a) Which of the following is correct?**

(i) $A_2$ is in $G_1$ and $A_6$ is in $G_2$

(ii) $A_2$ is in $G_2$ and $A_6$ is in $G_1$

(iii) $A_2$ and $A_6$ are both in $G_1$

(iv) $A_2$ and $A_5$ are both in $G_2$

**(b) Which of the following is correct?**

(i) $A_3$ is in $G_1$ and $A_5$ is in $G_2$

(ii) $A_3$ is in $G_2$ and $A_5$ is in $G_1$

(iii) $A_3$ is in $G_1$ and $A_7$ is in $G_2$

(iv) $A_3$ is in $G_2$ and $A_7$ is in $G_1$

**(c) Which of the following pairs is formed last?**

(i) ($A_3$, $A_7$) (ii) ($A_5$, $A_7$)

(iii) ($A_2$, $A_8$) (iv) ($A_4$, $A_6$)

**186. A, B, C, D (not in order) are on a straight road spaced equally. A man can walk with two different speeds but between any two successive points he walks with one of the two speeds. He walks at least once with each speed. Let the time taken by him to walk between (A, B); (B, C) and (C, D) be 1, 3 and 5 hours respectively.**

**(a) What is the ratio of his two speeds?**

(i) 1 : 2 (ii) 1 : 3

(iii) 2 : 3 (iv) cannot be determined

**(b) Which of the following is necessarily correct?**

(i) A is exactly between B and D

(ii) A is exactly between B and C

(iii) B is exactly between A and D

(iv) none of these

**187. (a) Out of 100 identical coins one coin is fake and weighs less than the others. If you are given a balance, in how many minimum number of measurements you can separate the fake coin?**

(i) 5 (ii) 6 (iii) 7 (iv) 8

**(b) Out of 36 identical coins, two coins are fake and weigh less than the others. If you are given a balance, in how many minimum number of measurements you can separate the fake coin?**

(i) 7 (ii) 8 (iii) 9 (iv) 10

**188. Suppose you have to weigh any integral number of weight upto 100 kg by manufacturing minimum number of standard weights, then**

**(a) what is the number of such weights?**

(i) 5 (ii) 6 (iii) 7 (iv) 8

**(b) what could be the maximum weight upto which any integral number of weights can be measured by using these standard weights?**

(i) 121 (ii) 123 (iii) 125 (iv) 127

**189. (a) A, B, C and D are four articles of different values. The price of a few articles of A is equal to that of the same number of articles comprising B and C while the price of a few articles of B is equal to that of the same number of articles comprising C and D. Which of the following is correct?**

(i) The price of a few articles of C is equal to that of the same number of articles comprising B and D

(ii) The price of a few articles of D is equal to that of the same number of articles comprising C and A

(iii) The price of a few articles of A is equal to that of the same number of articles comprising D and B

(iv) none of these

**(b) In part (a), assume there to be one more article E and an additional condition that the price of a few articles of D is equal to that of the same number of articles comprising C and E. Which of the following may be correct?**

(i) The price of a few articles of B may be equal to that of the same number of articles comprising A and E
(ii) The price of a few articles of D may be equal to that of the same number of articles comprising A and B
(iii) The price of a few articles of C may be equal to that of the same number of articles comprising B and E
(iv) none of these

**190. A, B, C bought 5 articles; the articles were of two kinds X or Y. Which of the following can be respectively the ratio of money spent by A, B and C?**

**(a)** (i) 2 : 3 : 5 (ii) 2 : 5 : 7
(iii) 3 : 5 : 7 (iv) none of these

**(b)** (i) 1 : 2 : 4 (ii) 1 : 2 : 3
(iii) 1 : 3 : 4 (iv) all of these

**191. A, B, C and D are four runners who started running simultaneously on a track. Let their speeds at the start be 10 m/s, 5 m/s, 15 m/s and 20 m/s respectively. They changed their speeds every second; A, B increased their speeds every second by 1 m/s and 2 m/s respectively while C, D decreased their speeds every second by 1 m/s and 2 m/s respectively.**

**(a) A overtook C**
(i) between 5 and 6 seconds
(ii) between 6 and 7 seconds
(iii) at the end of 6 seconds
(iv) at the end of 7 seconds

**(b) B overtook C between**
(i) 5 and 6 seconds (ii) 6 and 7 seconds
(iii) 7 and 8 seconds (iv) 8 and 9 seconds

**(c) B overtook D between**
(i) 6 and 7 seconds (ii) 7 and 8 seconds
(iii) 8 and 9 seconds (iv) 9 and 10 seconds

**192. A, B, C, D, E are five persons, each of whom takes care of one of other persons and no two persons take care of each other. It is known that if A takes care of B, then B does not take care of C, if B takes care of E, then D does not take care of A; if C takes care of A, then E does not take care of D. How many different cases are possible if**

**(a) A takes care of B?**
(i) 1 (ii) 2 (iii) 3 (iv) 4

**(b) B takes care of E?**
(i) 1 (ii) 2 (iii) 3 (iv) 4

**193. An article is sold in packing of**
**1 kg < *x* kg < *y* kg < 10 kg (*x*, *y* being integers)**
**while their respective costs are**
**Rs *p* < Rs 36 < Rs 76 < Rs *q* (*p*, *q* being integers)**
**It is known that with every additional kg of article, a successive discount of Rs 1 is given. Then**

**(a) *x* =**
(i) 2 kg (ii) 3 kg (iii) 4 kg (iv) 5 kg

**(b) *y* =**
(i) 6 kg (ii) 7 kg (iii) 8 kg (iv) 9 kg

**194. A porter can walk between two points A and B distance 1 km apart at 5 km/hr, 4 km/hr, 3 km/hr, 2 km/hr, 1 km/hr according as he carries no weight, 1 kg weight, 2 kg weight, 3 kg weight or 5 kg weight respectively.**

**(a) In what minimum amount of time can he transport 10 kg of a material from A to B?**
(i) 141 minutes (ii) 148 minutes
(iii) 153 minutes (iv) 160 minutes

**(b) In what minimum amount of time can he transport 5 kg of a material from A to B and 6 kg of the material from B to A if he starts walking from A?**
(i) 110 minutes (ii) 120 minutes
(iii) 130 minutes (iv) 140 minutes

**(c) If the porter has to transport large amount of heavy material from A to B, then which of the following will be the best option for him to transport them in minimum time?**
(i) He should carry 1 kg at a time
(ii) He should carry 2 kg at a time
(iii) He should carry 3 kg at a time
(iv) He should carry 4 kg at a time

**195. In Rs 100, I bought as many red marbles as possible and then with the money left, I bought as many blue marbles as possible and again with the money left, I bought as**

**many white marbles as possible and finally I bought 1 green marble exhausting all the money I had. The cost of white and green marbles are Rs 5 and Rs 2 respectively and the cost of red and blue marbles are integral number of rupees. Also I was able to buy only two blue marbles.**

**(a) What could be the number of red marble I bought?**
(i) 1 (ii) 1 or 2 (iii) 1 or 3 (iv) 1, 2 or 3

**(b) What could be the number of white marble I bought?**
(i) 1 (ii) 1 or 2 (iii) 1 or 3 (iv) 1, 2 or 3

**(c) What could be the maximum cost of a blue marble?**
(i) Rs 18 (ii) Rs 19 (iii) Rs 20 (iv) Rs 21

**196. My telephone is in strange habit of having two of its dialling number exchanged, for example, if I press 0, it may actually mean 1 and when I press 1, it then means 0.**

**(a) If I have to dial 21674, then the minimum number of wrong calls after which I can definitely end up dialling the desired number is**
(i) 34 (ii) 35 (iii) 44 (iv) 45

**(b) During my trial to dial a five digit number, I found that 83569 and 63598 are wrong calls while 95368 is the desired call, then which of the two numbers get exchanged while dialling?**
(i) 9 and 8 (ii) 6 and 9
(iii) 3 and 5 (iv) cannot be determined

**197. Shown alongside is a network of roads. The routes 1, 3, 5, 7 are of length 400 m while the routes 2, 9, 6, 10, 4, 8 are of length 200 m. Two persons start moving along the routes 1 → 2 → 3 → 4 → 5 → 6 → 7 → 8 → 9 → 3 → 10 repeatedly. If their speeds are 2 m/s and 1 m/s and if they start running simultaneously from O, then**

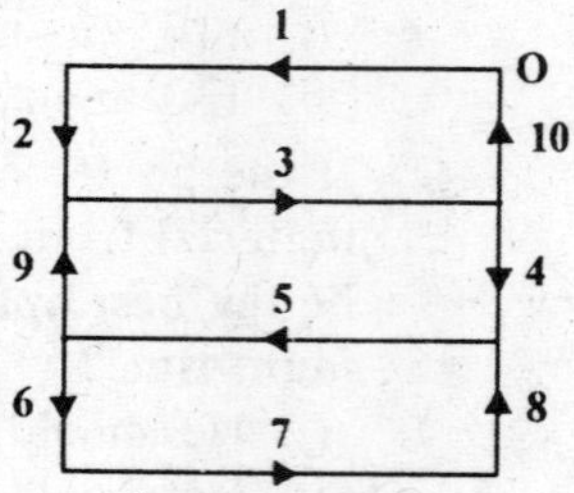


**(a) they will again meet after**
(i) 1200 seconds (ii) 1600 seconds
(iii) 1800 seconds (iv) 2000 seconds

(b) **they will keep meeting at**
(i) 2 different points on their tracks
(ii) 3 different points on their tracks
(iii) 4 different points on their tracks
(iv) 5 different points on their tracks

**198. A, B, C, D have respectively only Rs 500 note, Rs 100 note, Rs 50 note and Rs 20 note, the total amount held by any two of them not differing by more than Rs *n*.**

(a) **If the total number of notes held by them is known, then for what least value of *n*, the number of notes held by A cannot be known?**
(i) 250 (ii) 260 (iii) 280 (iv) 300

(b) **If *n* = 200 and the total number of notes held by them is 180, then the number of notes held by C will be**
(i) 42 (ii) 44
(iii) 48 (iv) cannot be determined

(c) **If *n* = 200 and the total number of notes held by them is 230, then the number of notes held by B will be**
(i) 25 (ii) 27
(iii) 28 (iv) cannot be determined

**199. A, B, C and D have equal amount of Rs 500 each, the notes being of denomination Rs 10, Rs 20, Rs 50 and Rs 100. Also each of them don't have a note of exactly one denomination, no two persons lacking the note of same denomination. Let the total notes of denomination Rs 10, 20, 50 and 100 held by the persons be 35, 35, 7 and 6 respectively while the total number of notes held by A, B, C, D be 22, 24, 19 and 18 respectively.**

(a) **A lacks in note of denomination**
(i) Rs 100 (ii) Rs 50
(iii) Rs 20 (iv) cannot be determined

(b) **B lacks in note of denomination**
(i) Rs 100 (ii) Rs 50
(iii) Rs 20 (iv) cannot be determined

(c) **C lacks in note of denomination**
(i) Rs 50 (ii) Rs 20
(iii) Rs 10 (iv) cannot be determined

**(d) D lacks in note of denomination**

(i) Rs 50 (ii) Rs 20
(iii) Rs 10 (iv) cannot be determined

**200. Consider a sequence of five single digit positive integers A, B, C, D and E where three of them are added and other two are subtracted.**

**A. Considering the value of all possible sequences to be different and three of A, B, C, D, E to be consecutive integers,**

**(a) how many different quintuplets (A, B, C, D, E) are possible?**

(i) 4 (ii) 6 (iii) 8 (iv) 10

**(b) how many such possible quintuplets do not contain 1?**

(i) 1 (ii) 2 (iii) 3 (iv) 4

**(c) which of the following number featured least of all in such possible quintuplets?**

(i) 2 (ii) 3 (iii) 4 (iv) 5

**(d) which of the following numbers would not appear in any of such possible quintuplets?**

(i) 2, 3, 4 (ii) 3, 4, 5 (iii) 5, 6, 7 (iv) 7, 8, 9

**B. Let A > B > C > D > E and the values of six of the sequences be positive while the values of others are negative.**

**(a) Which of the following is not possible?**

(i) A + D > B + C + E
(ii) A + E > B + C + D
(iii) B + C > A + D + E
(iv) all of these are possible

**(b) Which of the following can be uniquely determined?**

(i) A, E, B, C only (ii) A, E, C, D only
(iii) A, E, B, D only (iv) A, B, C, D, E

**(c) Which of the following necessarily holds?**

(i) A = B + C + D + E
(ii) A = B + C + E
(iii) A = B + C + D
(iv) none of these

**201.** **A, B, C, D are four persons each of whom can get a coin with a throw of a dice. Let A, B, C, D get a coin when the dice throws up (1, 3 or 5); (2, 5 or 6); (1, 2 or 4); (3, 4 or 6) respectively. Also let the coins received by them after certain number of times the dice is thrown be 5, 9, 6 and 8 respectively. Given that each number showed up once and no number turned up more than 4 times,**

**(a) the total number of times the dice was thrown is**
(i) 14 (ii) 15 (iii) 16 (iv) 17

**(b) the number of times 6 was thrown up by the dice is**
(i) 2 (ii) 3
(iii) 4 (iv) cannot be determined

**(c) the number of times 3 was thrown up by the dice is**
(i) 1 (ii) 2
(iii) 3 (iv) cannot be determined

**202.** **A, B, C, D are four persons, each of whom can get a coin according to following sequence of instructions:**

**I. If A and B have together an odd number of coins, then give a coin to C, otherwise not.**

**II. If A and C have together an odd number of coins, then give a coin to D, otherwise not.**

**III. If C and D have together an odd number of coins, then give a coin to B, otherwise not.**

**IV. If D and B have together an odd number of coins, then give a coin to A, otherwise not.**

**These set of four instructions are to be executed in the sequence it is given and a cycle completes after the execution of all four instructions after which another cycle starts. Initially only A has a coin and others none.**

**(a) After 10 cycles, how many coins will be with A?**
(i) 7 (ii) 8 (iii) 9 (iv) 10

**(b) After 15 cycles, how many coins will be with B?**
(i) 8 (ii) 9 (iii) 10 (iv) 11

**(c) After 20 cycles, how many coins will be with C?**
(i) 11 (ii) 12 (iii) 13 (iv) 14

**(d) After 25 cycles, how many coins will be with D?**
(i) 11 (ii) 12 (iii) 13 (iv) 14

**203. Two cannibals and three men want to cross a river by using a boat which can carry only two persons at a time. Also two cannibals will eat a man if they together find him alone. If both cannibals and men know how to row boat, then the minimum number of trips (a trip means going from one bank to the other by the boat) needed for all of them to cross the river without cannibals eating any of the men will be**

(i) 7 (ii) 9 (iii) 11 (iv) 13

**204. Five teachers A, B, C, D, E are engaged to take 3 classes I, II and III. Let (A, B); (B, C); (C, D); (D, E); (E, A) can teach Maths, Physics, Chemistry, Biology and English respectively. There are five periods in a day and each teacher takes only three classes, taking at least one class of each subject he knows. Each class is taught all subjects on every working day and each teacher takes one period of each class. Study the table below:**

| Period/Class | I | II | III |
|---|---|---|---|
| 1 | – | Chemistry | E |
| 2 | C | – | A |
| 3 | – | B | Chemistry |
| 4 | D | English | – |
| 5 | English | – | Physics |

**and answer the following questions:**

**(a) Class I is taught Physics and Chemistry respectively by**

(i) B and C (ii) B and D
(iii) C and D (iv) cannot be determined

**(b) Class II is taught Biology and Maths respectively by**

(i) D and A (ii) E and A
(iii) D and B (iv) E and B

**(c) Class III is taught English and Physics respectively by**

(i) A and B (ii) A and C
(iii) E and B (iv) E and C

**(d) The subjects class I is taught by A and E respectively are**

(i) Maths and English
(ii) Maths and Biology

(iii) English and Biology
(iv) cannot be determined

**(e) The subjects class II is taught by C and E respectively are**

(i) Physics and Biology
(ii) Physics and English
(iii) Chemistry and Biology
(iv) Chemistry and English

**205. There are five teachers A, B, C, D and E, each of whom can teach two of the following five subjects: Maths, Physics, Chemistry, Biology and English, no two teachers teaching the same pair of subjects. Each of them teaches in a school where they take three classes per day, teaching the subjects they know at least in one class. For a class of five subjects mentioned above, they get Rs 110, Rs 100, Rs 90, Rs 80 and Rs 70 respectively. On a day, each subject was taught thrice and A, B, C, D got Rs 310, Rs 250, Rs 280, Rs 220 respectively.**

**(a) Which of the following pair of subjects cannot be taught by any of the five teachers?**

(i) Maths, English (ii) English, Biology
(iii) Physics, Chemistry (iv) English, Chemistry

**(b) C teaches**

(i) Maths and Chemistry
(ii) Chemistry and Physics
(iii) Biology and Physics
(iv) Maths and Biology

**(c) Which of the following pair does not teach any common subject?**

(i) A, B (ii) A, E (iii) B, D (iv) D, E

**(d) Had A taught that subject twice which he actually taught once, then D would have got**

(i) Rs 10 less (ii) Rs 10 more
(iii) Rs 20 less (iv) Rs 20 more

**206. A, B, C, D, E are five teachers; each of whom can teach two of the following subjects: Maths, Physics, Chemistry, Biology and English. Each of them teaches in a school where they take three classes per day, teaching the**

**subjects they know at least once. For teaching Maths one gets Rs 100 per class and for teaching English one gets Rs 60 per class and for others, they get Rs 70, Rs 80 and Rs 90 per class.**

**On one day, A got Rs 210, B got Rs 240 and C got Rs 280. One of the subjects D and E teaches are Chemistry and Physics respectively and also their other subjects are not common. Had A taught that subject twice, he actually taught once, then A, B, C, D would have got respectively Rs 30 more, Rs 30 more, Rs *x* less and Rs 20 less.**

**(a)** $x =$

(i) 0 (ii) 10 (iii) 20 (iv) 30

**(b) For teaching Biology, how much money one would get per class?**

(i) Rs 70 or Rs 80 (ii) Rs 80 or Rs 90
(iii) Rs 70 or Rs 90 (iv) Rs 70 or Rs 80 or Rs 90

**(c) Which subject A teaches necessarily?**

(i) English (ii) Maths
(iii) Physics (iv) Chemistry

**(d) Who teaches Maths necessarily?**

(i) A (ii) B (iii) D (iv) E

**207. Consider a family of 8 persons: a couple and their three children, 2 boys and a girl, of which a boy and a girl are married and the girl has a baby (male). Let A, B, C, D, E, F, G, H denote all the persons as mentioned. It is given that**

**I. B, F, H are of same sex.**
**II. D, E, G are of same sex.**
**III. A, C are of same sex.**
**IV. There are all siblings in (A, D, F, G, H)**
**V. There are two couples in (A, B, C, D, E)**

**(a) Who is daughter-in-law?**

(i) C (ii) D (iii) F (iv) G

**(b) Who is daughter?**

(i) D (ii) E
(iii) G (iv) cannot be determined.

**(c) Who is unmarried son ?**

(i) A (ii) F
(iii) H (iv) cannot be determined.

**208.** **Two couples have a child each of opposite sex who are married to each other. Six persons are denoted by A, B, C, D, E, F or namely Tony, Bill, Harrison (all three males) and Monica, Jane and Sheila.**
**It is given that**
**Tony is married to E; Monica is married to F; Jane is married to D; Harrison is married to A and is not the father of C; C is daughter of Sheila.**

**(a) Tony is**
(i) B (ii) D
(iii) F (iv) cannot be determined.

**(b) E is**
(i) Sheila (ii) Monica
(iii) Jane (iv) cannot be determined.

**(c) C is married to**
(i) Tony (ii) Harrison
(iii) Bill (iv) cannot be determined.

**209.** **When first days of each month of a year was observed, it was found that there were three Sundays.**

**(a) Given that the year was a leap year, August starts with**
(i) Tuesday (ii) Wednesday
(iii) Friday (iv) Saturday

**(b) Which of the following day (first of each month) occurred only once?**
(i) Monday (ii) Tuesday
(iii) Wednesday (iv) Thursday

**(c) Given that the year was not a leap year, January starts with**
(i) Wednesday (ii) Thursday
(iii) Friday (iv) Saturday

**(d) Which of the following pair of months did not start with the same day?**
(i) March, November (ii) April, July
(iii) May, October (iv) September, December

**210.** **Five coins are taken, their faces are painted and numbers 0-9 are written on them, one number on one face. The five coins are then stacked together such that the numbers**

**0 and 1 appear on its upper and lower face respectively. Upper three coins and lower two coins are then reversed together and then again stacked (with upper two coins on the upper side) and the number 2 and 3 appears on the upper and lower face of the stack respectively. Now the upper two coins and lower three coins are similarly reversed and the numbers 4 and 5 appeared on the upper and lower face of the stack respectively. Again upper three coins are similarly reversed and the numbers 6 and 7 appeared on the upper and lower face respectively. Yet again the stack is divided into two portions, each portion is reversed similarly and finally the number 8 and 9 appeared on the upper and lower face of the stack respectively. Which number is written on the reverse face of a coin which one face bears the number**

**(a) 0?**

(i) 3 (ii) 4 (iii) 5 (iv) 7

**(b) 1?**

(i) 5 (ii) 6 (iii) 7 (iv) 8

**(c) 4?**

(i) 2 (ii) 6 (iii) 8 (iv) 9

**211. A, B, C, D, E and F are 6 consecutive numbers. When arranged as A C B D E F; D, F have to be moved (right or left) to make them in ascending order and when arranged as F D B C A E; A, C have to be moved to make them in ascending order. How many different possibilities of the order of numbers exist?**

(i) 4 (ii) 6 (iii) 8 (iv) 10

**212. The weight of 10 students increase consecutively from 51 to 60 kg. The average weight of girls is 3 kg less than that of boys. Also the weight of girls increase consecutively.**

**(a) The number of boys is**

(i) 4 (ii) 5 (iii) 6 (iv) 7

**(b) The heaviest girl weighs**

(i) 55 kg (ii) 56 kg (iii) 57 kg (iv) 58 kg

**213. A. A dice (which dots has been replaced by corresponding numbers) when seen from one corner, the**

numbers (2, 3, 4) are visible while from another corner, the numbers (1, 2, 6) are visible. The number opposite to 5 is

(i) 1 (ii) 2
(iii) 3 (iv) cannot be determined

B. Two identical dices (which dots have been replaced by corresponding numbers) are put on a table one over the other. It is observed that for three different types of their setting, the numbers (1, 2, 4), (2, 3, 5) and (3, 4, 6) out of pairs of numbers 1-6 are not visible.

(a) Which of the following cannot be the sum of digits on the opposite faces?
(i) 5 (ii) 6 (iii) 7 (iv) 8

(b) Which of the following may be on opposite faces?
(i) 2, 4 (ii) 2, 3
(iii) 3, 4 (iv) none of these

**214.**

| A | B | C | D | E | F |
|---|---|---|---|---|---|

By throwing a dice, a counter can be moved along the six blocks to and fro (as shown in the above figure), the change of positions being equal to the number shown by the dice. Initially the counter is outside and it starts moving from left to right (the number 1 on dice means it is to occupy the block A). After that the counter moves between A and F returning at the ends (these ends are not to be counted twice).

The dice is thrown five times successively and five different numbers are shown by it. Let the positions of dice after the throws of dice be A, B, C, D, D (not in order).

(a) After the initial throw of dice, the position of dice is at block
(i) A or B (ii) A or D (iii) B or C (iv) C or D

(b) The final position of dice is at
(i) A (ii) B (iii) C (iv) D

(c) The dice reached C after the dice showed the number
(i) 2 (ii) 3 (iii) 4 (iv) 5

(d) In five throws of dice, the number which did not show up was
(i) 1 (ii) 2 (iii) 3 (iv) 6

**215. An article comes in three packets of 2 kg, 3 kg and 4 kg. Three porters A, B and C carry 7, 9 and 14 packets respectively which corresponding total weights are 20, 30 and 50 kg. Every porter carries at least one packets of each types.**

**(a) If there are total 6 packets of 2 kg, then how many packets of 3 kg are there?**

(i) 6 (ii) 8 (iii) 10 (iv) 12

**(b) If there are total 12 packets of 3 kg, then how many packets of 2 kg does C carry?**

(i) 1 (ii) 2 (iii) 3 (iv) 4

**(c) If their are total 14 packets of 4 kg, then how many packets of 3 kg does B carry?**

(i) 2 (ii) 4
(iii) 6 (iv) cannot be determined.

**(d) If there are total 7 packets of 2 kg, then how many packets of 4 kg does B carry?**

(i) 3 (ii) 4 (iii) 5 (iv) 6

**216. A, B, C, D, E, F, G, H are divided into two groups of four elements each.**

**A. Two elements are chosen from each group to form another group. If the possible arrangements of third group can be {A, B, E, F} or {B, D, E, G} or {B, C, F, H}, then**

**(a) which of the following can be together in one of the first two groups?**

(i) A, E (ii) D, G (iii) C, H (iv) E, F

**(b) how many different forms of first two groups are possible?**

(i) 2 (ii) 3 (iii) 4 (iv) 6

**B. These groups are {A, B, C, D} and {E, F, G, H}. Two elements are chosen from each group to form another group X, this group containing A. The rest of elements forms another group Y. Two elements are again chosen from each of X and Y to form another group**

**(a) {A, G, C, D}. The different number of possible forms of group X is**

(i) 5 (ii) 6 (iii) 7 (iv) 9

(b) {A, G, C, E}. The different number of possible forms of group X is

(i) 9 (ii) 10 (iii) 11 (iv) 12

217. A, B, C, D, E, F, G, H, I are six delegates and three interpreters. Two of delegates speak French only, another two English only and the other two Russian only. Each interpreters speak only two of the languages. It is known that (A, B, I); (C, D, G) and (E, F, H) don't speak French, English and Russian respectively. Also known are that only one of (G, H), (G, I) and (I, H) speaks French, Russian and English respectively and each of A, C, E speaks only one language.

(a) How many possibilities for the delegates vis-a-vis their languages exist?

(i) 1 (ii) 2 (iii) 3 (iv) 4

(b) How many possibilities for the interpreters vis-a-vis their languages exist?

(i) 1 (ii) 2 (iii) 3 (iv) 4

218. A, B, C, D, E, F, G, H are eight delegates belonging to three countries, viz. England, France and Japan. England has two males and one female delegate, France has one male and two females delegates while Japan has one male and one female delegate. The triplets (A, B,C); (C, D, E) and (F, G, H) have a delegate belonging to each country and have at least one male and one female. Each of the pairs (A, D), (B, F) and (E, G) have one male and one female that belong to different countries. Also known is that H is female that doesn't belong to Japan.

(a) Which of the following belongs to England?

(i) A (ii) B (iii) C (iv) D

(b) Which of the following is female delegate of England?

(i) B (ii) D (iii) G (iv) H

(c) Which of the following is male delegate of France?

(i) A (ii) C (iii) E (iv) F

219. A, B, C, D, E are five letters which are to go in five envelopes F, G, H, I and J. (Each envelop being assigned to one letter).

**(a) In how many ways, the letters can be put in envelopes such that no letter goes in the right envelope?**

(i) 35 (ii) 44 (iii) 72 (iv) 90

**For (b), (c), and (d):**

**Let F, G, H, I, J and H, I, J, F, G not be the right envelopes for the letters A, B, C, D, E respectively. If it is known that the right envelopes for A is**

**(b) G, then in how many different ways the other letters can be tried to be put into right envelopes?**

(i) 5 (ii) 6 (iii) 7 (iv) 8

**(c) I, then in how many different ways the other letters can be tried to be put into right envelopes?**

(i) 3 (ii) 4 (iii) 5 (iv) 6

**(d) J, then all the corresponding envelopes of the letters can be known if it is given that**

(i) B goes in H (ii) C goes in I

(iii) D goes in F (iv) E goes in F

**220. A, B, C, D, E, F, G, H, I, J represent numbers through 0 to 9. When arranged as a sequence such that there are three triples of consecutive integers, no four consecutive letters representing consecutive numbers, it is found that only B > D > G > I can be the members not belonging to any of the triplets. If one of such sequence is I A F E H B D G C J, then**

**(a) A represents**

(i) 1 (ii) 2

(iii) 4 (iv) cannot be determined

**(b) 7 is represented by**

(i) B (ii) D

(iii) H (iv) none of these

**221. $X_1$, $X_2$ ......................, $X_{30}$ are 30 participants of a chess tournament. The match is first played between $X_1$ and $X_2$ and the winner plays with $X_3$ and then again winner plays with the next participant in the succession and so on. Let there be only 5 players who won at least one match, four of them won equal number of matches, nobody winning more that 10 matches. Also assume that no match is drawn.**

**(a) Which of the following cannot be the participant winning any of the matches?**

(i) $X_{11}$ (ii) $X_{12}$ (iii) $X_{13}$ (iv) $X_{14}$

**(b) Which of the following cannot be the participant winning any of the matches?**

(i) $X_{21}$ (ii) $X_{22}$ (iii) $X_{23}$ (iv) $X_{24}$

**(c) Let $X_{18}$ be one of the players who won at least one match. Which of the following is the player winning the last match of the tournament?**

(i) $X_{23}$ (ii) $X_{24}$ (iii) $X_{25}$ (iv) $X_{26}$

**222. There are four blood groups found in human being, viz. A, B, AB and O. Persons with any blood group can take blood from blood group O while persons with blood group AB can take blood from any blood group. Also persons of each blood group can take blood of same type. Let $P_1$, $P_2$, $P_3$, $P_4$, $P_5$, $P_6$ be six persons such that**

**A. (I) $P_1$ can take blood from $P_2$ but not $P_3$.**

**(II) $P_2$ can take blood from $P_3$ but not $P_4$.**
**Then the blood group of $P_1$ will be**

**(i) O (ii) A B (iii) A or B**

**(iv) the given conditions are not possible together.**

**B. (I) $P_1$ can take blood from $P_5$ or $P_3$ (both of different blood groups).**

**(II) $P_2$ can take blood from $P_1$ or $P_4$ (both of different blood groups).**

**(III) $P_3$ can donate blood to $P_2$ or $P_6$ (both of different blood groups).**

**(IV) $P_4$ can take blood from $P_5$ or the person with blood group B.**

**(V) $P_5$ cannot take blood from $P_2$ or the person with blood group A.**

**(a) What is the blood group of $P_1$?**

(i) A (ii) B
(iii) C (iv) cannot be determined

**(b) What is the blood group of $P_2$?**

(i) A (ii) B
(iii) AB (iv) cannot be determined

**(c) The blood group of which of the following person can be known?**

(i) $P_3$ (ii) $P_4$
(iii) $P_5$ (iv) $P_6$

**223. A B C D E F G H are four couples arranged in a line in the order given such that two of the couples are together and other two are not.**

**A. Let A, C, D and G be females.**

**(a) Which of the following cannot be a couple?**

(i) B, C (ii) D, E
(iii) F, G (iv) all of these may be a couple.

**(b) Which of the following cannot be a couple?**

(i) A, B (ii) D, B
(iii) E, A (iv) all of these may be a couple.

**B. Let B, E be males while D, G be females. If the couples who are together can be known from the given arrangement, then which of the following must be true?**

(i) C is a female and F is a male
(ii) C is a male and F is a female
(iii) Both C and F are of opposite sex and each can be a male or a female
(iv) None of these

**C. Let B be male and G be female. If from the given arrangements it can be inferred that although BC and GH may be a couple, both the cases cannot be possible together, then which of the following is necessarily true?**

(i) A should be a male and D should be a female
(ii) D should be a male and E should be a female
(iii) A and E should be of opposite sex although each can be a male or a female
(iv) D and F should be of same sex although both can be males or females.

**224. Let $A_i$ be the set of positive integers not more than 100 such that for all positive integers $n$,**

$$A_{n+1} = \begin{cases} A_n + A_{n-1} & \text{if } A_n + A_{n-1} \le 100 \text{ and} \\ A_n + A_{n-1} - 100 & \text{if } A_n + A_{n-1} > 100 \end{cases}$$

**(a) Let three of four consecutive terms of the sequence $A_i$ be equal. From the group of those terms, the unequal term will be the**

(i) first term (ii) second term
(iii) third term (iv) the case is not possible

**(b) Let $A_3 = 40$ and $A_6 = 100$. Then $A_0 =$**

(i) 30 (ii) 40 (iii) 50 (iv) 60

**(c) Let $A_4 = 30$ and $A_7 = 70$. Then $A_0 =$**

(i) 40 (ii) 70
(iii) 90 (iv) cannot be determined

**225. For all non-negative integers $n$, $x_n$ are integers such that $x_{n+1} = 2x_n$ if $x_n$ is odd.**

**$= 2x_n - 1$ if $x_n$ is even.**

**(a) If $x_{100} = \frac{2^{103}}{3} - 2$, then $x_0 =$**

(i) $\frac{2}{3}$ (ii) $\frac{4}{3}$ (iii) $\frac{5}{3}$ (iv) $\frac{7}{3}$

**(b) If $x_{100} = \frac{2^{102}}{3} - 1$, then $x_0 =$**

(i) $\frac{2}{3}$ (ii) $\frac{4}{3}$ (iii) $\frac{5}{3}$ (iv) $\frac{7}{3}$

**226. A sequence is to be made of elements A, B, C or D. Let $X_{n+1}$ can be A only if $X_n$ = B or C,**

**B only if $X_n$ = C or D,**

**C only if $X_n$ = D or A,**

**D only if $X_n$ = A,**

**where $X_n$ denotes the element at the $n$th position of the sequence.**

**(a) If the sequence is made out of only three of the given elements, then it may not contain**

(i) B or C (ii) C or D (iii) B or D (iv) B or C or D

**(b) Suppose a sequence starts from A and ends in A (no A's in between). What is the total number of such sequences?**

(i) 5 (ii) 6 (iii) 7 (iv) 8

(c) **Suppose a sequence (not more than nine elements) starts from C and ends in C (with no C's in between). How many such sequences are possible?**

(i) 6 (ii) 7 (iii) 8 (iv) 9

**227. A, B, C, D, E are five vertices of a pentagon (not in order) and each is assigned a distinct number from 11, 13, 15, 17 and 19. A counter (initially placed at A) moves from vertices to vertices clockwise counting each vertices once and temporarily halts at the vertex on which the total count is equal to the number assigned to the vertex from which it starts moving. Let four of the temporary halts be A E B C, in that order.**

(a) **Its next halt will be**

(i) A (ii) D
(iii) E (iv) cannot be determined

(b) **If 11 is assigned to A, then 19 is assigned to**

(i) B (ii) C (iii) D (iv) E

**228. A, B, C, D, E are five unequal positive numbers with E > A. Consider a sequence which *n*th term is given as**

$$t_{n+1} = t_n + A \quad \text{if } t_n + A \le E$$
$$= t_n + A - E \quad \text{if } t_n + A > E$$

**It is found that if any five consecutive terms are taken, then each of the given numbers is equal to one of the terms.**

(a) **Which of the following could not be the valid value of E/A?**

(i) 1.25 (ii) 2 (iii) 2.5 (iv) 5

(b) **How many values of E/A are possible if one of the given number is .5A?**

(i) 1 (ii) 2 (iii) 3 (iv) 4

(c) **If B + D = A, then C =**

(i) $\frac{2}{3}A$ (ii) $\frac{4}{3}A$

(iii) $\frac{1}{2}A$ (iv) cannot be determined

(d) If the least value is B and C + D = 2A, then B =

(i) $\frac{1}{4}A$ (ii) $\frac{1}{2}A$ (iii) $\frac{1}{3}A$ (iv) $\frac{2}{3}A$

**229.** Consider a set S of four numbers 1, 3, 5 and 7. Let S′ be the set of values of average of any four numbers from the set S where a number may be repeated once.

(a) The elements of set S′ could well be given by the average of any two different elements (although their value may be same) picked from the set {2, 3, 4, 5, 6, 7, 8, $x$, $y$, $z$,} where $x$, $y$, $z$ are distinct integers between 2 and 8. The set {$x$, $y$, $z$} does not contain

(i) 3 (ii) 4 (iii) 5 (iv) 6

(b) How many elements of set S′ are integer?

(i) 19 (ii) 20 (iii) 21 (iv) 22

(c) How many elements of distinct value are in the set S′?

(i) 9 (ii) 10 (iii) 11 (iv) 12

**230.** 21 stones are kept in a line at intervals of 1 m. Let A, B, C, D denote the positions of four stones, A being the first stone and AD > AC > AB. A man has to bring all stones at one point and he can carry only one stone at a time. Let $d_B$, $d_C$, $d_D$ be the distances covered by him when he has to bring all stones to the position of B, C, D respectively, the initial point of his journey being the point at which he has to bring all the stones.

(a) If B, C, D represent positions of consecutive stones, then $d_D + d_B - 2d_C =$

(i) 2 m (ii) 4 m (iii) 6 m (iv) 8 m

(b) If $d_B$ = 220 m, then the position of B is

(i) 10th stones (ii) 11th stones
(iii) 12th stones (iv) cannot be determined

(c) If the man can carry two stones at a time, then the minimum distance he has to carry to bring all stones to A (assuming that he starts his journey from A) is

(i) 210 m (ii) 220 m (iii) 230 m (iv) 240 m

**231.** A, B, C, D, E, F, G, H are eight persons: four males and four females. A committee of two males and two females is to be formed. Two particular males; two particular

**females; and a particular male and a particular female (from the remaining four persons) do not want to be in the committee together. Let four of such committees possible be (A, C, E, F); (D, F, G, H); (B, C, D, E) and (A, B, C, H). Also C is male and F is female, both of whom can be in committees with any person.**

**(a) How many such committees can be formed?**

(i) 14 (ii) 15 (iii) 16 (iv) 17

**(b) Who cannot be in a committee together with G?**

(i) A (ii) B
(iii) E (iv) cannot be determined

**(c) If A can be found in at most seven possible committees and H can be found in at most six possible committees, then which of the following will be incorrect?**

(i) A, B are of opposite sex
(ii) H, E are of opposite sex
(iii) D, G are of opposite sex
(iv) none of these

**232. A, B, C, D, E, F, G, H are four couples. A committee of four persons is to be formed having two men and two women such that it must not contain any couple. Let two of the ways in which a committee can be formed be (A, C, B, F) and (A, E, G, F).**

**(a) In how many different ways the committee can be formed?**

(i) 6 (ii) 8 (iii) 10 (iv) 12

**(b) If A is male and D is female, C is male and E is female, then which of the following are couples?**

(i) (A, D) and (C, G) (ii) (A, H) and (C, E)
(iii) (F, D) and (B, E) (iv) (F, H) and (B, G)

**233. A, B, C, D, E, F, G, H are eight persons divided into two groups of four persons, say $G_1$ and $G_2$. A committee of four persons are to be formed such that two persons from $G_1$ want to be chosen together while two persons from $G_2$ do not want to chosen together. Let four such committees possible be (A, E, G, H) ; (A, C, D, E); (B, C, D, F) and (B, F, G, H).**

(a) How many cases for the pair of people who want to be together exist?
(i) 3 (ii) 4 (iii) 5 (iv) 6

(b) How many cases for the pair of people who do not want to be together exist?
(i) 8 (ii) 10 (iii) 12 (iv) 16

(c) If A, E want to be together in a committee, then which of the following will not want to be together in the committee?
(i) (C, G) or (D, H)
(ii) (C, H) or (D, G)
(iii) (C, G), (C, H), (D, G) or (D, H)
(iv) may not be any of these

**234.** A, B, C, D, E, F, G, H are eight persons. A committee of a few persons are to be formed and each of them do not want to be chosen exactly with two of the other persons. Let five of the possible committee formed can be (B, C, H), (B, H, F), (A, B, G), (E, A, H) and (C, D, F).

(a) If a committee of four persons is to be formed, then how many distinct committees are possible?
(i) Two (ii) Four (iii) Six (iv) Eight

(b) If a committee of four persons is to be formed, then which of the following can be one of the possible committee?
(i) B, A, G, C (ii) B, A, F, G
(iii) B, H, F, C (iv) B, H, C, G

(c) D cannot be in a committee with
(i) A (ii) E (iii) G (iv) H

(d) E cannot be in a committee with
(i) C (ii) D (iii) F (iv) G

(e) G cannot be in a committee with
(i) C (ii) D (iii) E (iv) F

**235.** Six letters A, B, C, D, E and F are taken and they are assigned numbers 1, 2, 3, 4, 5, 6 respectively. The letters are arranged around a circle and it is required to have a cyclic sequence of A B C D E F (in clockwise manner). In any given sequence a letter can jump as many letters (in the clockwise sense) as the number assigned to that letter

**and such movement of any one letter constitute a move. A letter cannot make more than one move.**

**(a) If the initial sequence is D F C B E A (clockwise), then in how many moves, one can get the desired sequence?**

(i) 3 (ii) 4 (iii) 5 (iv) not possible

**(b) If the initial sequence is F E D C B A (clockwise), then in how many moves, one can get the desired sequence?**

(i) 3 (ii) 4 (iii) 5 (iv) not possible

**(c) Which of the following clockwise sequences is amenable to be modified into desired sequence?**

(i) B D C E A F (ii) C F D B A E

(iii) D A C E B F (iv) none of these

**236. Let the value of expression**

$$\frac{x_1 \cdot x_2 + x_4 \cdot x_5 + x_3 + x_2}{x_1 + x_2 + x_1 \cdot x_2 + x_1 \cdot x_4 + x_2 \cdot x_5}$$

**be independent of one of $x_i$ ($i$ = 1, 2, 3, 4, 5). Also if one of $x_i$ ($i$ = 1, 2, 3, 4, 5) is zero, then this value will be a constant equal to $c$ ($\neq 0$).**

**(a) The value of expression will be independent of**

(i) $x_1$ (ii) $x_2$ (iii) $x_4$ (iv) $x_5$

**(b) If one of $x_i$ is zero such that the value of expression is $c$ ($\neq 0$), then this $x_i$ is**

(i) $x_1$ (ii) $x_3$ (iii) $x_4$ (iv) $x_5$

**(c) The value of $c$ is**

(i) –1 (ii) $\frac{1}{2}$ (iii) 1 (iv) 2

**237. $A_0$ has two branches $A_1$ and $A_2$. $A_1$ has two branches $A_3$ and $A_4$ while $A_2$ also has two branches $A_5$ and $A_6$. Now $A_3$ has again two branches $A_7$ and $A_8$; $A_4$ has two branches $A_9$ and $A_{10}$; $A_5$ has two branches $A_{11}$ and $A_{12}$; $A_6$ has two branches $A_{13}$ and $A_{14}$; and so on.**

**(a) $A_{100}$ will be a direct branch of**

(i) $A_{48}$ (ii) $A_{49}$ (iii) $A_{50}$ (iv) $A_{51}$

**(b) If $A_{200}$ is a direct branch of $A_n$, then $A_n$ will be the direct branch of**

(i) $A_{47}$ (ii) $A_{48}$ (iii) $A_{49}$ (iv) $A_{50}$

**(c) Let $m, n, p$ be positive integers. If $A_m$ is a direct branch of $A_n$ and $A_n$ is a direct branch of $A_p$, then which of the following cannot be possible?**

$p =$

(i) $\frac{m-2}{4}$ (ii) $\frac{m-1}{4}$ (iii) $\frac{m+1}{4}$ (iv) $\frac{m+2}{4}$

**238. Consider a group of eight distinct elements. This group is divided into two exclusive subgroups, each containing four elements. Each of these subgroups are divided into two smaller subgroups, each containing two exclusive elements. Yet again, each of four subgroups are divided into two subgroups containing one exclusive element each. Let us name all the groups (and subgroups) as $G_1$, $G_2$ ....... $G_{15}$. Let**

**I. each of the following pair has one common element: ($G_1$, $G_6$), ($G_3$, $G_{14}$), ($G_7$, $G_{12}$), ($G_6$, $G_8$), ($G_2$, $G_{15}$), ($G_{13}$, $G_{10}$), ($G_4$, $G_{11}$), ($G_5$, $G_7$), ($G_9$, $G_{10}$), ($G_5$, $G_{14}$)**

**II. none of the following pair has any element in common: ($G_3$, $G_{10}$), ($G_6$, $G_9$), ($G_7$, $G_{11}$), ($G_4$, $G_{12}$), ($G_1$, $G_{13}$), ($G_2$, $G_{14}$), ($G_8$, $G_{15}$)**

**(a) Which of the following will have only one element?**

(i) $G_2$ (ii) $G_4$ (iii) $G_{11}$ (iv) $G_{13}$

**(b) Which of the following will have more than one element?**

(i) $G_1$ (ii) $G_3$ (iii) $G_8$ (iv) $G_9$

**(c) Which of the following will have more than two elements?**

(i) $G_5$ (ii) $G_6$

(iii) $G_{10}$ (iv) cannot be determined

**239. (a) Consider a grouped sequence in which the first group contains $A_1$; second contains ($A_2$, $A_3$); third contains ($A_4$, $A_5$, $A_6$) and so on. $A_{100}$ is found in**

(i) 12th group (ii) 13th group

(iii) 14th group (iv) 15th group

**(b) Had the groups in part (a) been $(A_1)$; $(A_2\ A_3, A_4)$; $(A_5, A_6, A_7, A_8, A_9)$ and so on, then $A_{1000}$ would have been found in**

(i) 31st group (ii) 32nd group
(iii) 33rd group (iv) 34th group

**240. Consider a sequence**

**(a) $(A_1)\ (A_3\ A_2)\ (A_4\ A_5\ A_6)\ (A_{10}\ A_9\ A_8\ A_7)\ (A_{11}\ A_{12}\ A_{13}\ A_{14}\ A_{15})$ ..... . The position of $A_{300}$ will be**

(i) 276th (ii) 277th
(iii) 300th (iv) none of these

**(b) $(A_1)\ (A_3\ A_2)\ (A_6\ A_5\ A_4)\ (A_{10}\ A_9\ A_8\ A_7)\ (A_{15}\ A_{14}\ A_{13}\ A_{12}\ A_{11})$. If $A_m$ and $A_{m+200}$ are adjacent to each other, then $m$ =**

(i) 4754 (ii) 4852 (iii) 4951 (iv) 5051

**(c) $(A_1)\ (A_4\ A_3\ A_2)\ (A_9\ A_6\ A_7\ A_8\ A_5)\ (A_{16}\ A_{11}\ A_{14}\ A_{13}\ A_{12}\ A_{15}\ A_{10})$ ........ . The position of $A_{200}$ will be**

(i) 192th (ii) 200th (iii) 204th (iv) 208th

**241. A, B, C, D, E are numbers 0, 1, 2, 3 and a negative sign '–'. When written in sequence the numbers are added except for the number preceded by '–' sign which is subtracted. Given A does not represent '–' and ABCDA = 3 and ACBEA = 4,**

**(a) C denotes**

(i) – (ii) 0 (iii) 1 (iv) 2

**(b) D denotes**

(i) – (ii) 1 (iii) 2 (iv) 3

**(c) E denotes**

(i) 0 (ii) 1 (iii) 2 (iv) 3

**242. A, B, C, D are four persons each of whom toss a coin simultaneously and the head or tail turned up by them are recorded. If any person throws head or tail successively thrice, then they get one point. Coins are tossed six times and each of them got exactly one point although in different toss number. Also both heads and tails are tossed successively thrice to get points. The table below shows few of heads (H) and tails (T) turned up by them:**

| TOSS NUMBER | A | B | C | D |
|---|---|---|---|---|
| 1 | T | T | H | H |
| 2 | – | – | – | – |
| 3 | – | – | – | – |
| 4 | – | T | T | – |
| 5 | T | T | – | T |
| 6 | T | – | T | T |

**(a) A got a point in toss number**
(i) 3 (ii) 4
(iii) 5 (iv) cannot be determined

**(b) B got a point in toss number**
(i) 3 (ii) 4 (iii) 5 (iv) 6

**(c) D got a point in toss number**
(i) 3 (ii) 4 (iii) 5 (iv) 6

**243. Four persons A, B, C, D, each tosses a coin simultaneously for five times and the head (H) and tail (T) are recorded each time. For five times, the record shows (4H), (3H, 1T), (2H, 2T), (1H, 3T), (4T) (not in order) tossed up by four persons. Also A tossed up 1H and 1T in first and fifth toss respectively; B tossed only 2H, and 1T in second and fourth toss; C tossed only 2H (one of which was in fourth toss) and 1T in third toss; while D tossed only 3H (one of which was in fourth toss) and 1T in second toss.**

**(a) How many times did A toss up H?**
(i) 1 (ii) 2 (iii) 3 (iv) 4

**(b) (2T, 2H) could not have been tossed in**
(i) first toss (ii) second toss
(iii) third toss (iv) fourth toss

**(c) If A, B, tossed up T in third toss, then in first, second and fifth toss, C tossed up**
(i) H, T, T respectively
(ii) T, H, T respectively
(iii) T, T, H respectively
(iv) cannot be determined

**(d) If A, C tossed up T and H respectively in second toss, then in first, third and fourth toss, B tossed up**
(i) H, H, T respectively
(ii) H, T, H respectively

(iii) T, H, H respectively
(iv) cannot be determined

**244. A, B, C, D, E, F are six persons (three males and three females) who toss a coin. If male tosses a coin, then he gets 1 or –1 point according as head or tail turns up and vice versa for female. Let a round consists of all of them tossing once. Let in round one, two and three, there be 2, 3 and 4 heads respectively while the respective points of A, B, C, D, E, F be 1, 1, –1, –1, 1, –1 for round one; –1, 1, 1, 1, –1, 1 for round two and 1, –1, 1, –1, 1, –1 for round three.**

**(a) Who is definitely a male?**
(i) A (ii) C (iii) E (iv) F

**(b) Who is definitely a female?**
(i) A (ii) B (iii) D (iv) E

**(c) Which of the following pair necessarily have a male and a female?**
(i) A, D (ii) B, E (iii) C, E (iv) D, F

**(d) In all three rounds, how many times did males toss up heads?**
(i) 4 (ii) 5
(iii) 6 (iv) cannot be determined

**245. A, B, C, D, E, F are three couples standing in a line at the interval of few steps (same/or any two adjacent persons). Each male takes two steps towards his spouse while each female takes one step towards her spouse. (Assume that span of step for each person to be same). Let the steps between**
**A, B be 13; A, C be 7; C, D be 11; B, F be 7; D, F be 10 and E, F be 12.**

**(a) What is the initial distance (in steps) between two adjacent persons?**
(i) 4 (ii) 5
(iii) 6 (iv) cannot be determined

**(b) Who are standing at the extreme?**
(i) B, E (ii) D, E (iii) A, F (iv) A, C

**(c) Who is male?**
(i) A (ii) B (iii) D (iv) E

**(d) Who is female?**
(i) A (ii) C (iii) D (iv) F

**(e) Who are necessarily a couple?**
(i) A, C (ii) B, D (iii) E, F (iv) D, E

**246. A, B, C, D, E, F (few males and few females) are standing at a point. They throw a dice and take as many steps as the number shown by the dice. The males move in east direction and the females in west direction. Also the span of step for each person are same and each of them threw up a different number. If A, E are 8 steps away; C, D are 7 steps away; B, F are 6 step away; E, F are 3 steps away; C is east to A; E is west to D; and F is east to E, then**

**(a) what is the number thrown by A?**
(i) 2 (ii) 3 (iii) 5 (iv) 6

**(b) who threw 4?**
(i) B (ii) C
(iii) D (iv) cannot be determined

**(c) the starting point is closest to**
(i) C (ii) D (iii) E (iv) F

**(d) who is female?**
(i) B (ii) C
(iii) D (iv) none of these

**(e) who is male?**
(i) A (ii) E
(iii) F (iv) none of these

**247. A, B, C, D, E, F, G, H are four couples seated around a round table with no couple sitting opposite to each other. Also only two males and only two females are sitting together. Now**

**(A, G) and (B, F) are couples;**
**A, a male, is sitting adjacent to E, a female;**
**F is sitting in between two males;**
**G is sitting in between a male and a female;**
**H is sitting adjacent to B;**
**D is sitting between two females;**
**C, a male, is sitting opposite to A.**

**(a) Which of the following is a couple?**
(i) D, H (ii) D, E
(iii) C, E (iv) cannot be determined

**(b) Who is sitting opposite to B?**
(i) A (ii) E
(iii) D (iv) none of these

**(c) Who is sitting in between two males?**
(i) E (ii) B
(iii) H (iv) none of these

**(d) Who is sitting in between two females?**
(i) A (ii) B
(iii) C (iv) none of these

**(e) Who is sitting opposite to D?**
(i) G (ii) H (iii) E (iv) F

**248. A, B, C, D, E , F are six persons who are to do a work. Efficiencies of all males and all females are same and that of a male is greater than that of a female. Let (A, B, D); (A, C, F) and (B, C, D, E) can do a work together in 42, 35 and 30 days respectively.**

**(a) Which of the following is necessarily true?**
(i) A female can do the whole work alone in 140 days.
(ii) A female can do the whole work alone in 210 days.
(iii) A male can do the whole work alone in 105 days.
(iv) none of these

**(b) Which of the following may not be a male?**
(i) A (ii) C (iii) F (iv) E

**(c) If B is a male, then how many females are there?**
(i) 1 (ii) 2
(iii) 3 (iv) cannot be determined

**(d) What could not be the number of males?**
(i) 3 (ii) 4
(iii) 5 (iv) all of these are possible

**249. There are two committees $G_1$ and $G_2$ to be formed in which the members are inducted by the toss of a coin. A male member gets in $G_1$ or $G_2$ according as he tosses up head or tail and a female member gets in $G_2$ or $G_1$ according as she tosses up head or tail.**

**A.** **Let there be seven persons: A, B, C, D, E, F and G, at least two of the persons are of both sex. Each of them tosses the coin once in a round and let there be four rounds. Let in four rounds, the number of times heads turn up be 2, 3, 4, 5 while $G_1$ comprises of (A, C, E): (C, D, F, G); (A, B, G) and (B, D, E, F) respectively.**

**(a) How many males are there?**

(i) 2 (ii) 3 (iii) 4 (iv) 5

**(b) Who will be definitely a male?**

(i) A (ii) B
(iii) D (iv) none of these

**(c) Who will be definetly a female?**

(i) C (ii) E
(iii) F (iv) none of these

**(d) If G is male, the which of the following will be a male?**

(i) D (ii) E
(iii) F (iv) cannot be determined

**(e) How many of the group (C, D, F, G) are males?**

(i) 1 (ii) 2 (iii) 3 (iv) 4

**(f) How many of the group (B, D, E, F) are males?**

(i) 1 (ii) 2 (iii) 3 (iv) 4

**250. Six persons A, B, C, D, E, F are initially grouped into two groups, $G_1$ and $G_2$ having three persons each. Each of them tosses a coin simultaneously and they remain in their own group if they turn up a head and change their group if they turn up a tail. After first toss $G_1$ has only one person. They also tossed three times successively after the first toss showing up head or tail as given in table below:**

| | A | B | C | D | E | F |
|---|---|---|---|---|---|---|
| IInd toss | – | T | H | – | H | T |
| IIIrd toss | H | – | T | T | – | T |
| IVth toss | T | H | – | H | H | –, |

**after which only C and D (initially both were in different groups) are found to be in their original groups. Given that after IInd toss, $G_2$ has only one person and after IIIrd toss, $G_1$ has only two persons, then**

**(a) which of the following was necessarily in $G_1$ initially?**
(i) A (ii) B (iii) E (iv) F

**(b) which of the following was necessarily in $G_2$ initially?**
(i) A (ii) B (iii) E (iv) F

**(c) after first toss, who was in $G_1$?**
(i) A (ii) C (iii) E (iv) F

**(d) after second toss, who was in $G_2$?**
(i) B (ii) C (iii) E (iv) F

**(e) the total number of heads turned up by which person cannot be determined?**
(i) A (ii) B (iii) E (iv) F

**(f) which of the following is correct?**
(i) In first toss, A, C, D, F turned up tail, head, head and head respectively
(ii) In second toss, A and D tossed up head and tail respectively
(iii) In third toss, both B and E tossed up tail
(iv) In fourth toss, C and F tossed up tail and head respectively

**251. A, B, C, D, E, F, G, H, I, J, K, L are divided into two groups, each having six letters. Within a group, each letter is assigned a number from 1 to 6. A dice is thrown and the letters in the groups assigned the number that is shown by the dice are exchanged. The dice is thrown successively six times, each time showing a different number. When it showed up 1 and 5, the letters K and I respectively changed their groups. Also when the dice showed up 3, 4 and 6, the first group has letters (K, B, L, D, H, E), (G, A, I, C, B, D) and (G, A, B, D, H, E) respectively.**

**(a) Which of the following must be assigned 2?**
(i) B (ii) D
(iii) F (iv) cannot be determined

**(b) If H is assigned 6, then C is assigned**
(i) 4 (ii) 5
(iii) 6 (iv) cannot be determined

**(c) If the dice showed 4 earlier than 6, then L is assigned**
(i) 3 (ii) 4
(iii) 6 (iv) cannot be determined

**(d) The position of throw of which of the following number shown up by the dice in the sequence of throw of dice can be known?**

(i) 2 (ii) 3 (iii) 4 (iv) 6

**252. A, B, C, D, E, F, G, H, I [a professor, an artist, a lawyer, a chemist, a doctor, an accountant, an engineer, an architect, an actor by profession (not in order)] are to be divided into three groups $G_1$, $G_2$ and $G_3$ of three persons each. Now each of the persons of the triplets (A, B, C), (D, E, F), (Chemist, Artist, Lawyer) are in different groups. Also G is architect, H is professor, I is engineer. Let A be in $G_3$, F in $G_2$, doctor in $G_1$, actor in $G_2$, lawyer in $G_1$. If A is not an accountant, B is chemist and (D, I) are in the same group, then**

**(a) the accountant is in group**

(i) $G_1$ (ii) $G_2$
(iii) $G_3$ (iv) cannot be determined

**(b) who is the lawyer?**

(i) C (ii) D
(iii) E (iv) cannot be determined

**(c) which of the following is correct?**

(i) Artist is in the same group as G.
(ii) C is in the same group as D.
(iii) E is in the same group as H.
(iv) none of these

**253. A, B, C, - - - - I are nine persons having four couples. They are to be divided into three groups of three members each. In each group, there is at least one male and one female with no couples in any of the group. Let two of the possible ways of grouping be**
**(A, H, E); (B, I, D) and (C, G, F) or**
**(A, F, I) ; (C, D, H) and (G, B, E)**
**If A, B, C, D, E are males and other females, then**

**(a) which of the following will be the bachelor?**

(i) A (ii) D
(iii) E (iv) cannot be determined

**(b) F will be married to**

(i) B (ii) D
(iii) E (iv) cannot be determined

**(c) which of the following is necessarily correct?**
(i) I is married to C and G to A
(ii) I is married to E and G to A
(iii) I is married to C and G to D
(iv) none of these

**254. A, B, C, D, E, F, G, H and I are nine persons. Let the group**
**(A, B, C, D) has two males and two females;**
**(E, F, G, H) has two males and two females;**
**(B, E, I, D) has three males and one female;**
**(C, I, D, H) has two males and two female.**

**(a) If A is male, then which of the following will also be a male?**
(i) B (ii) C
(iii) D (iv) any of these

**(b) If C is male, then which of the following must also be a male?**
(i) B (ii) E
(iii) D (iv) none of these

**(c) If F is a female, then which of the following must be a male?**
(i) E (ii) G
(iii) H (iv) none of these

**(d) If H is a female, then which of the following must be a male?**
(i) A (ii) B
(iii) G (iv) none of these

**255. A, B, C, D, E, F, G, H are four couples out of which a committee of four persons are to be formed having two males and two females. Let four of such committees be (A, B, C, F) having no couple; (C, E, G, H) having one couple; (B, D, E, G) having one couple; (A, D, F, H) having no couple.**

**(a) Which of the following is definitely a couple?**
(i) C, D (ii) C, H
(iii) A, E (iv) A, G

**(b) Which of the following is definitely a couple?**
(i) B, D (ii) B, H
(iii) E, F (iv) F, G

**(c) If A is male, then which of the following will definitely be a female?**

(i) E (ii) F

(iii) G (iv) cannot be determined

**(d) Suppose that above committees are not given and instead two committees $C_1$ and $C_2$ are given, of which $C_1$ has no couple while $C_2$ has one couple. Let $C'_1$ and $C'_2$ be the committees formed by other four persons not in the committees $C_1$ and $C_2$ respectively. Then**

(i) $C'_1$ has no couple (ii) $C'_2$ has one couple

(iii) Both (iv) None

**256. A, B, C, D, E, F, G, H are eight persons. A committee of four persons is to be formed having two males and two females. The committee can be**

**(B, C, G, H); (A, D, E, H); (C, E, F, G); (B, D, E, G) and (A, F, G, H), the first four having one couple each and the last one having none. If the number of males and females are not equal and there are**

**(a) two couples, then which of the following is not a couple?**

(i) B, H (ii) C, G

(iii) D, E (iv) cannot be determined

**(b) three couples, then which of the following must be a couple?**

(i) D, H (ii) B, G

(iii) C, E (iv) cannot be determined

**(c) three couples, then which of the following cannot be married?**

(i) A (ii) C

(iii) E (iv) H

**(d) three couples, then which of the following will be of different sex from others?**

(i) E (ii) F

(iii) G (iv) H

**257. A, B, C, D, E, F, G, H, I, J, K, L are six couples out of which a committee of four persons having one couple is to be chosen. Three of the couples want to be chosen together with their respective spouses, otherwise not, while other three do not want to be chosen together with their**

**respective spouses in the committee. Let three of such committees be (A, C, F, G), (B, D, H, J) and (E, I, K, L) and three committees which do not strictly conform to the above condition related to the choice of couples be (A, F, H, K) (B, D, I, L) and (C, E, G, J).**

**(a) Which of the following can be a couple?**

(i) A, F (ii) B, D
(iii) I, L (iv) none of these

**(b) If (C, J) is a couple, then which of the following is also a couple?**

(i) B, H (ii) D, I
(iii) E, L (iv) none of these

**(c) If (G, E) is a couple, then which of the following is also a couple?**

(i) F, K (ii) D, L
(iii) K, I (iv) none of these

**(d) If (F, K) is a couple, then which of the following must also be a couple?**

(i) B, H (ii) D, I
(iii) G, J (iv) none of these

**(e) If (A, C) is a couple, then which of the following must also be a couple?**

(i) B, H (ii) G, J
(iii) F, K (iv) none of these

**258. Five coins of different values (positive integers) are tossed simultaneously comprising a round. In each round, the sum of values of coins are taken, positive value is taken when head turns up and negative value is taken when tail turns up. Let in round one, two, three and four, 1, 2, 3, 4 heads turn up respectively while the sums are –5, –1, –3 and 7 respectively. Let the values of coins be $a < b < c < d < e$.**

**(a) How many times *a* turns up head?**

(i) 1 (ii) 2
(iii) 3 (iv) cannot be determined

**(b) How many times *b* turns up head?**

(i) 1 (ii) 2
(iii) 3 (iv) cannot be determined

**(c) The value of *c* is**

(i) 3 (ii) 4
(iii) 5 (iv) cannot be determined

**(d) The value of *e* is**

(i) 5 (ii) 6
(iii) 7 (iv) cannot be determined

**259. A, B, C, D, E are five dices each numbered 1–6. None of the dices have two opposite faces numbered with same pair of numbers. Let A, B, C, D, E have (3, 4) ; (2, 6) ; (3, 6) ; (1, 5) and (2, 4) respectively as a pair of number on their one of the opposite faces.**

**(a) All the numbering of opposite faces of which dice can be known?**

(i) A (ii) B (iii) C (iv) D

**(b) If the sums of numbers on opposite faces be equal for a dice, then this dice will be**

(i) A (ii) B (iii) C (iv) D

**(c) How many different possibilities for the numbering of dices exist?**

(i) 2 (ii) 3 (iii) 4 (iv) 5

**260. A. Two dices A and B each numbered 1–6 are tossed simultaneously thrice. The sum of numbers shown up are found to be 4, 9 and 8 while the sum of hidden numbers are found to be 6, 9 and 5 respectively. Then in one of the dice,**

**(a) 1 can be against**

(i) 2 (ii) 3 (iii) 4 (iv) 6

**(b) 2 can be against**

(i) 1 (ii) 3 (iii) 4 (iv) 5

**(c) 3 can be against**

(i) 1 (ii) 4 (iii) 5 (iv) 6

**(d) 4 can be against**

(i) 2 (ii) 3 (iii) 5 (iv) 6

**B. Two identical dices (having identical numbering from 1–6) are thrown up three times. The sum of numbers shown up are 4, 5 and 6 while the sum of hidden numbers are 8, 9 and 10 (may not be in order).**

**(a) When the sum of numbers shown up is 4, then the sum of hidden numbers cannot be**

(i) 8 (ii) 9
(iii) 10 (iv) can be any of these

**(b) 1 will be against**

(i) 4 (ii) 5
(iii) 6 (iv) cannot be determined

**(c) 3 will be against**

(i) 4 (ii) 5
(iii) 6 (iv) cannot be determined

**(d) When the sum of numbers shown up is 5, then the sum of hidden numbers cannot be**

(i) 8 (ii) 9
(iii) 10 (iv) can be any of these

**261. Consider a coin and a dice (numbered 1–6). The coin is tossed and the dice is thrown simultaneously. If head turns up, the number shown by dice is recorded and when tail turns up, the number opposite to that shown by dice is recorded. In eight tosses, let the numbers that turned up be**

**(a) 1, 2, 3, 4, 4, 5, 6, 6 and the numbers recorded be 1, 2, 2, 3, 4, 5, 5, 6, (not in order). If both head and tail turned up four times each, then which number is against 1?**

(i) 2 (ii) 3
(iii) 4 (iv) cannot be determined

**(b) 1, 1, 2, 2, 3, 4, 5, 6 and the number recorded be 1, 2, 4, 4, 5, 5, 6, 6 (not in order). If the head turned up only once which is when the dice showed up 5, then the number against it on the dice is**

(i) 1 (ii) 2
(iii) 3 (iv) cannot be determined

**262. Consider a dice (numbered 1–6) kept on a table and let X, Y be two perpendicular axes, each pointing perpendicular to one of its lateral faces (those other than top or bottom). A coin is tossed; if head turns up, then it is rotated through 90° clockwise along X axis as many times as the number**

**inscribed on the top surface and if tail turns up, then the same thing along Y axis.**
**Let initially it showed 1 and tosses showed up H, T, H, T (in sequence) while the numbers showed up were 2, 3, 4, 5 (may not be in order).**

**(a) Which number is against 1?**
(i) 2 (ii) 3 (iii) 4 (iv) 5

**(b) Which number is against 6?**
(i) 2 (ii) 3 (iii) 4 (iv) 5

**(c) Which number showed up after the first toss?**
(i) 2 (ii) 3 (iii) 4 (iv) 5

**263. Consider two dices A and B, both numbered 1–6. The dices are brought in contact face over face, the faces coming in contact having the same number inscribed on them. The numbers shown by the faces opposite to the hidden faces can be (3, 5) ; (1, 6) ; (2, 3) or (4, 1). (First of each pair correspond to A and second to B)**

**(a) In dice A, 6 cannot be against**
(i) 2 (ii) 3 (iii) 4 (iv) 5

**(b) In dice B, 4 cannot be against**
(i) 2 (ii) 3 (iii) 5 (iv) 6

**(c) When the two dices are brought together and A showed 5, then B showed**
(i) 2 (ii) 3
(iii) 4 (iv) cannot be determined

**(d) When the two dices are brought together and B showed 4, then A showed**
(i) 2 (ii) 5
(iii) 6 (iv) cannot be determined

**264. Consider an *x-y* coordinate system and a dice (numbered 1–6). An object is kept at an integeral point on the *x-y* plane which moves according as the number thrown up by the dice. For three numbers thrown up by the dice, it moves along direction parallel to *x* axis as many unit distance as the number shown up while for other three numbers thrown up, it moves likewise along direction parallel to *y* axis (The object moves in positive directions only).**

**Let after second and fourth throw of the dice, the positions of dice be (4, 3) and (10, 8) respectively. Let the initial position, position after second throw and that after sixth throw lie on a line. Also each number showed up exactly once.**

**(a) For which of the following number thrown up by the dice, the object moved in $x$ direction?**
(i) 1 (ii) 2 (iii) 3 (iv) 5

**(b) The distance between the initial and final position of the object is**
(i) 12 unit (ii) 15 unit
(iii) 18 unit (iv) none of these

**(c) Given that after first throw of the dice, it moved in $x$ direction, then the number thrown up after fifth toss was**
(i) 1 (ii) 2
(iii) 3 (iv) cannot be determined

265. **A. A dice has six distinct numbers (positive integers) inscribed on its faces, the sum of numbers on opposite faces being 36, 40 and 41. Another identical dice (with identical numbering) is brought and tossed together twice. The sum of numbers thrown up was found to be 33 and 39 while the sum of hidden numbers were 43 and 38 respectively.**

**(a) Let the difference between two numbers on the opposite faces be 5 and another two on the opposite faces be 14. The least number inscribed on the dice will be**
(i) 13 (ii) 14 (iii) 15 (iv) 16

**(b) The difference between two inscribed numbers may not be**
(i) 3 (ii) 5 (iii) 7
(iv) all numbers can be the difference

**(c) Which of the following will definitely be a difference between two of the inscribed numbers?**
(i) 2 (ii) 4
(iii) 6 (iv) none of these

**(d) If one of the sum of two inscribed numbers is 37, then which of the following must also be a sum of two numbers?**
(i) 42 (ii) 44 (iii) 45 (iv) 46

**B.** **A dice has six distinct numbers (positive integers) inscribed on its face, the sum of numbers on opposite faces being 11, 12 and 13. Another identical dice (with identical numbering) is brought and tossed together thrice. The sum of numbers thrown up was found to be 10, 11 and 15 while the sum of hidden numbers were 13, 14 and 9 respectively.**

**(a) The number not inscribed on the dice is**

(i) 4 (ii) 5 (iii) 6 (iv) 7

**(b) The numbers on the opposite faces which sum is 12 are**

(i) 3, 9 (ii) 4, 8
(iii) 5, 7 (iv) cannot be determined

**266. Consider two groups of players arranged in sequence as ($X_1$, $X_2$ ... $X_8$) and ($Y_1$, $Y_2$ ... $Y_8$). $X_1$ and $Y_1$ plays a game and if $X_1$ wins, it plays the next game with $Y_2$ and if $Y_1$ wins, it plays the next game with $X_2$. Now the winner of second game similarly plays with the third player of the opposite group and so on (i.e. the winner of *n*th game plays with (*n* + 1)th player of the opposite group).**

**(a) If $X_6$ did not play, then it necessarily implies that**

(i) $X_4$ played a game
(ii) $Y_4$ played a game
(iii) $Y_3$ played a game
(iv) none of these

**(b) If only 5 players of the first group had played the match, then how many players of the second group would have played?**

(i) 3 (ii) 4
(iii) 5 (iv) cannot be determined

**(c) If $X_3$, $Y_5$ and $X_7$ had played the match, which of the following would be correct?**

**I. If $Y_5$ had won a match, then $X_3$ would have played just one match.**

**II. If $Y_5$ had won a match, then $X_3$ would have played three matches.**

**III. If $Y_6$ had won a match, then $X_3$ would have played just one match.**

**IV. If $Y_6$ had won a match, then $X_3$ would have played three matches.**

(i) I or III (ii) II or IV
(iii) I or II (iv) III or IV

**267. A, B, C, D, E, F, G are seven persons: each of them can go out in pair with only two of the other persons. Let none of (A, B, C) or (E, F, G) go out together. Also let A can go with E; B with G and C with D.**

**(a) How many distinct possibilities exist?**
(i) 6 (ii) 7 (iii) 8 (iv) 9

**(b) A cannot go out with**
(i) D (ii) F
(iii) G (iv) can go out with any of these

**(c) B cannot go out with**
(i) D (ii) E
(iii) F (iv) can go out with any of these

**268. Six identical coins are taken and their faces are coloured with two different colours from four colours: red (R), blue (B), green (G) and yellow (Y), no coins being coloured with the same pair of colours.**

**A. The coins are tossed twice successively and it showed three heads (B, R, G) and three tails (B, R, Y); three heads (R, Y, B) and three tails (G, Y, Y).**

**(a) When both the coins which tails are coloured with Y, is taken, then one of the head must be coloured with**
(i) Red (ii) Blue
(iii) Green (iv) cannot be determined

**(b) If two of the heads are coloured with R, then one of these coins must be coloured with**
(i) Blue (ii) Green
(iii) Yellow (iv) cannot be determined

**(c) If two of heads are coloured with G, then one of these coins must be coloured with**
(i) Red (ii) Blue
(iii) Yellow (iv) cannot be determined

**(d) If two of the heads are coloured with B, then one of these coins must also be coloured with**

(i) red
(ii) Green
(iii) yellow
(iv) can be coloured with any of these

**B. Let the heads of two coins be coloured with red and other two coins with blue.**

**If a coin has its head and tail painted with**

**(a) green and red colour respectively, then the coin which head is coloured with blue cannot have its tail coloured with**

(i) red
(ii) green
(iii) yellow
(iv) can be coloured with any of these

**(b) yellow and green colour respectively, then the coin which head is coloured with red cannot have its tail coloured with**

(i) blue
(ii) green
(iii) yellow
(iv) can be coloured with any of these

**269. Six different coins of values Rs 1, Rs 2, Rs 3, Rs 4, Rs 5, Rs 6 are taken and their faces are coloured with two different colours from four colours: red, blue, green and yellow, no coins being coloured with same pair of colours. Let the sum of value of coins with red, green and yellow colours be 13, 12 and 11 respectively.**

**(a) Which of the coins of following given value could not be coloured with green?**

(i) Rs 2 (ii) Rs 3 (iii) Rs 4 (iv) Rs 5

**(b) Which of the coins of following given value could not be colored with yellow?**

(i) Rs 2 (ii) Rs 3 (iii) Rs 4 (iv) Rs 6

**(c) Which of the coins of following given value could not be coloured with blue?**

(i) Rs 1 (ii) Rs 2 (iii) Rs 3 (iv) Rs 4

**270. Consider a dice which faces are numbered 1– 6. Let three of the sum of numbers denoted by three faces having common vertex be 8, 9 and 10.**

**(a) 1 cannot be against**
(i) 3 (ii) 4 (iii) 5 (iv) 6

**(b) 2 cannot be against**
(i) 3 (ii) 4 (iii) 5 (iv) 6

**(c) 3 cannot be against**
(i) 2 (ii) 4 (iii) 5 (iv) 6

**(d) Which of the following such sum as 8, 9, 10 is not possible?**
(i) 6 (ii) 7
(iii) 13 (iv) all can be possible

**271. A dice which faces are numbered 1–6 is painted with six different colours: red, blue, green, yellow, black and white, a colour on each face. Now**
**2 is opposite to the face painted with yellow;**
**3 is opposite to the face painted with white;**
**5 is opposite to the face painted with red;**
**1 (not blue) is not opposite to 2 or to the face painted with blue;**
**4 (not green) is not opposite to 5 or to the face painted with green;**
**6 (not black) is not opposite to 3 or to the face painted with black.**

**(a) If 5 is painted with green, then which of the following will be correct?**
(i) 5 is opposite to 4 (ii) 3 is opposite to 1
(iii) 2 is opposite to 6 (iv) none of these

**(b) If 3 is painted with green, then which of the following will be correct?**
(i) 2 is opposite to 6 (ii) 5 is opposite to 1
(iii) 2 is opposite to 4 (iv) none of these

**(c) If 2 is painted with colour X, then the numbers of opposite faces cannot be determined. Then X is**
(i) blue (ii) green
(iii) black (iv) can be any of these

**272. Consider a dice which faces are numbered 1–6. Let all its edge be assigned a number which is sum of the pair of faces to which it is common and all such numbers are grouped in a set S.**

**(a) If S contains all the numbers from 3 to 11, then in how many different ways, the three pairs of numbers on opposite faces of the dice could have been chosen?**
(i) 3 (ii) 4 (iii) 5 (iv) 6

**(b) If S lacks exactly one number in 3 to 11, then it cannot be**
(i) 5 (ii) 6 (iii) 7 (iv) 8

**(c) If S lacks exactly one number in 3 to 11, then it can be**
(i) 9 (ii) 10
(iii) 11 (iv) any of these

**273. Consider four points $A_1$, $A_2$, $A_3$, $A_4$ on a circle (none of them being diametrically opposite) and their diametrically opposite point $A_5$, $A_6$, $A_7$, $A_8$ (not necessarily in order). The points are joined in sequence as $A_1$, $A_6$, $A_2$, $A_7$, $A_8$, $A_3$, $A_4$, $A_5$ dividing the circle successively in 2, 3, 5, 6, 9, 10 and 15 parts. Given that no three chords intersect at a point and $A_1$ is not adjacent to $A_3$ or $A_4$,**

**(a) $A_1$ will be diametrically opposite to**
(i) $A_5$ (ii) $A_6$ (iii) $A_7$ (iv) $A_8$

**(b) $A_2$ will be diametrically opposite to**
(i) $A_5$ (ii) $A_6$ (iii) $A_7$ (iv) $A_8$

**(c) $A_3$ will be diametrically opposite to**
(i) $A_5$ (ii) $A_6$ (iii) $A_7$ (iv) $A_8$

**(d) $A_4$ will be diametrically opposite to**
(i) $A_5$ (ii) $A_6$ (iii) $A_7$ (iv) $A_8$

**274. A, B, C, D, E are five persons, there being two couples in it. The average weight of two couples are 79 and 82 kg while that of women is 78 kg and all the five persons is 80 kg. Let the weight of C be 2 kg more than that of E and the weight of B be 8 kg more than that of A. Also the weight of each person is different and that of D is 78 kg.**

**(a) A is married to**
(i) B (ii) C (iii) D (iv) E

**(b) Who is unmarried?**
(i) B (ii) C (iii) D (iv) E

**275. A, B, C, D, E, F, G are two couples and three singles. Also there are three pairs of exclusive siblings: two brothers; two sisters; a brother and a sister. Let there be two couples in (B, C, E, G); two sisters in (A, D, F, G); a brother and a sister in (A, C, E, G). Also a male is married to one of the exclusive sisters who are unrelated to other four persons.**

**(a) B is married to**

(i) E (ii) C
(iii) G (iv) cannot be determined

**(b) Which of the following are two brothers (exclusive)?**

(i) A, B (ii) B, F
(iii) C, F (iv) cannot be determined

**(c) Which of the following are two sisters (exclusive)?**

(i) A, G (ii) D, G
(iii) F, G (iv) cannot be determined

**276. Consider two families, each family has a couple and their three children who are denoted by A, B, C, D, E, F, G, H, I and J. Each of the following quadruplets has two persons from one fam ily and two from the other family. Let**

**I. (A, B, D, E) has two pairs of siblings (two brothers of a family and two sisters of a family).**

**II. (C, G, D, J) has couple and a mother-daughter.**

**III. (E, G, F, I) has a mother-son and father-son.**

**IV. (A, J, E, H) has mother-daughter and a brother-sister.**

**(a) Which of the following is a couple?**

(i) C – J (ii) F – J
(iii) C – F (iv) none of these

**(b) Which of the following is father-son?**

(i) C – B (ii) G – E
(iii) F – A (iv) none of these

**(c) Which of the following is brother-sister?**

(i) B – H (ii) D – H
(iii) B – A (iv) D – E

**(d) Which of the following is father-daughter?**

(i) J – A (ii) C – H
(iii) F – E (iv) C – D

**277. Consider four sister and their husbands: A, B, C, D, E, F, G and H. The husband of any sister is elder to her but younger to her elder sister. Let there be two couples in (A, B, C, D) and agewise, G > A > F > B and E > C > H > D.**

**(a) Which of the following can be couples?**

(i) A, B (ii) A, C
(iii) A, D (iv) cannot be determined

**(b) Which of the following is correct?**

(i) G > E (ii) A > E
(iii) G > C (iv) none of these

**(c) How many different possibilities for group of four males exist?**

(i) 8 (ii) 16 (iii) 32 (iv) 64

**278. A, B, C, D, E, F, G, H are four couples. Four of them speak truth and another four lie (Do not assume that one speaking lie will say a male to be a female or vice versa). A, B, C, D, E, F, G, H say they are respectively married to F, G, H, F, A, C, D, B.**

**(a) How many couples can be definitely known?**

(i) zero (ii) one
(iii) two (iv) three

**(b) If only one female speaks lie, then which of the following will speak lie?**

(i) A (ii) B (iii) C (iv) D

**(c) If all males speak lie, then which of the following will be correct?**

(i) (B, G) and (C, F) are couples
(ii) (B, H) and (D, F) are couples
(iii) (C, F) and (G, D) are couples
(iv) none of these

**279. A, B, C, D, E, F, G are seven persons of a family: a parent, their three children of whom two are married. Four of them speak truth and three of them lie (Do not assume that one speaking lie will say a male to be a female or vice versa). Now**

**I. A says he is brother of C.**
**II. B says he is married to D.**
**III. C says she is married to G.**

**IV. D says she is married to A.**
**V. E says she is daughter of F.**
**VI. F says he is brother of B.**
**VII. G says she is sister of E.**

**(a) C is married to**

(i) A (ii) B
(iii) F (iv) cannot be determined

**(b) D is married to**

(i) A (ii) B
(iii) F (iv) cannot be determined

**(c) Which of the following are sisters?**

(i) D – E (ii) D – G
(iii) E – G (iv) cannot be determined

**(d) Who is daughter-in law?**

(i) D (ii) E
(iii) G (iv) cannot be determined

**280. Letters of a word (meaningful or absurd) are to be transformed into another word by exchanging the positions of two letters at a time. A process consists of exchanging the positions of two letters. What is the minimum number of process needed to transform**

**(a) 'IGNRDAE' into 'READING'?**

(i) 3 (ii) 4 (iii) 5 (iv) 6

**(b) 'AEGEMNANTM' into 'MANAGEMENT'?**

(i) 8 (ii) 9 (iii) 10 (iv) 11

**281.**

| | | | |
|---|---|---|---|
| $A_1$ | $A_2$ | $A_3$ | $A_4$ |
| $A_5$ | $A_6$ | $A_7$ | $A_8$ |
| $A_9$ | $A_{10}$ | $A_{11}$ | $A_{12}$ |
| $A_{13}$ | $A_{14}$ | $A_{15}$ | $A_{16}$ |

**Shown above are 16 men and women forming 8 couples arranged in 4 × 4 rows and column. Let each row and column has at least one couple.**

**Let the spouses of $A_1$, $A_6$, $A_{11}$, $A_{16}$ be in their respective rows and the spouses of $A_4$, $A_7$, $A_{10}$, $A_{13}$ in their respective columns.**

**(a) If ($A_1$, $A_2$) is a couple, then which of the following will necessarily be a couple?**

(i) $(A_4, A_8)$ (ii) $(A_5, A_{13})$
(iii) $(A_9, A_{11})$ (iv) $(A_{15}, A_{16})$

**(b) If $(A_5, A_6)$ is a couple, then which of the following will necessarily be a couple?**

(i) $(A_2, A_{10})$ (ii) $(A_3, A_7)$
(iii) $(A_4, A_{12})$ (iv) $(A_9, A_{13})$

**(c) If $(A_7, A_{15})$ is a couple, then which of the follwoing will necessarily be a couple?**

(i) $(A_1, A_3)$ (ii) $(A_4, A_8)$
(iii) $(A_5, A_{13})$ (iv) $(A_9, A_{11})$

**(d) If $(A_4, A_{12})$ is a couple, then which of the following will necessarily be a couple?**

(i) $(A_1, A_{10})$ (ii) $(A_5, A_{13})$
(iii) $(A_7, A_{15})$ (iv) $(A_{14}, A_{16})$

**282. A, B, C, D, E, F, G, H, I are nine balls, three each of colours: red, blue and green. In the arrangement shown (the sequence of letters), no two balls of same colours are placed together. Let none of (A, D, G, H) be blue, (C, E, F, I) be red.**

**(a) How many different possible cases exist?**

(i) 6 (ii) 8 (iii) 9 (iv) 12

**(b) The colour of which of the balls can be definitely known?**

(i) B (ii) D
(iii) E (iv) none of these

**(c) The colour of which of the balls can be definitely known?**

(i) G (ii) F
(iii) I (iv) none of these

**283. A, B, C, D, E, F, G, H, I are 9 persons, three of them are bosses of three departments, another three secretaries, and last three clerks. Each boss has one secretary and each secretary has one clerk to assist in work. Let each of triplets (A, E, I); (C, D, H); (B, F, G) has one boss, one secretary and one clerk belonging to different departments.**

**(a) How many different possibilities of their position (vis-a-vis their posts and department) exist?**

(i) 216 (ii) 256 (iii) 432 (iv) 512

**(b) If C is A's (boss) secretary, then which of the following cannot be possible?**
(i) B is E's (secretary) boss
(ii) I is F's (secretary) clerk
(iii) I is D's (clerk) boss
(iv) G is H's (clerk) secretary

**(c) If B is D's (clerk) secretary, then which of the following cannot be possible?**
(i) H is A's (secretary) boss
(ii) C is I's (clerk) secretary
(iii) F is E's (clerk) boss
(iv) all of these are possible

**284. A, B, C, D are four letters which are to go in four envelopes E, F, G, H (Each envelope assigned to one letter).**

**(a) In how many ways, the letters can be put in envelopes such that no letter goes in the right envelope?**
(i) 8 (ii) 9 (iii) 10 (iv) 12

**(b) If A, B, C, D can be put in envelopes E, G, F, H respectively or H, F, G, E respectively such that no letter goes in the right envelope, then it can be concluded that**
(i) there can be only two distinct possibilities for corresponding envelopes of the letters
(ii) two pairs can be chosen such that if letters of each pair is mutually exchanged, then all the letters will be in the right envelopes
(iii) Both (iv) None

**285. A, B, C, D, E, F, G, H are eight persons who are to sit in a row, side by side. Two of them want to sit together; another two do not want to sit together; yet another two do not want to sit at ends; and out of last two one wants to sit in the group of first four persons and the other wants to sit in the group of last four persons. Let two of the arrangements in which they can be seated be**

**B E F A C D G H and G H C A F D B E.**

**(a) If B, E want to be together, then which of the following can be the two persons who do not want to sit at ends?**
(i) F, A (ii) F, C (iii) F, D (iv) C, A

**(b) If B, E want to be together, then how many different cases of pairs of two persons who do not want to sit together can exist?**

(i) 2 (ii) 3 (iii) 4 (iv) 5

**(c) If A, F want to be together, then how many different cases of pairs of two persons who do not want to sit together can exist?**

(i) 1 (ii) 2 (iii) 3 (iv) 4

**(d) If C, A want to be together, then how many different cases of pairs of two person who do not want to sit together can exist?**

(i) 1 (ii) 2 (iii) 3 (iv) 4

**286. A, B, C, D, E, F, G, H are four couples. Two couples want to sit together whereas another two couples do not want to sit together. Let two of the arrangements in which they can be seated by A G B E F H D C and G B E D H H F C A.**

**(a) Which of the following will be a spouse of the couple who want to sit together?**

(i) B and D (ii) B and H
(iii) D and H (iv) E and H

**(b) Which of the following will be a spouse of the couple who do not want to sit together?**

(i) A and C (ii) A and F
(iii) C and G (iv) F and G

**(c) Which of the following is correct?**

(i) If D is a spouse of the couple who do not want to sit together, then the other spouse is B.
(ii) If E is a spouse of the couple who do not want to sit together, then the other spouse is A.
(iii) If F is a spouse of the couple who do not want to sit together, then the other spouse is D.
(iv) If G is a spouse of the couple who do not want to sit together, then the other spouse is C.

**287. A, B, C, D, E are five flats and each of them is shared by two peoples from $P_1$, $P_2$, $P_3$, $P_4$ and $P_5$. Each of the person has shares in exactly two flats and no two persons share same two flats. Let**

**$P_1$ has a share in A and shares the other flat with $P_3$; $P_2$ has a share in B and shares the other flat with $P_5$; and C is not shared by $P_4$, D is not shared by $P_1$ and E is not shared by $P_2$.**

**(a) If ($P_3$, $P_4$) share a flat, then the other flat $P_4$ shares will be**

(i) A (ii) B (iii) D (iv) E

**(b) If ($P_4$, $P_5$) share a flat, then the other flat $P_4$ shares will be**

(i) A (ii) B (iii) D (iv) E

**288. A schedule of final exam for undergraduates of science stream is prepared. There are four compulsory subject: English, Physics, Chemistry and Maths and one elective subject from Biology, Computer Science and Economics. The exam is to be culminated in fortnight starting on Monday of first week and ending on Saturday of the next week, there being no exam on Sunday. Now**

**I. there is a gap of 3 days between the schedules of Maths and English;**

**II. there is a gap of 1 week between the schedules of Physics and Maths;**

**III. there is exam on each day of the week except Sunday;**

**IV. there is no gap between the schedules of Biology and that of the subject that just precedes it;**

**V. the schedule Computer science follows that of Chemistry.**

**(a) Two of the exams fall on**

(i) Monday (ii) Tuesday
(iii) Friday (iv) Saturday

**(b) How many days are between the schedules of English and Economics?**

(i) 1 (ii) 2
(iii) 4 (iv) cannot be determined

**(c) How many days are between the schedules of Economics and Biology?**

(i) 2 (ii) 4
(iii) 5 (iv) cannot be determined

**(d) The schedule of which of the following subjects can be uniquely determined?**

(i) English (ii) Biology
(iii) Economics (iv) none of these

**(e) In how many different ways, the schedule of all exams are possible?**

(i) 4 (ii) 6 (iii) 7 (iv) 8

**289. Six multiple choice questions are asked numbered 1– 6 which answers are one of A, B, C or D. Three students gave responses as A B C D C A; C A A B B C and D B A C B C where the sequence represent responses to questions 1 to 6 in order. Also all three of them gave three correct answers and each question is given a correct answer by at least one student.**

**(a) The correct response for which of the question can be determined?**

(i) Second (ii) Third
(iii) Fifth (iv) Sixth

**(b) Which of the following can be the correct responses for the first and fourth questions respectively?**

(i) (A, B) or (C, D) (ii) (A, B) or (D, B)
(iii) (A, C) or (C, D) (iv) (A, C) or (D, B)

**(c) If there are three questions having same answers, then it can be**

(i) A or B (ii) A or C
(iii) B or C (iv) A, B or C

**(d) How many distinct cases for the correct responses of the questions exist?**

(i) 4 (ii) 6 (iii) 8 (iv) 10

**(e) For how many cases of part (d), D is an answer for at least one of the questions?**

(i) 2 (ii) 3 (iii) 4 (iv) 5

**290. Consider a 13 – gon which vertices are $A_1$, $A_2$, $A_3$, ... $A_{13}$.**

**(a) Let there be exactly one vertex between $A_i$ and $A_{i+1}$ ( $1 \le i \le 12$). Then $A_1$ is between**

(i) $A_7$ and $A_8$ (ii) $A_8$ and $A_9$
(iii) $A_9$ and $A_{10}$ (iv) $A_{10}$ and $A_{11}$

**(b) Let there be exactly two vertices between $A_i$ and $A_{i+1}$ $(1 \le i \le 12)$. Then $A_1$ is between**

(i) $A_5$ and $A_9$ (ii) $A_5$ and $A_{10}$
(iii) $A_6$ and $A_{10}$ (iv) $A_6$ and $A_{11}$

**(c) Let there be exactly *i* vertices between $A_i$ and $A_{i+1}$ $(1 \le i \le 12)$. Then $A_1$ is between**

(i) $A_5$ and $A_{10}$ (ii) $A_5$ and $A_{11}$
(iii) $A_5$ and $A_{12}$ (iv) the case is not possible

**291. 10 identical coins are arranged such that six of them touch other three coins, two of them touch other four coins and remaining two of them touch *n* other coins. The coins are named A to J. Now A touches J, G and C only; I touches B, D and F only; and H touches B, C, F and G only.**

**(a) The value of *n* is**

(i) 3 (ii) 4 (iii) 5 (iv) 6

**(b) How many coins does E touch?**

(i) 3 (ii) 4
(iii) *n* (iv) cannot be determined

**(c) C does not touch**

(i) F (ii) G (iii) J (iv) D

**292. A, B, C, D, E, F are three couples: Teacher, Doctor, Lawyer, Accountant, Actor and Dancer by profession (not in order). Now**
**Teacher is female not married to C (male);**
**Doctor is female not married to D (male);**
**Accountant is male not married to B (female).**

**(a) If A, E, F are respectively married to dancer, actor and lawyer respectively, then A cannot be**

(i) Accountant (ii) Teacher
(iii) Doctor (iv) the case is not possible

**(b) If F is married to actor and lawyer is married to dancer, then A is married to**

(i) B (ii) E
(iii) F (iv) cannot be determined

**(c) If F is married to dancer and A is married to lawyer, then E is married to**

(i) Teacher (ii) Actor
(iii) Accountant (iv) cannot be determined

**(d) For part (c), actor is married to**
(i) B (ii) C
(iii) E (iv) cannot be determined

**293. A, B, C, D, E are five persons each living in one of five houses P, Q, R, S, T (located in a row) which are painted with five different colours, viz. red, blue, green, yellow and white. Now**
**A lives in the house adjacent to red and blue houses;**
**B lives in the house adjacent to S;**
**C lives in the house adjacent to T and white house (both different);**
**D lives in the house adjacent to P and**
**E lives in the house adjacent to Q and green house (both different).**

**(a) Who lives in the centre?**
(i) A (ii) C
(iii) E (iv) cannot be determined

**(b) If A lives in Q, then which of the following is correct?**
(i) T is painted yellow, R green and Q white
(ii) T is painted green, R white and Q yellow
(iii) T is painted green, R yellow and Q white
(iv) none of these

**(c) Which of the following must be at the ends?**
(i) T and green house
(ii) Q and white house
(iii) R and yellow house
(iv) none of these

**294. A, B, C, D are four persons; Accountant, Artist, Doctor and Professor by profession (not in order). Each of them have different sums of money. Let**
**Professor has Rs 100 more than D;**
**Accountant has Rs 100 less than C;**
**Artist has double the money A has and**
**Doctor has Rs 200 less than B.**

**(a) A has**
(i) Rs 100 (ii) Rs 200
(iii) Rs 300 (iv) cannot be determined

**(b) The money with B cannot be**
(i) Rs 300 (ii) Rs 400 (iii) Rs 500 (iv) Rs 600

**(c) If the professor has Rs 500, then the accountant has**
(i) Rs 200 (ii) Rs 300
(iii) Rs 400 (iv) cannot be determined

**(d) The money with D cannot be**
(i) Rs 100 (ii) Rs 200 (iii) Rs 300 (iv) Rs 400

**295. Consider four persons A, B, C, D: doctor, lawyer, painter and Wrestler by profession (not in order). Now the income of wrestler is half the sum of that of C and D; the income of doctor is half the sum of that of A and B; and the income of painter is half that of D.**

**(a) The ratio of incomes of A and B cannot be equal to**
(i) 1 : 2 (ii) 1 : 3 (iii) 3 : 5 (iv) 5 : 3

**(b) If the income of A is thrice that of B, then A, B, C, D are respectively**
(i) painter, wrestler, doctor and lawyer
(ii) wrestler, painter, lawyer and doctor
(iii) wrestler, lawyer, painter and doctor
(iv) painter, wrestler, lawyer and doctor

**(c) For which of the following case, the ratio of incomes of A and C will be 5 : 4?**
**Doctor, Wrestler, Painter, Lawyer are respectively**
(i) C, B, A, D (ii) C, B, A, D
(iii) D, A, B, C (iv) D, B, A, C

**(d) For which of the following case, the ratio of incomes of A and C will be 3 : 2?**
**Doctor, Wrestler, Painter, Lawyer are respectively**
(i) C, B, A, D (ii) D, A, B, C
(iii) D, A, C, B (iv) D, B, C, A

**(e) For which of the following case, the ratio of incomes of A and C will be 5 : 2?**
**Doctor, Wrestler, Painter, Lawyer are respectively**
(i) C, A, B, D (ii) C, B, A, D
(iii) D, B, A, C (iv) D, B, C, A

**296. A, B, C, D, E are five persons: Professor, doctor, lawyer, artist and chemist by profession (not in order). Also A's income is Rs 10,000 more than that of professor and**

**Rs 10,000 less than that of lawyer; B's income is Rs 10,000 less than that of doctor and Rs 30,000 less than that of artist; and D's income is Rs 10,000 less than that of chemist and Rs 10,000 more than that of E. Also the income of each person is different.**

**(a) A is**

(i) Doctor (ii) Chemist
(iii) Artist (iv) cannot be determined

**(b) C is**

(i) Professor (ii) Chemist
(iii) Doctor (iv) cannot be determined

**(c) D is**

(i) Lawyer (ii) Artist
(iii) Doctor (iv) cannot be determined

**(d) E is**

(i) Professor (ii) Lawyer
(iii) Artist (iv) cannot be determined

**297. A, B, C, D are four persons: artist, lawyer, doctor and chemist by profession. All of them have different amount of money. Let**

**A. Artist has Rs 100 more than one of C or D.**
**Chemist has Rs 100 less than one of A or D.**
**Lawyer has Rs 100 less than one of B or C.**
**Doctor has Rs 100 more than one of B or A.**

**A has Rs 100 more than one of artist or chemist.**
**B has Rs 100 more than one of doctor or artist.**
**C has Rs 100 less than one of lawyer or doctor.**
**D has Rs 100 more than one of chemist or lawyer.**

**(a) The difference between the amounts of A and D is**

(i) Rs 100 (ii) Rs 200
(iii) Rs 300 (iv) cannot be determined

**(b) The difference between the amounts of A and C is**

(i) Rs 100 (ii) Rs 200
(iii) Rs 300 (iv) cannot be determined

**(c) The difference between the amounts of artist and lawyer is**

(i) Rs 100 (ii) Rs 200
(iii) Rs 300 (iv) cannot be determined

**(d) The difference between the amounts of artist and chemist is**

(i) Rs 100 (ii) Rs 200
(iii) Rs 300 (iv) cannot be determined

**B. Lawyer has Rs 100 more than one of B, D and Rs 100 less than the other;**
**Doctor has Rs 100 more than one of C, A and Rs 100 less than the other;**
**Chemist has Rs 100 less than one of lawyer, artist.**

**(a) The difference in amount of Doctor and Chemist is**

(i) Rs 100 (ii) Rs 200
(iii) Rs 300 (iv) cannot be determined

**(b) The difference in amount of A and C is**

(i) Rs 100 (ii) Rs 200
(iii) Rs 300 (iv) cannot be determined

**(c) The difference in amount of B and D is**

(i) Rs 100 (ii) Rs 200
(iii) Rs 300 (iv) cannot be determined

**298. A, B, C, D are four persons: artist, lawyer, teacher and doctor by profession (not in order) who live exclusively in one of the floors (ground, first, second and top). Also each of them like exactly one of colours: red, blue, green and yellow. Let**
**A likes blue; B is lawyer; Teacher likes yellow; Artist lives on second floor; Doctor lives just above A; and one who likes green lives on the ground floor:**

**(a) B lives on**

(i) ground floor (ii) first floor
(iii) second floor (iv) top floor

**(b) Teacher lives on**

(i) first floor (ii) second floor
(iii) top floor (iv) cannot be determined

**(c) Which of the following is correct?**

(i) Doctor likes red and artist likes blue.
(ii) Doctor likes blue and artist likes red.
(iii) C likes red and D likes yellow.
(iv) C likes yellow and D likes red

**299.** **A, B, C, D are four persons: artist, lawyer, teacher and doctor by profession (not in order) who live exclusively in one of the floors (ground, first, second and top). Also each of them like exactly one of colours: red, blue, green and yellow. Let**

**A, B, C, D be not artist, lawyer, doctor, teacher respectively;**

**A, B, C, D do not like yellow, blue, green, red respectively;**

**A, B, C, D do not live an second, top first and ground floor respectively;**

**teacher, artist, doctor, lawyer do not like red, yellow green, blue respectively.**

**teacher, artist, doctor, lawyer, do not live on ground, second, first and top floor respectively;**

**one who likes green, yellow, blue, red do not live on first top, ground floor respectively.**

**(a) How many possibilities for A, B, C, D vis-a-vis professions and choice of colour exist?**

(i) 24 (ii) 36

(iii) 48 (iv) 72

**(b) If A is lawyer and C likes red, then D lives on**

(i) first floor (ii) second floor

(iii) top floor (iv) cannot be determined

**(c) If A is lawyer and D likes green, then C lives on**

(i) ground floor (ii) second floor

(iii) top floor (iv) cannot be determined

**(d) If B is artist and C likes red, then D lives on**

(i) ground floor (ii) second floor

(iii) top floor (iv) cannot be determined

**(e) If B is artist and D likes green, then C lives on**

(i) ground floor (ii) second floor

(iii) top floor (iv) cannot be determined

**300.** **A, B, C and D are four persons: doctor, actor, lawyer and professor (not in order) who like exactly two of the four colours: red, blue, green and yellow. Also each colour is liked exactly by two persons. Let**

**Doctor likes red but not blue;**
**Actor likes blue but not yellow;**
**Lawyer likes yellow but not green;**
**Professor likes green but not red;**

**(a) A likes red but not blue;**
**B likes red but not yellow;**
**C likes blue but not red and**
**D likes yellow but not green.**

**Which of the following is necessarily correct?**

(i) Doctor likes green and lawyer likes blue.
(ii) Actor likes red and C likes yellow.
(iii) A likes yellow and D likes red.
(iv) none of these

**(b) A likes red but not green;**
**B likes yellow but not blue;**
**C likes blue but not red and**
**D likes green but not yellow.**

**The proffession of all the persons (A, B, C, D) can be uniquely known if it is given that A is**

(i) Actor (ii) Doctor
(iii) Lawyer (iv) none of these

**(c) A likes red but not yellow;**
**B likes blue but not green;**
**C likes yellow but not red and**
**D likes green but not blue.**

**Which of the following will be correct?**

(i) A cannot be lawyer
(ii) B cannot be actor
(iii) C cannot be professor
(iv) D cannot be doctor

**301. A four digit number is chosen. A multiple of 100 (less than thousand) is added successively four times to it, the last sum still being a four digit number. Let two of the numbers in the original number and successive sums be (4, 7), (3, 6), (4, 9), (5, 6) and (1, 4) respectively. Given that none of the digits in original number or the first sum are repeated, then**

**(a) the multiple of 100 which is added to the numbers is**
(i) 300 (ii) 400 (iii) 500 (iv) 600

**(b) in the original sum, 7 is**
(i) first digit
(ii) second digit
(iii) one of last two digits
(iv) cannot be determined

**(c) in the first successive sum, 3 is**
(i) first digit
(ii) second digit
(iii) one of last two digits
(iv) cannot be determined

**(d) in the third successive sum, 5 is**
(i) first digit
(ii) second digit
(iii) one of last two digits
(iv) cannot be determined

**302. Let the sum of 4 four-digit numbers *abcd*, *dabc*, *cdab* and *bcda* be five-digit number *aeecd* where *a*, *b*, *c*, *d* and *e* are distinct single digit numbers. Then**

**(a) *b* =**
(i) 4 (ii) 5 (iii) 7 (iv) 8

**(b) which is the least number?**
(i) *a* (ii) *c* (iii) *d* (iv) *e*

**(c) which is the greatest number?**
(i) *a* (ii) *b* (iii) *c* (iv) *d*

**303. *a*, *b*, *c*, *d*, *e*, *f*, *g*, *h*, *i* are 9 single digit non-negative integers. Four of them are distinct integers from (4, 6, 7, 8, 9) and three of them are distinct integers from (1, 2, 3, 5). If the sum of three numbers *abc*, *def* and *ghi* is a four digit number *aaaa*, then the number not represented by the nine given letters is**

**(a)** (i) 6 (ii) 7 (iii) 8 (iv) 9
**(b)** (i) 1 (ii) 2 (iii) 3 (iv) 5

**304. Let *ABC*, *BCA*, *CAB*, *ACB*, *CBA* be 6 three-digit integers. Two of them are chosen and their sum is found to be 1150. Another two of them are chosen and their sum is**

**found to be 1231. The sum of remaining two is found to be 139*x* (a four-digit integer). Then**

**(a)** $x =$

(i) 1 (ii) 3 (iii) 5 (iv) 7

**(b) which of the following is not a member of the set** $\{A, B, C\}$**?**

(i) 4 (ii) 5 (iii) 6 (iv) 7

**305.** $A, B, C, D, E, F$ **are six distinct single digit positive integers such that**

$ABC + DEF = 1056$

$BCA + EFD = 1569$ **and**

$CAB + FDE = n05$

**where** $n$ **is single digit integer. Then**

**(a)** $n =$

(i) 6 (ii) 7 (iii) 8 (iv) 9

**(b) which of the following is not an admissible value of** $(A, D)$**?**

(i) (5, 4) (ii) (6, 3) (iii) (7, 2) (iv) (8, 1)

(Order within bracket does not matter)

**(c) if** $n$ **is different from all of** $A, B, C, D, E$ **and** $F$**, then which of the following number is not a member of the set** $\{A, B, C, D, E, F\}$**?**

(i) 1 (ii) 2 (iii) 3 (iv) 4

**(d) how many distinct possible solutions of the value set of letters are possible?**

(i) 32 (ii) 40 (iii) 56 (iv) 64

**306.** $A, B, C, D$ **are four distinct single digit positive integer such that** $AB + BC + CD = 170$ **and** $BD + DC + CA = 218$ **where the combination of letters denote 2-digit numbers.**

**(a)** $A + B + C + D$ **cannot be equal to**

(i) 22 (ii) 23 (iii) 24 (iv) 25

**(b)** $D - B =$

(i) 1 (ii) 2

(iii) 3 (iv) cannot be determined

**(c)** $B - A =$

(i) −1 (ii) 1

(iii) 2 (iv) cannot be determined

**307.** **Let $A, B, C, D$ are distinct single digit positive intgers such that $A \times D + CB = 136$ and $C \times B + AD = 112$**
**where $CB$ and $AD$ are two-digit numbers.**

**(a)** $A$ **cannot be equal to**
(i) 5 (ii) 7 (iii) 8 (iv) 9

**(b)** $B$ **cannot be equal to**
(i) 2 (ii) 4 (iii) 6 (iv) 8

**(c)** **How many possible distinct values of $D$ is possible?**
(i) 1 (ii) 2 (iii) 3 (iv) 4

**(d)** **Had $C \times B + AD = 113$ instead of 112, then which of the following would have been greatest?**
(i) $A$ (ii) $B$ (iii) $C$ (iv) $D$

**308.** **Let $A, B, C, D, E, F, G, H, I$ be 9 distinct single digit positive positive integers.**
**Let $ABC + DEF + GHI = x$**
**where $ABC$, $DEF$ and $GHI$ are 3 three-digit integers. Let for particular values of $x$, there exist 216 distinct values of $(A, B, C \dots H, I)$. The minimum of such values of $x$ will be divisible by**
(i) 41 (ii) 43 (iii) 47 (iv) 53

**309.** **Consider first nine single digit positive integers. They are divided into three triplets. Three three-digit numbers are formed by the arrangements of integers of each triplets separately. Let the sum of two of the three-digit numbers be equal to the third number.**

**(a)** **If there is no carry in the sum of the two three-digit numbers, then how many distinct ways of division of the given nine numbers into three triplets are possible?**
(i) 0 (ii) 1 (iii) 2 (iv) 3

**(b)** **If there is one carry (1) in the sum of the two three-digit numbers, then how many distinct ways of division of the given nine numbers into three triplets are possible?**
(i) 0 (ii) 1 (iii) 2 (iv) 3

(c) If there are two carries (1, 1)in the sum of the two three-digit numbers, then how many distinct ways of division of the given nine numbers into three triplets are possible?

(i) 0 (ii) 1 (iii) 2 (iv) 3

(d) If there is one carry (2) in the sum of the two three-digit numbers, then how many distinct ways of division of the given nine numbers into three triplets are possible?

(i) 0 (ii) 1 (iii) 2 (iv) 3

**310.** **A three-digit number when multiplied by 3, 4, 5 have numbers (0, 3, 2), (0, 3, 7) and (0, 3, 8) repectively in the product.**

**(a) The first digit of the three-digit number is**

(i) 5 (ii) 6 (iii) 7 (iv) 8

**(b) The second digit of the three-digit number is**

(i) 4 (ii) 6 (iii) 8 (iv) 9

**311.** **Consider two three-digit numbers (having non zero digits) which sum is 466. Let the digits of each numbers be different and one of the digits of first number be equal to one of the digits of second number.**

**(a) How many different possibilities of pair of such numbers exists?**

(i) 22 (ii) 23 (iii) 24 (iv) 25

**(b) In how many different possibilities, the first digit of one number is equal to the third digit of the second number?**

(i) 3 (ii) 4 (iii) 5 (iv) 6

**(c) In how many different possibilities, the first digit of one number is equal to the second digit of the second number?**

(i) 3 (ii) 4 (iii) 5 (iv) 6

**312.** **Let *x* be a three-digit number (less than 300). The sum of digits of *x*, 2*x* and 3*x* are 10, 11 and 21 respectively.**

**(a) How many distinct possibilities for *x* exist?**

(i) 3 (ii) 4 (iii) 5 (iv) 6

**(b) How many such number ($x$) exist between 200 and 300?**

(i) 1 (ii) 2 (iii) 3 (iv) 4

**(c) How many such numbers ($x$) will be divisible by 11?**

(i) 0 (ii) 1 (iii) 2 (iv) 30

**313. Let $xy \times yx = xxab$. Then**

**(a) $x$ =**

(i) 5 (ii) 6 (iii) 7 (iv) 8

**(b) $a$ =**

(i) 2 (ii) 3 (iii) 4 (iv) 6

**(c) $b$ =**

(i) 3 (ii) 4 (iii) 5 (iv) 6

**314. Let $xy \times z = -\,8\,-$**

**$yz \times x = 2\,-\,-$ and**

**$zx \times y = -\,1$**

**where $x, y, z$ are distinct single digit positive integers. Then**

**(a) $z$ =**

(i) 5 (ii) 6

(iii) 8 (iv) cannot be determined

**(b) which of the following is correct?**

(i) When $x$ is least, then $y$ is most

(ii) When x is least, then z is most

(iii) When $y$ is least, then $x$ is most

(iv) When $y$ is most, then $z$ is least

**315. A. Let $3x \times y7 = 1a\,3b$**

**where $x, y, a, b$ are single digit positive integers. Then**

**(a) $x$ cannot be equal to**

(i) 4 (ii) 6 (iii) 7 (iv) 9

**(b) $y$ cannot be equal to**

(i) 3 (ii) 4 (iii) 5 (iv) 6

**(c) $a$ cannot be equal to**

(i) 3 (ii) 6 (iii) 8 (iv) 9

**(d) $b$ cannot be equal to**

(i) 2 (ii) 3 (iii) 4 (iv) 8

**B.** **Let** $w87 \times 15w = x92yz$

**where** $w, x, y, z$ **are single digit positive integers. Then**

**(a)** $x =$

(i) 3 (ii) 4 (iii) 5 (iv) 7

**(b)** $y =$

(i) 1 (ii) 3 (iii) 4 (iv) 5

**316. Let the sum and product of two two-digit integers** $ab$ **and** $bx$ **be** $xy$ **and** $y0x$ **respectively where** $a, b, x, y$ **are distinct single digit positive integers. Then**

**(a)** $a =$

(i) 1 (ii) 2 (iii) 3 (iv) 4

**(b)** $b =$

(i) 2 (ii) 3 (iii) 4 (iv) 6

**(c)** $x =$

(i) 3 (ii) 4 (iii) 5 (iv) 6

**(c)** $y =$

(i) 6 (ii) 7 (iii) 8 (iv) 9

**317. Let** $A, B, C$ **be single digit positive integers such that when** $ABCCC$ **... (it being a multiple digit number having any number of** $C$**) is divided by 37, it leaves a constant remainder. Given** $C < 6$**,**

**(a)** $A =$

(i) 1 (ii) 2

(iii) 3 (iv) cannot be determined

**(b)** $B =$

(i) 1 (ii) 2

(iii) 3 (iv) cannot be determined

**(c) the remainder is**

(i) 12 (ii) 13

(iii) 21 (iv) cannot be determined

**318. Let** $11 \times xy = aby$ **and**

$13 \times xy = 8ya$

**Then**

**(a)** $a =$

(i) 5 (ii) 6 (iii) 7 (iv) 8

**(b)** $b =$

(i) 4 (ii) 5 (iii) 6 (iv) 7

**319. Consider three two-digit integers, their sum being less than 200. Sum of three of them with one of them having its digits interchanged are 147, 156 or 165.**

**(a) The sum of three numbers is**

(i) 129 (ii) 138
(iii) 171 (iv) cannot be determined

**(b) The sum of first digits of the three considered numbers is equal to**

(i) 11 (ii) 12
(iii) 13 (iv) cannot be determined

**(c) The sum of last digits of the three considered numbers is equal to**

(i) 16 (ii) 17
(iii) 18 (iv) cannot be determined

**320. Sum of three two-digit integers is 35 while sum of product of them, taken two at a time, is 406.**

**(a) The least number is**

(i) 10 (ii) 11
(iii) 12 (iv) cannot be determined

**(b) The greatest number is**

(i) 13 (ii) 14
(iii) 15 (iv) cannot be determined

**321. Consider a three-digit integer. The digits in product when it is multiplied by 2 are *a*, 6, 9 (not in order) and when multiplied by 3, are *a*, 1, 3, 5 (not in order).**

**(a) The three-digit integer must be divisible by**

(i) 13 (ii) 17 (iii) 19 (iv) 23

**(b) In the product of 3 and the number, *a* is at**

(i) unit-digit place (ii) ten-digit place
(iii) hundred-digit place (iv) thousand-digit place

**322. Consider a three-digit integer which when multiplied by 2 have *x*, 3 and 9 (not in order)in its product. The three-digit number is reshuffled so that no digit occupy its previous place and when it is multiplied by 2, then the product contains either *x*, 1, 2 and 9 or *x*, 1, 3 and *y*.**

(a) $x =$

(i) 2 (ii) 4

(iii) 6 (iv) cannot be determined

(b) $y =$

(i) 4 (ii) 6

(iii) 8 (iv) cannot be determined

**323. Let $x$, $y$, $z$ be three four-digit numbers such that $z = x + y$ and the digits of $x$, $y$, $z$ are (3, 4, 7, 8), (2, 5, 6, 9) and ($a$, 3, 5, 6) respectively**

**(a) $a =$**

(i) 0 (ii) 3 (iii) 6 (iv) 9

**(b) In $x$, 4 is at**

(i) unit-digit-place (ii) ten-digit place

(iii) hundred-digit place (iv) thousand-digit place

**(c) In $y$, 9 is at**

(i) unit-digit place (ii) ten-digit place

(iii) hundred-digit place (iv) cannot be determined

**(d) In $z$, 5 is at**

(i) ten-digit place

(ii) hundred-digit place

(iii) thousand-digit place

(iv) cannot be determined

**324. Consider a four digit integer (all digits different) divisible by 7. When the middle two digits are exchanged, it get divisible by 11 and when the outer two digits are exchanged, it is still divisible by 7.**

**(a) The difference in first and last digit will be**

(i) 3 (ii) 4

(iii) 7 (iv) cannot be determined

**(b) The difference in values of middle digits will be**

(i) 3 (ii) 4

(iii) 7 (iv) cannot be determined

**(c) If the digit at unit digit place is 0, then the digit at ten-digit place is**

(i) 1 (ii) 2 (iii) 3 (iv) 4

**325. $ABCD$ is a four-digit number such that $A + B - D = 9$ and $B + C = 10$, $A, B, C, D$, being distinct.**

**(a) The number must be divisible by**

(i) 3 (ii) 5

(iii) 7 (iv) cannot be determined

**(b) The number must be divisible by**

(i) 13 (ii) 17

(iii) 19 (iv) cannot be determined

**326. Let 12$xy$49 be a perfect square. Then**

**(a)** $x =$

(i) 1 (ii) 3 (iii) 5 (iv) 7

**(b)** $y =$

(i) 2 (ii) 4 (iii) 6 (iv) 8

**327. Let $uvwxyz$ be the first six digit of $(123456789)^2$. Then**

**(a)** $x =$

(i) 2 (ii) 4 (iii) 7 (iv) 9

**(b)** $y =$

(i) 1 (ii) 3 (iii) 6 (iv) 8

**(c)** $z =$

(i) 2 (ii) 3 (iii) 4 (iv) 5

**328. Let**

$$\begin{array}{r} A\ B\ C \\ +\ 4\ C\ D \\ \hline D\ A\ B \end{array}$$

**where $A$, $B$, $C$, $D$ are distinct non zero single digit integers. Then how many distinct values of**

**(a) A are possible?**

(i) 2 (ii) 3 (iii) 4 (iv) 5

**(b) B are possible?**

(i) 3 (ii) 4 (iii) 5 (iv) 6

**(c) C are possible?**

(i) 2 (ii) 3 (iii) 4 (iv) 5

**(d) D are possible?**

(i) 2 (ii) 3 (iii) 4 (iv) 5

**329.** Let

$$\begin{array}{cccc} & A & B & C \\ + & 2 & C & 8 \\ + & D & E & B \\ \hline 1 & A & 1 & E \end{array}$$

**where $A, B, C, D, E$ are distinct single digit integers.**

**(a)** $B + C - E =$

(i) 2 (ii) 7
(iii) 12 (iv) cannot be determined

**(b)** $E + 5D =$

(i) 35 (ii) 37
(iii) 39 (iv) cannot be determined

**330.** Let

$$\begin{array}{cccc} & A & 1 & B \\ + & 3 & C & D \\ + & E & F & 2 \\ \hline 1 & 6 & 6 & 5 \end{array}$$

**where $A, B, C, D, E, F$ are six distinct integers from 4 to 9.**

**(a) Which of the following cannot be equal to $B$ or $D$?**

(i) 4 (ii) 5 (iii) 6 (iv) 7

**(b) How many cases for ($A, B, C, D, E, F$) exist?**

(i) 16 (ii) 24 (iii) 32 (iv) 40

**331.** **$A, B, C, D$ are four distinct single digit positve integers such that**

$$\begin{array}{ccccc} & A & B & C & D \\ + & B & C & D & A \\ + & C & D & A & B \\ \hline 1 & ? & D & C & A \end{array}$$

**(a)** ? =

(i) A (ii) B (iii) C (iv) D

**(b)** $C + A =$

(i) 5 (ii) 6 (iii) 7 (iv) 8

**332. Let *a*, *b*, *c* be three single digit positive integers such that** $ab \times bc \times ca = 98da2$

**(a)** $a =$

(i) 3 (ii) 4 (iii) 6 (iv) 8

**(b)** $b =$

(i) 4 (ii) 6 (iii) 7 (iv) 8

**(c)** $c =$

(i) 3 (ii) 4 (iii) 6 (iv) 8

**(d)** $d =$

(i) 4 (ii) 5 (iii) 7 (iv) 8

**333. Let *a*, *b*, *c*, *d* be four distinct single digit integers such that**

$$\begin{array}{cccc} & a & b & c \\ & \times & d & 7 \\ \hline c & b & d & a \end{array}$$

**Then**

**(a)** $a =$

(i) 1 (ii) 3 (iii) 8 (iv) 9

**(b)** $b =$

(i) 2 (ii) 4 (iii) 5 (iv) 8

**(c)** $c =$

(i) 3 (ii) 4 (iii) 7 (iv) 9

**(c)** $d =$

(i) 1 (ii) 2 (iii) 3 (iv) 4

**334. Let *A*, *B*, *C*, *D* be four distinct single digit integers such that**

$$\begin{array}{ccccccc} & A & B & C & 9 & 4 & 7 \\ & & & & & \times & B \\ \hline D & B & D & 3 & B & C & A \end{array}$$

**Then**

**(a)** $A =$

(i) 1 (ii) 2 (iii) 6 (iv) 8

**(b)** $C =$

(i) 2 (ii) 4 (iii) 7 (iv) 8

**(c)** $D =$

(i) 1 (ii) 2 (iii) 3 (iv) 4

**335. *A*, *B*, *C*, *D* are four single digit distinct positive integers such that**

$$\begin{array}{r} C\ A\ B \\ \times\ B\ A \\ \hline B\ 2\ D\ 4\ 0 \end{array}$$

**Then**

**(a)** $A =$

(i) 4 (ii) 5 (iii) 6 (iv) 8

**(b)** $B =$

(i) 4 (ii) 5 (iii) 6 (iv) 8

**(c)** $C =$

(i) 6 (ii) 7 (iii) 8 (iv) 9

**(d)** $D =$

(i) 1 (ii) 3 (iii) 4 (iv) 7

**336. Let *A*, *B*, *C*, and *D* be non-negative integers such that**

$$\begin{array}{r} A\ B\ C \\ \times\ A\ B \\ \hline B\ D\ D\ B \end{array}$$

**(a)** $A =$

(i) 1 (ii) 2

(iii) 3 (iv) cannot be determined

**(b)** $B =$

(i) 5 (ii) 6

(iii) 8 (iv) cannot be determined

**(c)** $C =$

(i) 1 (ii) 3

(iii) 6 (iv) cannot be determined

**(d)** $D =$

(i) 0 (ii) 2

(iii) 4 (iv) cannot be determined

**337.**

$$\begin{array}{r} A\ B\ 6 \\ \times\ D\ A \\ \hline 2\ B\ 9\ C\ C \end{array}$$

**where $A$, $B$, $C$, $D$ are four distinct single digit integers.**

**(a)** $A =$

(i) 1 (ii) 2 (iii) 3 (iv) 4

**(b)** $B =$

(i) 4 (ii) 5 (iii) 7 (iv) 8

**(c)** $C =$

(i) 2 (ii) 4 (iii) 6 (iv) 8

**(d)** $D =$

(i) 1 (ii) 2 (iii) 3 (iv) 4

**338. A, B, C are three distinct single digit integers such that**

$$\begin{array}{r} A\ 6\ B \\ \times\ 4\ C \\ \hline 1\ B\ C\ 8\ A \end{array}$$

**(a)** $A =$

(i) 1 (ii) 2 (iii) 3 (iv) 4

**(b)** $B =$

(i) 4 (ii) 7 (iii) 8 (iv) 9

**(c)** $C =$

(i) 4 (ii) 7 (iii) 8 (iv) 9

**339. Let**

$$\begin{array}{r} 1\ a\ b \\ \times\ c\ 7 \\ \hline 6\ a\ 0\ a \end{array}$$

**where $a$, $b$, $c$ are three distinct single digit integers. Then**

**(a)** $a =$

(i) 6 (ii) 7 (iii) 8 (iv) 9

**(b)** $b =$

(i) 3 (ii) 4 (iii) 7 (iv) 8

**(c)** $c =$

(i) 3 (ii) 4 (iii) 5 (iv) 6

**340. Let $a$, $b$, $c$ be three single digit possitive integers such that**

$$\begin{array}{r} a\ b\ 6 \\ \times\ 7\ a \\ \hline 2\ b\ 9\ c\ c \end{array}$$

**(a)** $b =$

(i) 3 (ii) 4 (iii) 5 (iv) 8

**(b)** $c =$

(i) 2 (ii) 4 (iii) 6 (iv) 8

**341. Let**

$$\begin{array}{r} 5\ a\ 6 \\ \times\ 2\ b \\ \hline c\ b\ 2\ d\ e \end{array}$$

**where $a$, $b$, $c$, $d$ and $e$ are distinct single digit numbers other than 2, 5 and 6.**

**(a) There is an ambiguity about the values of**

(i) $(a, b)$ (ii) $(b, e)$ (iii) $(a, d)$ (iv) $(b, c)$

**(b) If none of the digits is equal to 0, then which of the following is greatest?**

(i) $a$ (ii) $b$ (iii) $d$ (iv) $e$

**(c) If none of the digits is equal to 0, then $a$ =**

(i) 1 (ii) 3 (iii) 4 (iv) 7

**342. Consider all numbers formed by the permutation of digits of a three-digit integer (all digits being distinct and non zero). The numbers are divided into three exclusive pairs which sums are 827, 980 and 1079.**

**(a) Which of the following can be one of the digit of a number?**

(i) 1 (ii) 2

(iii) 5 (iv) none of these

**(b) Which of the following cannot be any of the digit of a number?**

(i) 3 (ii) 4 (iii) 6 (iv) 7

**(c) If one of the numbers of sums 980, 1079 are $ABC$ and $CBA$ respectively, then the another number of sum 1079 is**

(i) $BAC$ (ii) $ACB$

(iii) $BCA$ (iv) cannot be determined

**343. Consider a two-digit number $x$ and a three-digit number $y$ and the number in which the places of three digits are reversed, $\bar{x}$ and $\bar{y}$ respectively. Let three of $x + y$, $x + \bar{y}$, $\bar{x} + y$ and $\bar{x} + \bar{y}$ be 713, 731 and 911 (not in order).**

**(a) The middle digit of the three-digit number is**
(i) 5 (ii) 6 (iii) 7 (iv) 8

**(b) The sum of digits of two-digit number is**
(i) 8 (ii) 9 (iii) 10 (iv) 11

**(c) The sum of digits of three-digit number is**
(i) 18 (ii) 20 (iii) 21 (iv) 23

**344. Let $x$, $y$ be two two-digit positive integers such that the value of $x \div y = .807228915$ upto nine decimal places.**

**(a) The digit at unit digit place of $x$ is**
(i) 3 (ii) 5 (iii) 6 (iv) 7

**(b) The digit at ten digit place of $x$ is**
(i) 2 (ii) 4 (iii) 6 (iv) 7

**(c) The digit at unit digit place of $y$ is**
(i) 3 (ii) 5 (iii) 7 (iv) 9

**(d) The digit at ten digit place of $y$ is**
(i) 2 (ii) 5 (iii) 6 (iv) 8

**345. A. Consider two three-digit numbers which sum is 1000. If the product of these numbers is 2165 $xy$, then**

**(a) $x =$**
(i) 1 (ii) 3 (iii) 7 (iv) 8

**(b) $y =$**
(i) 1 (ii) 4 (iii) 6 (iv) 9

**B. Consider two three-digit numbers which product is 31411. If one number is greater than 300, then**

**(a) their sum must be divisible by**
(i) 3 (ii) 4 (iii) 6 (iv) 8

**(b) their difference must not be divisible by**
(i) 3 (ii) 4 (iii) 5 (iv) 7

**346. Let $x$, $y$ be two three-digit integers which difference is less than 40 such that**

$x \times 90 + 1 = y \times 101$

**(a) The middle digit of $x$ will be**
(i) 3 (ii) 4
(iii) 5 (iv) cannot be determined

**(b) Which of the following cannot be a digit of $y$?**
(i) 1 (ii) 2 (iii) 3 (iv) 4

**347. Let $x$, $y$ be two four-digit numbers. Let the digits of $x$ and $y$ be (5, 6, 8, 9) and (6, 7, 8, 9) respectively while the digits of their sum be (1, 2, 5, 6, 8).**

**(a) How many different cases for pair of numbers at the unit-digit place exist?**
(i) 3 (ii) 4 (iii) 5 (iv) 6

**(b) How many different cases for pair of numbers at the unit-digit place exist if, in the sum, the digit at unit-digit place is 5?**
(i) 0 (ii) 1 (iii) 2 (iv) 3

**(c) If 2 is at unit-digit place in sum, then which of the following pair of numbers cannot have the same digit place in the numbers $x$ and $y$?**
(i) 6, 7 (ii) 9, 6 (iii) 8, 7 (iv) 5, 9

**(d) If 9 is at unit-digit place in both $x$ and $y$, then which of the following pair of numbers cannot have the same digit place in the numbers?**
(i) 5, 6 (ii) 6, 7 (iii) 7, 8 (iv) 6, 8

**(e) The position of which of the digit in the sum is fixed?**
(i) 1 (ii) 6
(iii) 8 (iv) none of these

**348. Let $a$, $b$, $c$ be three single digit integers such that $ab \times bc \times ca = 11xxy4$. Then**

**(a) $x =$**
(i) 5 or 6 (ii) 6 or 7 (iii) 7 or 8 (iv) 5 or 8

**(b) $y =$**
(i) 3 or 5 (ii) 5 or 7 (iii) 7 or 3 (iv) 9 or 5

**(c) $a + b + c =$**
(i) 13 (ii) 14
(iii) 15 (iv) cannot be determined

**(d) Let $a$ be the least number. Which of the following is correct?**
(i) If $x - y = 1$, then $b > c$
(ii) If $x - y = 2$, then $b < c$
(iii) If $x - y = 3$, then $b < c$
(iv) If $x - y = 4$, then $b > c$.

**349. Let the digits of a four-digit number be (5, 6, 8, 9) and the digits of product of the number and 7 be (2, 6, 8, 9, 9)**

**(a) In the number, 8 is at**

(i) unit digit place
(ii) ten digit place
(iii) hundred digit place
(iv) thousand digit place

**(b) In the product, 8 is at**

(i) unit digit place
(ii) ten digit place
(iii) hundred digit place
(iv) thousand digit place

**350. The sum of digits of the product**

**(a) 81 × 123456789 is**

(i) 54 (ii) 63 (iii) 72 (iv) 81

**(b) 81 × 12345678987654321 is**

(i) 72 (ii) 81 (iii) 90 (iv) 99

**351. Let $x00000y00002z$ be divisible by 81 where $x$, $y$, $z$ are distinct non zero single digit integers.**
**The value of**

**(a) $x$ is**

(i) 1 (ii) 2
(iii) 4 (iv) cannot be determined

**(b) $y$ is**

(i) 1 (ii) 2
(iii) 3 (iv) cannot be determined

**(c) $z$ is**

(i) 1 (ii) 3
(iii) 4 (iv) cannot be determined

**352. Let the sum of digits of product of 7 and $AB$, $BC$ and $CA$ be 14, 9 and 11 respectively where $A$, $B$, $C$ are three single digit positive integers.**

**(a) A cannot be equal to**

(i) 3 (ii) 5 (iii) 6 (iv) 7

**(b) C cannot be equal to**

(i) 3 (ii) 5 (iii) 6 (iv) 7

**(c) Which of the following must be equal to one of $A$, $B$ or $C$?**

(i) 3 (ii) 5 (iii) 6 (iv) 7

(d) If $B + C = 9$, then $A + B =$
(i) 10 (ii) 11 (iii) 12 (iv) 13

**353.** ***A*, *B*, *C* are three two-digit numbers which sum of digits are also two-digit numbers. Let the sum of digits of ($A + B - C$), ($B + C - A$) and ($C + A - B$) be 6, 11 and 13 respectively. The sum of digits of**

**(a)** ***A*** **will be**
(i) 11 (ii) 12 (iii) 13 (iv) 14

**(b)** ***B*** **will be**
(i) 11 (ii) 12 (iii) 13 (iv) 14

**(c)** ***C*** **will be**
(i) 11 (ii) 12 (iii) 13 (iv) 14

**(d)** **($A + B + C$) will be**
(i) 12 (ii) 19
(iii) 21 (iv) cannot be determined

**354. Consider a four digit number which digits are (3, 5, 8, 9) (may not be in order) and its products with three single digit integers *x*, *y*, *z* which digits are (0, 1, 4, 7, 9); (0, 1, 7, 9, 9) and (1, 2, 5, 6, 8) respectively. Then**

**(a)** $x =$
(i) 3 (ii) 4 (iii) 5 (iv) 6

**(b)** $y =$
(i) 4 (ii) 5 (iii) 7 (iv) 8

**(c)** $z =$
(i) 4 (ii) 5 (iii) 7 (iv) 8

**(d) In the number, 3 is at**
(i) unit digit place
(ii) ten digit place
(iii) hundred digit place
(iv) thousand digit place

**(e) In the number, 5 is at**
(i) unit digit place
(ii) ten digit place
(iii) hundred digit place
(iv) thousand digit place

**355. Consider a three digit number. The digits of its product with two single digit integers $x$ and $y$ are(1, 3, 4, 9) and (0, 1, 2, 9) respectively. Then**

**(a)** $x =$

(i) 2 (ii) 4 (iii) 6 (iv) 8

**(b)** $y =$

(i) 3 (ii) 5 (iii) 6 (iv) 9

**(c) the digits of which place of three-digit number can be determined?**

(i) unit (ii) ten
(iii) hundred (iv) all

**356. Let $w$, $x$, $y$, $z$ be four three-digit integers which digits are (2, 5, 9); (4, 6, 7); (1, 6, 7) and (5, 8, 9) respectively. The sum of two of them is equal to that of another two. Also 2 in $w$ and 1 in $y$ occupy the same digit place in their respective numbers.**

**(a) Which of the following is correct?**

(i) $w + x = y + z$
(ii) $w + y = x + z$
(iii) $w + z = x + y$
(iv) cannot be determined

**(b) The middle digit of $w$ is**

(i) 2 (ii) 5
(iii) 9 (iv) cannot be determined

**(c) The middle digit of $x$ is**

(i) 4 (ii) 6
(iii) 7 (iv) cannot be determined

**(d) The middle digit of $y$ is**

(i) 1 (ii) 6
(iii) 7 (iv) cannot be determined

**(e) The middle digit of $z$ is**

(i) 5 (ii) 8
(iii) 9 (iv) cannot be determined

**357. Let the digits of the product of a 4-digit integer and 13 be 2, 4, 5, 7 and 9.**

**(a) How many distinct cases for 4-digit integer exist?**

(i) 4 (ii) 5 (iii) 6 (iv) 7

**(b) In how many of these cases, the first digit will be 2?**
(i) 1 (ii) 2 (iii) 3 (iv) 4

**(c) In how many of these cases, the first digit will be 4?**
(i) 1 (ii) 2 (iii) 3 (iv) 4

**(d) In how many of these cases, the first digit will be 7?**
(i) 1 (ii) 2 (iii) 3 (iv) 4

**(e) In how many of these cases, the first digit will be 9?**
(i) 1 (ii) 2 (iii) 3 (iv) 4

**358. $x$, $y$, $z$ are three 3-digit numbers. Let the digits of $x + y$, $y + z$ and $z + x$ be (0, 9, 9), (5, 7, 8) and (2, 4, 7) respectively. Also the sum of $x$, $y$ and $z$ is a four digit number with three of its digits as 1 and fourth being one of 0, 2 and 4.**

**(a) Which of the following will be one of the digit of $(x + y + z)$?**
(i) 0 (ii) 2
(iii) 4 (iv) cannot be determined

**(b) Which is the least of $x$, $y$ and $z$?**
(i) $x$ (ii) $y$
(iii) $z$ (iv) cannot be determined

**(c) Which is the most of $x$, $y$ and $z$?**
(i) x (ii) y
(iii) z (iv) cannot be determined

**(d) The digit at hundred place of $x$ cannot be**
(i) 3 (ii) 5
(iii) 6 (iv) all of these are possible

**(e) The digit at hundred place of $y$ cannot be**
(i) 3 (ii) 5
(iii) 6 (iv) all of these are possible

**359. Let A be a four digit number such that the digits of A + 3678 = 2, 5, 6, $x$ (not in order) and A + 4321 = 1, 6, 7, $y$ (not in order). Then**

**(a) the difference of $x$ and $y$ will be**
(i) 2 (ii) 3 (iii) 4 (iv) 6

**(b) the first digit of A will be**
(i) 1 (ii) 2 (iii) 3 (iv) 4

**(c) the second digit of A will be**
(i) 3 (ii) 5 (iii) 6 (iv) 8

**(d) the third digit of A will be**
(i) 3 (ii) 4 (iii) 5 (iv) 6

**360. Consider three 3-digit number which digits are (3, 5, 7) (4, 6, 8) and (1, 7, 9) while the digits of their sums, taken two at a time, are (1, 2, 3, 8), (1, 1, 5, 8) and (1, 3, 4, 9) (not in order). Let *S* be the sum of the three digits. Then**

**(a) the second digit of S is**
(i) 6 (ii) 7 (iii) 8 (iv) 9

**(b) the third digit of S is**
(i) 5 (ii) 6 (iii) 7 (iv) 8

**(c) the fourth digit of S is**
(i) 4 (ii) 5 (iii) 6 (iv) 7

**(d) the sum of digits of S is**
(i) 19 (ii) 21 (iii) 22 (iv) 23

# Keys to Problems

| | | |
|---|---|---|
| **1.** | | (i) |
| **2.** | (a) | (i) |
| | (b) | (iv) |
| **3.** | (a) | (ii) |
| | (b) | (iii) |
| **4.** | (a) | (iii) |
| | (b) | (iii) |
| **5.** | (a) | (i) |
| | (b) | (i) |
| | (c) | (ii) |
| **6.** | (a) | (i) |
| | (b) | (i) |
| | (c) | (iii) |
| **7.** | | (i) |
| **8.** | (a) | (i) |
| | (b) | (iv) |
| **9.** | (a) | (ii) |
| | (b) | (ii) |
| **10.** | (a) | (iv) |
| | (b) | (i) |
| | (c) | (ii) |
| **11.** | (a) | (iv) |
| | (b) | (iii) |
| **12.** | (a) | (iv) |
| | (b) | (i) |
| | (c) | (ii) |
| **13.** | (a) | (ii) |
| | (b) | (ii) |
| | (c) | (iv) |
| **14.** | (a) | (iii) |
| | (b) | (i) |
| **15.** | (a) | (i) |
| | (b) | (iii) |
| | (c) | (i) |
| **16.** | (a) | (iii) |
| | (b) | (ii) |
| **17.** | (a) | (iii) |
| | (b) | (iv) |
| | (c) | (iii) |
| **18.** | (a) | (i) |
| **19.** | (a) | (ii) |
| | (b) | (ii) |
| **20.** | (a) | (iv) |
| | (b) | (iii) |
| **21.** | | (iv) |
| **22.** | (a) | (ii) |
| | (b) | (iv) |
| **23.** | | (i) |
| **24.** | | (ii) |
| **25.** | (a) | (iv) |
| | (b) | (iii) |
| | (c) | (iii) |
| **26.** | (a) | (iv) |
| | (b) | (i) |
| **27.** | | (i) |
| **28.** | (a) | (ii) |
| | (b) | (i) |
| **29.** | (a) | (iii) |
| | (b) | (ii) |
| | (c) | (ii) |
| **30.** | (a) | (iii) |
| | (b) | (iii) |
| **31.** | (a) | (iv) |
| | (b) | (iii) |
| | (c) | (iv) |
| | (d) | (iv) |
| | (e) | (i) |
| **32.** | (a) | (ii) |
| | (b) | (iv) |
| | (c) | (ii) |
| | (d) | (i) |
| | (e) | (i) |
| **33.** | (a) | (ii) |
| | (b) | (ii) |
| | (c) | (i) |
| **34.** | (a) | (i) |
| | (b) | (i) |
| | (c) | (i) |
| | (d) | (i) |
| **35. A.** | (a) | (ii) |
| | (b) | (iv) |
| **B.** | (a) | (ii) |
| | (b) | (i) |
| | (c) | (iii) |
| **C.** | (a) | (iv) |
| | (b) | (iii) |
| | (c) | (ii) |
| **36.** | (a) | (i) |
| | (b) | (ii) |
| | (c) | (ii) |
| **37. A.** | (a) | (ii) |
| | (b) | (i) |
| | (c) | (i) |
| **B.** | (a) | (iii) |
| | (b) | (ii) |
| **38.** | (a) | (i) |
| | (b) | (i) |
| | (c) | (i) |
| **39.** | (a) | (ii) |
| | (b) | (i) |
| | (c) | (iii) |
| **40.** | (a) | (iii) |
| | (b) | (i) |
| | (c) | (i) |
| **41.** | (a) | (ii) |
| | (b) | (iv) |
| | (c) | (iii) |
| **42.** | (a) | (ii) |
| | (b) | (iv) |
| | (c) | (i) |
| | (d) | (ii) |

**43.** (a) (iii)
(b) (iii)
(c) (iv)
**44.** (a) (iii)
(b) (i)
(c) (ii)
(d) (ii)
**45.** (a) (iv)
(b) (iii)
**46.** (a) (i)
(b) (iv)
(c) (iii)
(d) (iii)
**47.** (a) (ii)
(b) (i)
(c) (iii)
(d) (iv)
**48.** (a) (iii)
(b) (i)
(c) (i)
**49. A.** (a) (iv)
(b) (i)
**B.** (iii)
**50.** (iv)
**51.** (iii)
**52.** (a) (i)
(b) (i)
**53.** (a) (iv)
(b) (ii)
(c) (ii)
(d) (i)
(e) (ii)
**54.** (a) (iii)
(b) (ii)
**55.** (a) (ii)
(b) (iv)
**56.** (a) (iv)
(b) (iii)
**57.** (a) (iv)
(b) (iii)
(c) (iv)
**58. A.** (a) (iii)
(b) (iv)
(c) (iii)
**B.** (ii)
**59.** (a) (ii)
(b) (iv)
(c) (i)
(d) (iii)
**60.** (a) (iii)
(b) (iii)
**61.** (a) (iii)
(b) (iii)
(c) (i)
(d) (ii)
**62. A.** (a) (iii)
(b) (i)
(c) (iv)
(d) (iv)
**B.** (a) (ii)
(b) (iii)
**63.** (a) (iv)
(b) (i)
(c) (i)
**64.** (a) (iii)
(b) (ii)
**65.** (a) (i)
(b) (i)
(c) (i)
**66.** (a) (iii)
(b) (iv)
(c) (i)
**67. A.** (a) (ii)
(b) (ii)
**B.** (a) (ii)
(b) (iii)
(c) (iv)
(d) (i)
**68.** (a) (ii)
(b) (i)
**69.** (a) (iii)
(b) (ii)
**70. A.** (a) (i)
(b) (iii)
(c) (iv)
**B.** (a) (iv)
(b) (iv)
**71.** (a) (iv)
(b) (i)
(c) (i)
(d) (ii)
**72.** (a) (iv)
(b) (iv)
**73.** (a) (iii)
(b) (i)
(c) (i)
**74.** (a) (iv)
(b) (ii)
(c) (ii)
**75.** (a) (iii)
(b) (iii)
(c) (ii)
(d) (i)
**76.** (a) (iii)
(b) (ii)
(c) (i)
**77.** (a) (i)
(b) (iii)
(c) (iv)
**78.** (a) (iii)
(b) (ii)
**79.** (a) (iii)
(b) (iv)
(c) (i)
**80.** (a) (iv)
(b) (iv)
(c) (iv)
(d) (iv)
**81.** (a) (ii)
(b) (iv)

(c) (ii)
(d) (iv)
82. (a) (iv)
(b) (iv)
83. (a) (iv)
(b) (iv)
(c) (iv)
84. (a) (i)
(b) (iii)
85. (a) (iv)
(b) (iii)
86. (a) (i)
(b) (iv)
(c) (i)
87. (a) (ii)
(b) (ii)
(c) (ii)
88. (a) (i)
(b) (iii)
(c) (ii)
89. (a) (ii)
(b) (ii)
(c) (ii)
90. (a) (iii)
(b) (ii)
(c) (ii)
91. (a) (iii)
(b) (iii)
(c) (i)
92. (a) (iv)
(b) (iv)
93. (a) (ii)
(b) (ii)
(c) (i)
(d) (iii)
94. (a) (iv)
(b) (ii)
95. (a) (i)
(b) (iii)
(c) (iii)
96. A. (a) (i)
B. (a) (i)
(b) (ii)
(c) (iii)
97. (a) (iv)
(b) (iv)
(c) (iv)
98. (a) (iv)
(b) (iv)
99. (a) (ii)
(b) (i)
(c) (iii)
(d) (iv)
100. (a) (iii)
(b) (iii)
101. (a) (iii)
(b) (iii)
(c) (ii)
102. (a) (i)
(b) (ii)
(c) (iv)
103. (a) (iv)
(b) (iv)
(c) (i)
104. A. (a) (iii)
(b) (ii)
(c) (iv)
(d) (i)
(e) (ii)
B. (a) (iii)
(b) (ii)
(c) (iv)
105. (a) (iii)
(b) (ii)
(c) (i)
(d) (i)
(e) (iv)
106. (a) (iii)
(b) (iii)
(c) (i)
(d) (iv)
(e) (ii)
(f) (ii)
107. (a) (i)
(b) (ii)
(c) (ii)
(d) (iv)
108. (a) (i)
(b) (ii)
(c) (ii)
(d) (iii)
(e) (i)
109. (a) (iv)
(b) (iii)
(c) (iii)
(d) (iii)
110. (a) (iv)
(b) (i)
(c) (iv)
(d) (iv)
(e) (i)
(f) (ii)
111. (a) (i)
(b) (iii)
(c) (ii)
(d) (iv)
(e) (iii)
112. (a) (ii)
(b) (ii)
(c) (i)
(d) (ii)
(e) (iv)
113. (a) (iii)
(b) (iv)
(c) (iii)
(d) (iv)
114. (a) (iii)
(b) (ii)
(c) (i)
(d) (iii)

**115.** (a) (iv)
(b) (ii)
**116.** (a) (iii)
(b) (ii)
(c) (ii)
(d) (iv)
**117.** (a) (ii)
(b) (ii)
(c) (iv)
(d) (iii)
**118.** (a) (i)
(b) (ii)
(c) (iii)
(d) (iii)
(e) (iv)
**119.** (a) (iii)
(b) (iv)
(c) (iv)
**120.** (a) (iii)
(b) (iii)
(c) (i)
(d) (i)
(e) (i)
**121. A.** (a) (i)
(b) (iii)
(c) (i)
**B.** (a) (ii)
(b) (iii)
**122.** (a) (iii)
(b) (iv)
(c) (iii)
(d) (iv)
**123.** (a) (iv)
(b) (iv)
**124.** (a) (i)
(b) (iv)
(c) (iv)
(d) (ii)
**125.** (a) (iv)
(b) (i)
(c) (iv)
(d) (i)
(e) (i)
**126.** (a) (iii)
(b) (ii)
(c) (iv)
(d) (ii)
**127.** (a) (iii)
(b) (iii)
(c) (iv)
(d) (ii)
(e) (ii)
**128.** (a) (i)
(b) (iv)
**129.** (a) (iii)
(b) (iv)
(c) (iii)
(d) (iii)
(e) (ii)
**130.** (a) (ii)
(b) (iv)
(c) (ii)
**131.** (a) (iv)
(b) (i)
(c) (iii)
(d) (iv)
**132.** (a) (i)
(b) (iii)
(c) (iv)
**133.** (a) (ii)
(b) (i)
(c) (iii)
(d) (iv)
**134.** (a) (iv)
(b) (iv)
(c) (iv)
**135.** (a) (iii)
(b) (ii)
(c) (ii)
(d) (ii)
(e) (ii)
**136.** (a) (iii)
(b) (iv)
(c) (iii)
(d) (iv)
(e) (iv)
**137.** (a) (ii)
(b) (i)
(c) (iii)
(d) (i)
(e) (ii)
**138.** (a) (i)
(b) (iii)
(c) (i)
(d) (i)
(e) (ii)
(f) (iii)
**139.** (a) (i)
(b) (iv)
(c) (iv)
(d) (iii)
(e) (iii)
**140.** (a) (ii)
(b) (i)
(c) (iii)
(d) (ii)
**141.** (a) (i)
(b) (ii)
(c) (i)
**142.** (a) (ii)
(b) (ii)
(c) (iii)
**143.** (a) (iii)
(b) (iv)
(c) (ii)
(d) (iii)
**144.** (a) (i)
(b) (iv)
(c) (iii)
(d) (ii)

**145.** (a) (iii)<br>(b) (ii)<br>(c) (ii)

**146.** (a) (i)<br>(b) (iii)<br>(c) (iii)<br>(d) (iii)

**147.** (a) (iv)<br>(b) (ii)

**148.** (a) (ii)<br>(b) (iii)<br>(c) (iii)

**149.** (a) (i)<br>(b) (iii)

**150.** (a) (ii)<br>(b) (i)<br>(c) (iv)

**151.** (a) (iii)<br>(b) (iv)<br>(c) (iv)<br>(d) (iii)<br>(e) (i)

**152.** (a) (i)<br>(b) (iii)<br>(c) (ii)<br>(d) (i)

**153.** (a) (i)<br>(b) (iii)<br>(c) (i)<br>(d) (iii)

**154.** (a) (iv)<br>(b) (iv)<br>(c) (ii)

**155.** (a) (iv)<br>(b) (i)<br>(c) (iv)

**156.** (a) (iii)<br>(b) (iii)<br>(c) (ii)

**157.** (a) (iii)<br>(b) (iv)<br>(c) (iv)<br>(d) (i)

**158.** (a) (iv)<br>(b) (iv)

**159.** (a) (i)<br>(b) (i)<br>(c) (i)

**160.** (a) (i)<br>(b) (ii)<br>(c) (iv)<br>(d) (iv)

**161.** (a) (i)<br>(c) (iii)<br>(c) (iii)<br>(d) (ii)

**162.** (a) (iii)<br>(b) (iv)<br>(c) (ii)<br>(d) (ii)<br>(e) (iv)

**163.** (a) (i)<br>(b) (ii)

**164.** (a) (i)<br>(b) (i)<br>(c) (iv)

**165.** (a) (iii)<br>(b) (iv)<br>(c) (i)<br>(d) (i)<br>(e) (i)

**166.** (a) (i)<br>(b) (iv)<br>(c) (iv)

**167.** (a) (ii)<br>(b) (ii)<br>(c) (iii)<br>(d) (i)

**168.** (a) (iv)<br>(b) (ii)<br>(c) (iv)<br>(d) (iii)

**169.** (a) (ii)<br>(b) (i)

**170.** (a) (iii)<br>(b) (iii)<br>(c) (i)<br>(d) (iv)<br>(e) (iv)

**171.** (a) (iii)<br>(b) (i)<br>(c) (i)

**172.** (a) (i)<br>(b) (ii)

**173.** (a) (iii)<br>(b) (iv)<br>(c) (ii)

**174.** (a) (ii)<br>(b) (ii)

**175.** (a) (ii)<br>(b) (ii)<br>(c) (ii)

**176.** (a) (ii)<br>(b) (i)<br>(c) (iii)

**177.** (a) (iii)<br>(b) (i)<br>(c) (i)

**178.** (a) (i)<br>(b) (iii)<br>(c) (iv)

**179.** (a) (i)<br>(b) (ii)<br>(c) (ii)

**180.** (a) (iv)<br>(b) (iv)<br>(c) (iv)<br>(d) (iv)<br>(e) (iv)

**181.** (a) (ii)

(b) (iii)
(c) (ii)
(d) (i)
(e) (ii)

**182.** (a) (i)
(b) (iii)
(c) (i)

**183.** (a) (i)
(b) (iii)
(c) (iii)
(d) (iii)

**184.** (a) (iii)
(b) (ii)
(c) (ii)

**185.** (a) (iii)
(b) (ii)
(c) (iv)

**186.** (a) (iv)
(b) (iv)

**187.** (a) (i)
(b) (i)

**188.** (a) (i)
(b) (i)

**189.** (a) (iv)
(b) (i)

**190.** (a) (iv)
(b) (iv)

**191.** (a) (iii)
(b) (iii)
(c) (iii)

**192.** (a) (ii)
(b) (ii)

**193.** (a) (iii)
(b) (ii)

**194.** (a) (i)
(b) (i)
(c) (iii)

**195.** (a) (i)
(b) (ii)
(c) (iv)

**196.** (a) (ii)
(b) (iii)

**197.** (a) (i)
(b) (i)

**198.** (a) (iii)
(b) (ii)
(c) (iii)

**199.** (a) (iv)
(b) (iv)
(c) (ii)
(d) (iii)

**200. A.** (a) (iii)
(b) (i)
(c) (iii)
(d) (i)

**B.** (a) (iii)
(b) (iv)
(c) (iii)

**201.** (a) (i)
(b) (iii)
(c) (iv)

**202.** (a) (ii)
(b) (ii)
(c) (i)
(d) (iii)

**203.** (i)

**204.** (a) (i)
(b) (i)
(c) (ii)
(d) (i)
(e) (iv)

**205.** (a) (iv)
(b) (ii)
(c) (i)
(d) (ii)

**206.** (a) (iii)
(b) (iii)
(c) (i)
(d) (ii)

**207.** (a) (ii)
(b) (iii)
(c) (iv)

**208.** (a) (i)
(b) (i)
(c) (iii)

**209.** (a) (ii)
(b) (i)
(c) (ii)
(d) (iii)

**210.** (a) (iii)
(b) (iii)
(c) (iv)

**211.** (ii)

**212.** (a) (ii)
(b) (ii)

**213. A.** (a) (ii)

**B.** (a) (ii)
(b) (iv)

**214.** (a) (ii)
(b) (iv)
(c) (i)
(d) (iii)

**215.** (a) (ii)
(b) (i)
(c) (ii)
(d) (iii)

**216. A.** (a) (iv)
(b) (iii)

**B.** (a) (iv)
(c) (iii)

**217.** (a) (iv)
(b) (i)

**218.** (a) (i)
(b) (iv)
(c) (iv)

**219.** (a) (ii)
(b) (i)
(c) (ii)
(d) (iv)

220. (a) (i)
(b) (iv)
221. (a) (iv)
(b) (iii)
(c) (ii)
222. A. (a) (iv)
B. (a) (iv)
(b) (iii)
(c) (iii)
223. A. (a) (ii)
(b) (ii)
B. (ii)
C. (iv)
224. (a) (ii)
(b) (ii)
(c) (i)
225. (a) (iv)
(b) (ii)
226. (a) (iv)
(b) (i)
(c) (iv)
227. (a) (i)
(b) (i)
228. (a) (ii)
(b) (ii)
(c) (iv)
(d) (iii)
229. (a) (i)
(b) (iii)
(c) (ii)
230. (a) (ii)
(b) (ii)
(c) (ii)
231. (a) (iii)
(b) (ii)
(c) (iv)
232. (a) (i)
(b) (iv)
233. (a) (ii)
(b) (i)
(c) (iii)
234. (a) (i)
(b) (iv)
(c) (iv)
(d) (i)
(e) (iv)
235. (a) (i)
(b) (ii)
(c) (ii)
236. (a) (ii)
(b) (iv)
(c) (iii)
237. (a) (ii)
(b) (iii)
(c) (iv)
238. (a) (iv)
(b) (ii)
(c) (i)
239. (a) (iii)
(b) (ii)
240. (a) (ii)
(b) (iii)
(c) (ii)
241. (a) (iv)
(b) (iv)
(c) (i)
242. (a) (iv)
(b) (iii)
(c) (iv)
243. (a) (iii)
(b) (iv)
(c) (ii)
(d) (iv)
244. (a) (ii)
(b) (ii)
(c) (iv)
(d) (ii)
245. (a) (ii)
(b) (ii)
(c) (iii)
(d) (i)
(e) (i)
246. (a) (iv)
(b) (iv)
(c) (iv)
(d) (ii)
(e) (iii)
247. (a) (ii)
(b) (ii)
(c) (i)
(d) (i)
(e) (ii)
248. (a) (iii)
(b) (iv)
(c) (i)
(d) (ii)
249. (a) (iii)
(b) (ii)
(c) (i)
(d) (ii)
(e) (ii)
(f) (iii)
250. (a) (i)
(b) (iv)
(c) (ii)
(d) (iii)
(e) (ii)
(f) (i)
251. (a) (iv)
(b) (iii)
(c) (i)
(d) (iv)
252. (a) (iii)
(b) (iv)
(c) (iii)
253. (a) (iii)
(b) (ii)
(c) (i)
254. (a) (i)
(b) (ii)

(c) (i)
(d) (ii)

**255.** (a) (ii)
(b) (i)
(c) (ii)
(d) (iii)

**256.** (a) (i)
(b) (i)
(c) (i)
(d) (ii)

**257.** (a) (iv)
(b) (i)
(c) (iv)
(d) (i)
(e) (iv)

**258.** (a) (ii)
(b) (iv)
(c) (i)
(d) (i)

**259.** (a) (iv)
(b) (i)
(c) (i)

**260. A.** (a) (iii)
(b) (ii)
(c) (iii)
(d) (iv)

**B.** (a) (i)
(b) (iv)
(c) (i)
(d) (iv)

**261.** (a) (ii)
(b) (iii)

**262.** (a) (ii)
(b) (iii)
(c) (i)

**263.** (a) (iii)
(b) (iv)
(c) (i)
(d) (iii)

**264.** (a) (ii)
(b) (ii)
(c) (iv)

**265. A.** (a) (i)
(b) (iv)
(c) (i)
(d) (iv)

**B.** (a) (iii)
(b) (i)

**266.** (a) (iv)
(b) (ii)
(c) (iii)

**267.** (a) (ii)
(b) (i)
(c) (i)

**268. A.** (a) (iii)
(b) (ii)
(c) (iii)
(d) (ii)

**B.** (a) (i)
(b) (iv)

**269.** (a) (i)
(b) (ii)
(c) (iv)

**270.** (a) (iv)
(b) (iii)
(c) (ii)
(d) (iv)

**271.** (a) (iv)
(b) (iii)
(c) (i)

**272.** (a) (ii)
(b) (i)
(c) (ii)

**273.** (a) (ii)
(b) (iv)
(c) (i)
(d) (iii)

**274.** (a) (ii)
(b) (iii)

**275.** (a) (iv)
(b) (iv)
(c) (ii)

**276.** (a) (ii)
(b) (i)
(c) (i)
(d) (ii)

**277.** (a) (ii)
(b) (iii)
(c) (ii)

**278.** (a) (ii)
(b) (i)
(c) (iii)

**279.** (a) (iii)
(b) (iv)
(c) (iii)
(d) (i)

**280.** (a) (ii)
(b) (i)

**281.** (a) (iv)
(b) (iv)
(c) (i)
(d) (ii)

**282.** (a) (iii)
(b) (ii)
(c) (iii)

**283.** (a) (iii)
(b) (iv)
(c) (iv)

**284.** (a) (ii)
(b) (iii)

**285.** (a) (iv)
(b) (iii)
(c) (iv)
(d) (iv)

**286.** (a) (ii)
(b) (i)
(c) (iv)

**287.** (a) (ii)
(b) (i)

**288.** (a) (iv)

(b) (i)
(c) (iv)
(d) (ii)
(e) (iv)

**289.** (a) (i)
(b) (i)
(c) (iv)
(d) (ii)
(e) (ii)

**290.** (a) (i)
(b) (ii)
(c) (iv)

**291.** (a) (i)
(b) (ii)
(c) (iv)

**292.** (a) (iv)
(b) (ii)
(c) (iii)
(d) (i)

**293.** (a) (i)
(b) (i)
(c) (iii)

**294.** (a) (ii)
(b) (iv)
(c) (i)
(d) (iii)

**295.** (a) (i)
(b) (ii)
(c) (i)
(d) (iii)
(e) (iv)

**296.** (a) (i)
(b) (ii)
(c) (ii)
(d) (ii)

**297. A.** (a) (ii)
(b) (iv)
(c) (iv)
(d) (ii)

**B.** (a) (ii)
(c) (i)
(c) (iii)

**298.** (a) (i)
(b) (i)
(c) (i)

**299.** (a) (i)
(b) (ii)
(c) (ii)
(d) (iii)
(e) (iii)

**300.** (a) (iv)
(b) (i)
(c) (i)

**301.** (a) (iv)
(b) (ii)
(c) (ii)
(d) (ii)

**302.** (a) (iv)
(b) (ii)
(c) (ii)

**303.** (a) (iv)
(b) (iv)

**304.** (a) (ii)
(b) (ii)

**305.** (a) (ii)
(b) (i)
(c) (iii)
(d) (i)

**306.** (a) (iv)
(b) (iii)
(c) (iii)

**307.** (a) (iii)
(b) (iv)
(c) (ii)
(b) (iv)

**308.** (ii)

**309.** (a) (i)
(b) (i)
(c) (i)
(d) (i)

**310.** (a) (iii)
(b) (ii)

**311.** (a) (iv)
(b) (iii)
(c) (iv)

**312.** (a) (ii)
(b) (iii)
(c) (ii)

**313.** (a) (ii)
(b) (i)
(c) (ii)

**314.** (a) (iv)
(b) (i)

**315. A.** (a) (iii)
(b) (iv)
(c) (ii)
(d) (iii)

**B.** (a) (iii)
(b) (i)

**316.** (a) (ii)
(b) (ii)
(c) (iii)
(d) (iii)

**317.** (a) (i)
(b) (ii)
(c) (i)

**318.** (a) (iii)
(b) (ii)

**319.** (a) (ii)
(b) (ii)
(c) (iii)

**320.** (a) (i)
(b) (i)

**321.** (a) (iv)
(b) (iii)

**322.** (a) (iv)
(b) (iii)

**323.** (a) (ii)
(b) (i)
(c) (i)
(d) (iv)

**324.** (a) (iii)
(b) (iv)

(c) (iv)

**325.** (a) (iii)

(b) (i)

**326.** (a) (iv)

(b) (ii)

**327.** (a) (ii)

(b) (i)

(c) (iv)

**328.** (a) (iv)

(b) (iv)

(c) (ii)

(d) (iii)

**329.** (a) (i)

(b) (iii)

**330.** (a) (ii)

(b) (i)

**331.** (a) (i)

(b) (iv)

**332.** (a) (i)

(b) (i)

(c) (iii)

(d) (ii)

**333.** (a) (ii)

(b) (ii)

(c) (iv)

(d) (ii)

**334.** (a) (ii)

(b) (iv)

(c) (i)

**335.** (a) (ii)

(b) (iii)

(c) (iv)

(d) (i)

**336.** (a) (ii)

(b) (iii)

(c) (iii)

(b) (i)

**337.** (a) (iii)

(b) (iv)

(c) (ii)

(d) (ii)

**338.** (a) (iii)

(b) (ii)

(c) (iv)

**339.** (a) (iii)

(b) (ii)

(c) (i)

**340.** (a) (iii)

(b) (iv)

**341.** (a) (iii)

(b) (iv)

(c) (iv)

**342.** (a) (iv)

(b) (iv)

(c) (iv)

**343.** (a) (iii)

(b) (i)

(c) (iii)

**344.** (a) (iv)

(b) (iii)

(c) (i)

(d) (iv)

**345. A.** (a) (i)

(b) (i)

**B.** (a) (ii)

(b) (ii)

**346.** (a) (ii)

(b) (iv)

**347.** (a) (iv)

(b) (iii)

(c) (i)

(d) (ii)

(e) (i)

**348.** (a) (ii)

(b) (i)

(c) (ii)

(d) (iv)

**349.** (a) (iii)

(b) (iv)

**350.** (a) (iv)

(b) (iii)

**351.** (a) (iv)

(b) (ii)

(c) (iv)

**352.** (a) (iii)

(b) (iii)

(c) (i)

(d) (ii)

**353.** (a) (iv)

(b) (iii)

(c) (ii)

(d) (i)

**354.** (a) (i)

(b) (ii)

(c) (iii)

(d) (iv)

(e) (iii)

**355.** (a) (i)

(b) (i)

(c) (i)

**356.** (a) (ii)

(b) (iv)

(c) (iv)

(d) (iv)

(e) (iv)

**357.** (a) (iv)

(b) (ii)

(c) (ii)

(d) (i)

(e) (ii)

**358.** (a) (i)

(b) (iii)

(c) (iv)

(d) (iii)

(e) (ii)

**359.** (a) (ii)

(b) (ii)

(c) (iv)

(d) (ii)

**360.** (a) (iv)

(b) (iii)

(c) (iii)

(d) (iv)

# Analytical Reasoning for CAT

# Solutions

# Analytical Reasoning for CAT

# Solutions

1. **The correct option is (iii). EXPLANATION:**
   Note that $n$ must be of the form $3k + 1$ ($k$ being a natural number) and subsequently the sum of digits of the given number reduced by 1 must be divisible by 3 which only 1438 satisfies.

2. (a) **The correct option is (i). EXPLANATION:**
   Note that a cycle of counting ends after $(2n - 1)$ count at $A_2$ and then again the counting starts in a similar fashion.
   $\therefore$ the count $(2n - 1)$ or its multiple will always come on $A_2$.

   (b) **The correct option is (iv). EXPLANATION:**
   By the some logic as given in part (a), count $100n$ or $50(2n - 1) + 50$ will end on 50th lamppost from $A_1$, i.e., $A_{50}$.

3. (a) **The correct option is (ii). EXPLANATION:**
   Competence can be alternatively seen as the probability of getting things done. Let the probabilities that A, B, C deals with the situation be $p$, $q$ and $r$. Then the probability that B and C deal with the situation together is
   $1 - (1 - q)(1 - r) = q + r - q\,r$ ...(i)
   Now, by the conditions of the given problem,
   $p = q + r - q\,r$ and $q = p + r - p\,r$
   Adding we get $r(2 - p - q) = 0$

$\therefore$ either $r = 0$ or $p + q = 2$

$\because$ $p, q \le 1$ $\therefore$ either $r = 0$ $p = q = 1$.

**(b) The correct option is (iii). EXPLANATION:**

By the condition of the given problem,

$2p = q + r - q\,r$ and $2q = p + r - p\,r$ [using equation (i)]

Subtraction gives $2(p - q) = -(p - q) + (p - q)\,r$

$\Rightarrow p - q = 0$ or $r = 3$. But $r \le 1$

$\therefore p = q$ and $p = r - p\,r \quad \Rightarrow r = \dfrac{p}{1-p}$

Now $r = \dfrac{p}{1-p} > p \quad \Rightarrow$ statement II

Statement III $\Rightarrow \quad r < 2p \quad \Rightarrow \dfrac{p}{1-p} < 2p$

$\Rightarrow 1 < 2 - 2p \Rightarrow p < \dfrac{1}{2}$

Also $r < 1 \Rightarrow \dfrac{p}{1-p} < 1 \Rightarrow p < \dfrac{1}{2} \Rightarrow$ statement III.

**4. (a) The correct option is (iii). EXPLANATION:**

Let $B_i$ (i = 1 to 6) denote boys such that

$B_1$ — — —
$B_2$ — —
$B_3$ — — —
$B_4$ — —
$B_5$ —
$B_6$ —

where blanks signify girlfriends.

Note that there can be 10 boyfriends made by the girls. Now

(i) is not possible since only other four girls can have a boyfriend each but not the sixth one.

(ii) is not possible because if two girls have three boyfriends and one girl has two boyfriends, then only two out of remaining three girls can have a boyfriend since number of boyfriends made is ten.

(iii) is possible since four girls have two boyfriends each and the remaining two girls can have a boyfriend each.

**(b) The correct option is (iii). EXPLANATION:**

(i) is possible because if one girl has five boyfriends, then the other five girls can have one boyfriends each.

(ii) is also possible as two girls can have $B_1$, $B_2$ and $B_3$ as common boyfriends and other four girls can have a boyfriends each.

(iii) is not possible because if three girls have two boyfriends each, then there can be four boyfriends made by other three girls (which is only possible if one more girl has two boyfriends).

**5.** Note that the sequence (in decreasing order of ages of siblings) can be ABCD, CABD, ACBD, ACDB, CADB, CDAB and in terms of M, F (male, female): MMFF, MFMF, MFFM, FFMM, FMFM and FMMF. These can be arranged as possibilities:

MMFF → ABCD, CABD, ACBD, ACDB, CADB
MFMF → ABCD, CABD, ACBD, CDAB
MFFM → ACDB, CADB, CDAB
FFMM → CDAB
FMFM → CADB, ACDB
FMMF → ABCD, CABD, ACBD

**(a) The correct option is (i). EXPLANATION:**
Note that from all given options, only (i) satisfies it.

**(b) The correct option is (i) EXPLANATION:**
Note that from all given options, only (i) satisfies it.

**(c) The correct option is (ii). EXPLANATION:**
Note that from all given options, only (ii) satisfies it.

**6.** The situations just before the number of males and females become equal can be

| Cases | M/F | → M/F | → M/F | → M/F |
|---|---|---|---|---|
| I | $\frac{m+3}{m}$ | $\frac{m+1}{m-1}$ | $\frac{m-2}{m-1}$ | $\frac{m-3}{m-3}$ |
| II | $\frac{m+2}{m}$ | $\frac{m-1}{m}$ | $\frac{m-2}{m-2}$ | |
| III | $\frac{m+1}{m}$ | $\frac{m}{m-2}$ | $\frac{m-3}{m-2}$ | $\frac{m-4}{m-4}$ |

(Note that M, F denote male, female and $\frac{m+3}{m}$ signifies that the number of males is ($m$ + 3) while that of females is $m$ and so on)

∴ the least number of males who went out of the room can be only $n - m +$ (3, 2 or 4)

Also the least number of females who went out of the room can be 2, 3 or 4 only.

For $m = 10$, $n = 40$; 27 men could left the room initially leaving 13 men which will then correspond to case I.

**So the correct options for (a), (b) and (c) are (i), (i) and (iii) respectively.**

7. **The correct option is (i). EXPLANATION:**
   $A_1$ can be married to $A_4$, $A_5$ or $A_6$;
   $A_2$ can be married to $A_5$ or $A_6$ and
   $A_3$ can be married to $A_6$ only.
   ∴ $A_2$ will be married to $A_6$, $A_2$ will be married to $A_5$ and $A_1$ will be married to $A_4$.

8. The couples can be
   ($A_1$, $A_3$), ($A_2$, $A_5$), ($A_4$, $A_6$) or ($A_1$, $A_4$), ($A_2$, $A_5$), ($A_3$, $A_6$) or ($A_1$, $A_4$), ($A_2$, $A_6$), ($A_3$, $A_5$) or ($A_1$, $A_5$), ($A_2$, $A_4$), ($A_3$, $A_6$)

   (a) **The correct option is (i): EXPLANATION:**
   Note that from all given options, only (i) satisfies it.

   (b) **The correct option is (iv). EXPLANATION:**
   All the couples can be specified if it is given that one of the following is a couple: ($A_1$, $A_3$), ($A_1$, $A_5$), ($A_2$, $A_4$), ($A_2$, $A_6$), ($A_3$, $A_5$), ($A_4$, $A_6$) and there will be ambuiguities about other couples if it is given that one of the following is a couple: ($A_1$, $A_4$), ($A_2$, $A_5$), ($A_3$, $A_6$).

   $$\therefore \text{ the required probability } = \frac{6}{3+6} = \frac{2}{3}$$

9. The distribution can be only like

| A | B | C | D |
|---|---|---|---|
| 3 | 2 | 5 | 4 |
| 4 | 3 | 1 | 6 |
| 2 | 5 | 6 | 1 |
| 5 | 4 | 2 | 3 |

(last two rows exchangeable)

or

| A | B | C | D |
|---|---|---|---|
| 3 | 2 | 5 | 4 |
| 4 | 3 | 1 | 6 |
| 6 | 5 | 2 | 1 |
| 1 | 4 | 6 | 3 |

(last two rows exchangeable)

(a) **The correct option is (ii). EXPLANATION:** Self explained from the above chart.

(b) **The correct option is (ii). EXPLANATION:** From above chart, there can be only four required ways.

10\. (a) **The correct option is (iv). EXPLANATION:** The positions of a, b, c, d, after first four processes are respectively

| | | | | | | | | | |
|---|---|---|---|---|---|---|---|---|---|
| | a | | | a | | | | a | |
| b | | c, | c | | d | and | d | | b |
| | d | | | b | | | | c | |

Note that after every three processes, the configuration is restored. Therefore after 99 processes, the configuration remains as original and after next process, position 3 will be occupied by d.

(b) **The correct option is (i). EXPLANATION:** The position of a, b, c, d, after first four processes are respectively.

| | | | | | | | | | | | | |
|---|---|---|---|---|---|---|---|---|---|---|---|---|
| | b | | | d | | | c | | | | a | |
| c | | d, | a | | c, | b | | a | and | d | | b |
| | a | | | b | | | d | | | | c | |

It is evident that after every four processes, the original configuration is restored. Therefore after 100 processes, position 1 will be occupied by a.

(c) **The correct option is (ii). EXPLANATION:** After every subprocess, the configurations will be respectively

| | | | | | | | | | | | | | | |
|---|---|---|---|---|---|---|---|---|---|---|---|---|---|---|
| | b | | | b | | | b | | | b | | | c | |
| d | | a, | d | | c, | a | | c, | c | | a, | b | | a, |
| | c | | | a | | | d | | | d | | | d | |

| | | | | | | | | | |
|---|---|---|---|---|---|---|---|---|---|
| | d | | | d | | | | d | |
| b | | a, | b | | c | and | c | | b |
| | c | | | a | | | | a | |

Therefore the whole process is equivalent to the exchange of letters at first and third positions.

**11. (a) The correct option is (iv). EXPLANATION:**

Let us start from a, i.e., consider a to be the required alphabet. Then the reverse sequence in which it exchanged its place would be g e i h b c d f a.

If we consider b to be required alphabet, then corresponding reverse sequence would be c d f a g e i h b.

Therefore the required alphabet cannot be determined.

**(b) The correct option is (iii). EXPLANATION:**

Note the cyclic sequence we got in part (a), i.e., a f d c b h i e g in which any letter can start exchanging its position in the cyclic sequence as written. If e exchanged its position after four exchanges, then after five, six and seven exchanges, it will be g, a and f respectively.

**12.** Let $p$th row and $q$th column get same numbering by both the pupils. Then

$(p - 1)\ m + q = (q - 1)\ n + p$ ...(i)

**(a) The correct option is (iv). EXPLANATION:**

Putting $m = 21$ and $n = 41$ in (i), we have

$(p - 1)\ 21 + q = (q - 1)\ 41 + p$

$\Rightarrow 40q - 20p = 20$

$\Rightarrow 2q - p = 1$ ...(ii)

Now $p \leq 41$ and $q \leq 21$

$\therefore$ the number of distinct values of $(p, q)$ satisfying (ii) will be 21.

**(b) The correct option is (i). EXPLANATION:**

Putting $m = 20$ and $n = 40$ in (i), we have

$(p - 1)\ 20 + q = (q - 1)\ 40 + p$

$\Rightarrow 39q - 19p = 20$

$\Rightarrow 19\ (q - p) + 20q = 20$

$\Rightarrow 20\ (q - 1) = 19\ (p - q)$

which is only possible when $q - 1 = 0$ and $p = q = 1$

or $q - 1 = 19$ and $p - q = 20$

i.e., $q = 20$ and $p = 40$

$\therefore$ only two cases are possible.

**(c) The correct option is (ii) EXPLANATION:**

Putting $m = n$ in (i) and using the fact that 17th block for two kinds of numbering is same, we get

$(p - 1)\ m + q = (q - 1)\ m + p = 7$ for a paritcular value of $(p, q)$. Therefore $(p - q)\ m = p - q$, i.e. $p = q$ since $m > 1$ and consequently we have $(p - 1)\ m + p = 17$

$$\Rightarrow p = \frac{17+m}{1+m}$$

$\therefore$ $m = 7$ and 15 are only valid for the integeral value of $p$.

**13.** In one day, the boss can do, with one secreatary absent,

$\frac{1}{2}\left(\frac{1}{6}, \frac{1}{4}, \frac{1}{3}, \frac{1}{2}\right)$ part of the job $\equiv \frac{1}{12}, \frac{1}{8}, \frac{1}{6}, \frac{1}{4} \equiv$

$\frac{2}{24}, \frac{3}{24}, \frac{4}{24}, \frac{6}{24}$

Now for job to be finished,

$$\frac{2w+3x+4y+6z}{24} = 1 \Rightarrow 2w + 3x + 4y + 6z = 24 \qquad \text{...(i)}$$

where $w, x, y, z$ are number of days for which secretaries A, B, C, D remain absent respectively.

**(a) The correct option is (ii). EXPLANATION:**
From (i), $x$ cannot be odd as others are even.

**(b) The correct option is (ii). EXPLANATION:**
Note that if each secretary remained absent for at least one day, then the least value of $w, x, y, z$ must be 1. Also as $x$ cannot be odd therefore its least value will be 2. The possible values of $(w, x, y, z)$ can be (4, 2, 1, 1); (2, 2, 2, 1); (1, 4, 1, 1) or (1, 2, 1, 2).
Therefore the boss can finish work in 6, 7 or 8 days.

**(c) The correct option is (iv). EXPLANATION:**
For the given condition to satisfy, one of $w, x, y, z$ must be zero and sum of other three must be equal to 6. But there can be more than one solution as
$w = 1, \quad x = 0, \quad y = 4$ and $z = 1$ or
$w = 0, \quad x = 2, \quad y = 3$ and $z = 1$.

**14.** Let (A, B), (A, C), (A, D), (B, C), (B, D) and (C, D) shared $x_1, x_2, x_3, x_4, x_5$ and $x_6$ apples respectively between them. Then

$x_1 + x_2 + x_3 = 26$

$x_1 + x_4 + x_5 = 22$

$x_2 + x_4 + x_6 = 18$

$x_3 + x_5 + x_6 = 14$

**(a) The correct option is (iii). EXPLANATION:**
Note that 26 + 14 = 22 + 18
$\Rightarrow x_1 + x_2 + x_3 + x_3 + x_5 + x_6 = x_1 + x_4 + x_5 + x_2 + x_4 + x_6$
$\Rightarrow 2x_3 = 2x_4 \quad \Rightarrow x_3 = x_4$

**(b) The correct option is (i). EXPLANATION:**
Note that $22 + 18 + 14 - 26 = 2\,(x_4 + x_5 + x_6)$
$\Rightarrow 18 = 2\,(x_4 + x_5 + x_6)$
$\Rightarrow x_4 + x_5 + x_6 = 9$

**15.** Let $c_1A_1 + c_2A_2 + c_3A_3 + c_4A_4 = 0$
where $c_1, c_2, c_3, c_4$ are constants to be determined.
From the given data,
$c_1 + 2c_2 + 3c_3 + 4c_4 = 0$ and ...(i)
$4c_1 + 5c_2 + 6c_3 + 8c_4 = 0$ and ...(ii)
(ii) $-2 \times$ (i) yields
$2c_1 + c_2 = 0$ and ...(iii)
(ii) − (i) yields
$3(c_1 + c_2 + c_3) + 4c_4 = 0$
$\Rightarrow 3(-c_1 + c_3) + 4c_4 = 0$ [Using (iii)] ...(iv)

$\therefore$ putting the values of $c_2$ and $c_4$ from (iii) and (iv) in original equation, we have

$$c_1A_1 - 2c_1A_2 + c_3A_3 - \frac{3}{4}(c_3 - c_1)A_4 = 0$$
$\Rightarrow 4c_1A_1 - 8c_1A_2 + 4c_3A_3 - 3c_3A_4 + 3c_1A_4 = 0$
$\Rightarrow c_1(3A_4 + 4A_1 - 8A_2) + c_3(4A_3 - 3A_4) = 0$ ...(v)

**(a) The correct option is (i) EXPLANATION:**
$\because 4A_3 = 3A_4 \therefore 3A_4 + 4A_1 - 8A_2 = 0 \Rightarrow A_1 = 1$

**(b) The correct option is (iii) EXPLANATION:**
For $A_3 = A_4 = 0$, $4A_1 = 8A_2 \Rightarrow A_1 = 2A_2$

**(c) The correct option is (i) EXPLANATION:**
The case is possible only when $4A_1 - 8A_2 = -4A_3$
$\Rightarrow A_3 = 2A_2 - A_1$.

**16.** Let $n$ be the least number, then
$S = n + n + 1 + \ldots\ n + 8 +$ number in the centre
$= 9n + 36 +$ number in the middle.
$\therefore 10n + 36 \le S \le 10n + 44$

**(a) The correct option is (iii). EXPLANATION:**

$\because$ $n$ is an integer, $\therefore$ it has to be equal to 41 if $446 \leq S \leq 454$.

**(b) The correct option is (ii). EXPLANATION:**

$10n + 36 \leq S \leq 10n + 44$

$\Rightarrow 10(n + 3) + 6 \leq S \leq 10(n + 4)$

$\therefore$ S cannot be of the form $10k + 5$

**17. (a) The correct option is (iii). EXPLANATION:**

The distribution of money can be shown as below:

| $A_1$ | $A_2$ | $A_3$ | $A_4$ |
|---|---|---|---|
| 1 | $k$ | $k$ | $k$ |
| $k'$ | $m$ | $k'$ | $k'$ |

$\because$ the total amount remains constant

$\therefore 1 + 3k = m + 3k'$

$\Rightarrow m = 1 + 3(k - k')$

$\therefore$ $m$ can equal to 1, 4, 7 ...

**(b) The correct option is (iv). EXPLANATION:**

The distribution of money can be shown as below:

| $A_1$ | $A_2$ | $A_3$ | $A_4$ | Total amount |
|---|---|---|---|---|
| 0 | $m_1$ | $m_1$ | $m_1$ | $= 3m_1$ |
| $m_2$ | 3 | $m_2$ | $m_2$ | $= 3(m_2 + 1)$ |
| $m_3$ | $m_3$ | 6 | $m_3$ | $= 3(m_3 + 2)$ |
| $m_4$ | $m_4$ | $m_4$ | 9 | $= 3(m_4 + 3)$ |

$\because$ $A_4$ can retain 9 coins $\quad\therefore m_3 > 9$ and

$\because$ $A_3$ can retain 6 coins $\quad\therefore m_4 > 6$

$\therefore$ the least number of coins $= 3(m_3 + 2)$

$= 3 \cdot 12$ ($\because$ the least value of $m_3$ is 10)

$= 36$

**(c) The correct option is (iii). EXPLANATION:**

The initial distribution of money is shown as below:

| $A_1$ | $A_2$ | $A_3$ | $A_4$ | Total amount |
|---|---|---|---|---|
| $a$ | $a + 3$ | $a + 6$ | $a + 9$ | $4a + 18$ |

For $a$ to be distributed among $A_2$, $A_3$ and $A_4$, minimum value of $a = 9$. Similarly, when

$A_2$ distributes, minimum value of $a = 12$

$A_3$ distributes, minimum value of $a = 15$

$A_4$ distributes, minimum value of $a = 9$

∴ the least value of a should be 15 as each person is able to distribute his money by the conditions given in the problem.

**18. The correct option (ii). EXPLANATION:**
$S_1 \equiv \{x + b + \alpha,\quad \beta + y + c,\quad a + \gamma + z\} \equiv \{p_1, p_2, p_3\}$ say.
$S_2 \equiv \{x + \beta + a,\quad b + y + \gamma,\quad \alpha + c + z\} \equiv \{q_1, q_2, q_3\}$ say.
Now $p_1 + p_2 + p_3 = q_1 + q_2 + q_3$.
If two of $p$'s are equal to two of $q$'s, then the third ones must be equal.

**19.** The possible arrangements are
$(X_1, X_3)$, $(X_2, X_5)$, $(X_4, X_6)$,

| | $X_1$ | $X_2$ | $X_3$ |
|---|---|---|---|
| | $X_4$ | $X_6$ | $X_5$ |
| or | $X_4$ | $X_5$ | $X_6$ |
| | $X_5$ | $X_4$ | $X_6$ |
| | $X_6$ | $X_4$ | $X_5$ |

**(a) The correct option is (ii). EXPLANATION:**
From the various possible arrangements shown above, there are two possible arrangements for $(X_1, X_4)$.

**(b) The correct option is (ii). EXPLANATION:**
If the pairs $(X_1, X_3)$, $(X_1, X_5)$, $(X_1, X_6)$, $(X_2, X_6)$ or $(X_4, X_6)$ are given, then all other pairs can be determined, while if the pairs $(X_1, X_4)$, $(X_2, X_4)$, $(X_2, X_5)$, $(X_3, X_5)$ or $(X_3, X_6)$ are given, then all other pairs cannot be determined. Therefore, required probability

$$= \frac{\text{Total number of favourable cases}}{\text{Total number of possible cases}} = \frac{5}{10}$$

**20.** Cases which are not possible: $(X_1, X_2)$; $(X_1, X_3)$; $(X_1, X_5)$; $(X_1, X_6)$; $(X_2, X_3)$; $(X_2, X_4)$; $(X_2, X_5)$; $(X_3, X_4)$; $(X_3, X_6)$; $(X_4, X_6)$ and $(X_5, X_6)$.

Cases which can be possible: $(X_1, X_4)$; $(X_2, X_6)$ or $(X_3, X_5)$

**So the correct options for (a) and (b) are (iv) and (iii) respectively.**

21. **The correct option is (iv). EXPLANATION:**
We have
— — — $2X_1$ — $2X_2$ — $2X_3$
where blanks denote the positions of the race. Now $X_2$, $X_1$ cannot be at second or third position (as the speed of each person is less than twice of that of the person just behind him)
$\therefore$ we may have
$X_1\ X_2\ X_4\ X_3\ X_5$ or $X_1\ X_4\ X_2\ X_3\ X_5$
$\therefore$ $X_1$ may not be just behind $X_2$ and
$X_2$ may not be just behind $X_3$.

22. $5a_1 + 6a_2 + 10a_3 = 5a_4 + 6a_5 + 10a_6$
$\Rightarrow$ $5(a_1 - a_4) + 6(a_2 - a_5) + 10(a_3 - a_6) = 0.$
$\because$ all the differences are intergers $\therefore$ $a_2 - a_5 = \pm 5$
and $a_1 - a_4$ must be even, i.e. $a_1 - a_4 = \pm 2$ or $\pm 4$.
$\because$ the difference between extreme terms is 5
$\therefore$ $(a_2, a_5)$ are exteme terms. Also the difference between any other terms must be less than 4. $\therefore$ $a_1 - a_4 = \pm 4$ is rejected. For $a_1 - a_4 = \pm 2$
$\pm 10 \pm 30 + 10\ (a_3 - a_6) = 0$
$\Rightarrow$ $a_3 - a_6 = \pm 2$ or $\pm$ 4
But $a_3 - a_6 = \pm 4$ is not possible
$\therefore$ $a_3 - a_6 = \pm 2$ and hence middle terms cannot be determined.
**So the correct options for (a) and (b) are (ii) and (iv) respectively.**

23. **The correct option is (i). EXPLANATION:**
Let $m$, $n$ be the number of male delegates from guest and host countries respectively. Then
$m(10 - n) + n(8 - m) = 40$
$m(10 - 2n) + 8n = 40$
$\Rightarrow$ $2m(5 - n) = 8(5 - n)$
$\therefore$ either $n = 5$ or $m = 4$ which implies that delegates of one of the country have equal number of males and females.

24. **The correct option is (ii). EXPLANATION:**
Let the original sitting arrangement be A B C, then after first exchange of seats, it can be B C A or C A B. If any two of

them exchange their places, then one of them will be at his original position.

25. (a) **The correct option is (iv). EXPLANATION:**
The positions of ball can be given sequentially as
C — — C — — C — — C — — C — — C — — C
where 12 blanks are to be filled by A, B and D.
∴ D would have held the ball for 12 – (3 + 5) = 4 times.

(b) **The correct option is (iii). EXPLANATION:**
The positions of ball can be given sequentially as
C — — C — — C — — C — — C — — C — — CD
So D would have held the ball 12 – 8 + 1 = 5 times.

(c) **The correct option is (iii). EXPLANATION:**
The positions of ball can be given sequentially as
CD — — D — — D — — D — — D — — D — — D — — D
where 14 blanks are to be filled by 3A, 5B and 6C.
∴ the maximum number of times D would have held the ball is 8.

26. (a) **The correct option is (iv). EXPLANATION:**
Let after *n*th process their shares are given as:

| A | B | C | D |
|---|---|---|---|
| $x_n$ | $x'_n$ | $x''_n$ | $x''_n$ |

where $x_n + x'_n + x''_n + x''_n = 100$

After $(n + 1)$th process, share of A will be

$$\frac{x'_n + x''_n + x''_n}{3}, \text{ i.e. } \frac{100 - x_n}{3}$$

$$\therefore x_{n+1} = \frac{100 - x_n}{3} \text{ and}$$

$$x_1 = \frac{100 - 10}{3} = 30, \quad x_2 = \frac{70}{3} = 23.3$$

$$x_3 = \frac{86.7}{3} = 28.9 \simeq 29, \quad x_4 = \frac{71}{3} \simeq 23.7$$

$$x_5 = \frac{86.7}{3} = 28.8 \simeq 29$$

**(b) The correct option is (i). EXPLANATION:**
For large number of times,
$x'''_n = x'''_{n+1}$

$$\therefore x'''_n = \frac{100 - x'''_n}{3}$$

$\Rightarrow 4x'''_n = 100$
$\Rightarrow x'''_n = 25$

**27. The correct option is (i). EXPLANATION:**
The boy spends same amount $x, x, x, \ldots$ every day.
Then on 30th day he spends 100%,

on 29th day he spends $\frac{1}{2} \cdot 100\%$ (= 50%) and so on.

As on $(30 - n)$th day he spends $\frac{1}{n+1} \times 100\%$

$\therefore$ one of the value of $x_1, \ldots\ldots x_{30}$ can be 4 only (for $n = 24$).

**28. (a) The correct option is (ii). EXPLANATION:**
Let the cost of A, B and C be $a$, $b$ and $c$ respectively.
Then $a^2 = b^2 + 57 = c^2 + 10x$
$\Rightarrow a^2 - b^2 = 57 = 19 \cdot 3$
$\therefore a + b = 19$ and $a - b = 3$ or
$a + b = 57$ and $a - b = 1$
$\Rightarrow (a = 11, b = 8)$ or $(a = 29, b = 28)$
If $a = 23$, then $10x = (29 - c)(29 + c)$
Checking $c = 21 \Rightarrow x = 40$, not valid
If $a = 11$, then $10x = (11 - c)(11 + c)$
Checking $c = 1$, $x = 12$, not valid
$c = 9$, $x = 4$ which is valid.

**(b) The correct option is (i). EXPLANATION:**
Now $b = 8$ and $c = 9$. $\therefore$ their difference is 1.

**29.** Note that only exclusive pairs are
$(F_5, F_6) \rightarrow$ deficient in vitamin A,
$(F_2, F_3) \rightarrow$ deficient in vitamin B and
$(F_1, F_7) \rightarrow$ deficient in vitamin C.
$\therefore F_4$ will be deficient in vitamin D.

**So the correct options for (a), (b) and (c) are (iii), (ii) and (ii) respectively.**

**30.** The different ways in which foods of total calories 1000 kcal can be bought are A + 2C, 2B + C, 2A + 2B and 3A + C.

Note that $\overline{A+2C} + \overline{2A+2B} = \overline{2B+C} + \overline{3A+C}$

Also 41 + 29 = 32 + 38

$\because$ $\overline{2A+2B}$ is an integer $\therefore$ it can be equal to 32 or 38.

CASE I. 2A + 2B = 32

Then A + 2C = 38 and

$$\left\{\begin{array}{l}2B+C=29\\3A+C=41\end{array}\right. \text{ or } \left.\begin{array}{l}2B+C=41\\3A+C=29\end{array}\right\}$$

$$\Rightarrow \left.\begin{array}{l}2C-B=22\\2B+C=29\end{array}\right\} \text{ or } \left.\begin{array}{l}2C-B=22\\2B+C=41\end{array}\right\}$$

RJECTED as B is not an integer

$\Rightarrow$ C = 17, B = 12 and A = 4 RETAINED

CASE II. 2A + 2B = 38

Then A + 2C = 32 and

$$\left\{\begin{array}{l}2B+C=29\\3A+C=41\end{array}\right. \text{ or } \left.\begin{array}{l}2B+C=41\\3A+C=29\end{array}\right\}$$

$$\Rightarrow \left\{\begin{array}{l}2C-B=13\\2B+C=29\end{array}\right. \text{ or } \left.\begin{array}{l}2C-B=13\\2B+C=41\end{array}\right\}$$

C = 11, B = 9 and A = 10 RETAINED

RJECTED as B is not an integer

**So the correct options for (a) and (b) are (iii).**

**31.** Let the cost of articles P, Q, R be $x$, $y$ and $z$ respectively, and the money A, B, C initially had be $a$, $b$, $c$ respectively. Then

$$\frac{x}{4}+\frac{y}{3}+\frac{2z}{5}=a, \frac{x}{4}+\frac{y}{2}+\frac{z}{5}=b \text{ and } \frac{x}{2}+\frac{y}{6}+\frac{2z}{5}=c.$$

Also, $a$, $b$, $c$ = 90, 100, 120. (may not be in order.)

Now $\frac{x}{4}-\frac{y}{6}=c-a$

$$\frac{5}{6}y = 2b - c \qquad \Rightarrow y = \frac{6}{5}(2b - c)$$

$$\text{and } \frac{x}{4} = c - a + \frac{(2b-c)}{5} \qquad \Rightarrow x = \frac{4}{5}(4c - 5a + 2b)$$

For $x$ to be positive, $c$ has to 120.
For $a = 100$, $b = 90$,

$$x = \frac{4}{5}(480 - 500 + 180) \text{ or } \frac{4}{5}(480 - 500 + 180)$$

$$= 128 \text{ or } 120$$

Subsequently, $y = \frac{6}{5}(180 - 120)$ or $\frac{6}{5}(200 - 120)$

$\Rightarrow$ $y = 72$ or $96$
and $z = 110$ or $94$.

$\therefore$ (P, Q, R) $\equiv$ (128, 72, 110) or (120, 96, 94) according as (A, B, C) $\equiv$ (100, 90, 120) or (90, 100, 120).

**So the correct options for (a), (b), (c), (d) and (e) are (iv), (iii), (iv), (iv) and (i) respectively.**

**32.** Note that if $x$ be the price of most expensive article, then the prices of articles are $x$, $x - 10$, $x - 20$ and $x - 30$.
If P, Q, R, S also denote the money they respectively have, then P = $4x - 60$.
Note that the difference between the amount held by any two of them is either 50, 100 or 150 only.

$\therefore$ R, S = $\overline{3(x-30)} + \overline{x-20}$, $3\overline{x} + \overline{x-10}$ or vice versa.

The fourth amount must be $4x - 160$ which must be Q.

CASE I. If R = $\overline{3(x-30)} + \overline{x-20}$, then

Q = $\overline{x} + \overline{x-20} = 4x - 160$

$\Rightarrow x = 70$ and
(A, B, C, D) $\equiv$ (60, 40, 70, 50)

CASE II. If S = $\overline{3(x-30)} + \overline{x-20}$, then

Q = $x - 30 + x - 10 = 4x - 160$

$\Rightarrow x = 60$ and
(A, B, C, D) $\equiv$ (40, 60, 30, 50)

**So the correct options for (a), (b), (c), (d) and (e) are(ii), (iv), (ii), (i) and (i) respectively.**

**33. (a) The correct option is (ii). EXPLANATION:**
The car could have covered only 99 miles by going along the path A B C A again and again.
$\therefore$ it would have passed B just once to cover 100 miles as $3 \times 32 + 4 = 100$.

**(b) The correct option is (ii). EXPLANATION:**
First 96 miles can be travelled along ABCA while the last five miles can be travelled as

A C B D C A

**(c) The correct option is (i). EXPLANATION:**
The car could have gone for $i$ =
1 as $(A\ B\ C\ A\ \dots\ A)_{30\text{ miles}} \rightarrow B$
2 as $(A\ C\ B\ A\ \dots\ A)_{30\text{ miles}} \rightarrow CB$
So it may not pass through D.

**34.** The marks of topper and second topper will be E + 30 and D + 20 respectively while the marks of student getting the least number will be C – 20 or A – 30.

Case I. Let A = E + 30, then A will be the topper and E will be the one getting the least marks. Also $C - 20 \neq D$ $\therefore$ D + 20 = B and the ranks of the students will be A B C D E or A B D C E (rejected as A – E = 30 and B – D = 20, C – E = 20)

Case II. Let A = D + 20, then

— A C D — (30), not possible.

**The correct options for (a), (b), (c) and (d) are (i).**

**35. A. (a) The correct option is (ii). EXPLANATION:**
Note that (A, B, C, F) are married to persons of the group (D, E, G, H). $\because$ each column has exclusively A, B, C or F $\therefore$ each of them will have a couple. Also all couples may be in a row.

**(b) The correct option is (iv). EXPLANATION:**
The possible couples can be
(F, H), (B, E), (C, G) or (F, G), (B, E), (C, H) or (F, E), (B, H), (C, G).

**B.** Note that only exclusive pairs satisfying the given relation are (A, E), (B, D), (C, G) and (F, H).

**So the correct options for (a), (b) and (c) are (ii), (i) and (iii) respectively.**

**C. (a) The correct option is (iv). EXPLANATION:**

Note that if BH is a couple, then CE has to be a couple. Now either AG or FH has to be a couple which is not possible.

**(b) The correct option is (iii). EXPLANATION:**

When AD is a couple, then either CE or CH can be a couple. But if CE is a couple, then either BH and FH has to be a couple, an impossible case, or BE and FG has to be a couple which is again an impossible case.

If CH is a couple, then other couples can be BE and FG.

**(c) The correct option is (ii). EXPLANATION:**

When AE is a couple, then GF, BH and CD cannot be couples. G can be married to B or C. If BG is a couple, then either CD or FG has to be a couple which is not possible. If GC is a couple, then other couples will be BD and FH.

**36.** We can have the following arrangements:

| | | |
|---|---|---|
| First Group: | (A, D), (B, F), (C, E) | |
| Third Group: | (A, B), (C, D), (E, F) | |
| Second Group: | (A, F), (B, C), (D, E) | ✓ |
| | (A, F), (B, E), (C, D) | × |
| | (A, C), (B, D), (E, F) | × |
| | (A, C), (B, E), (D, F) | ✓ |
| | (A, E), (B, C), (D, F) | ✓ |
| | (A, E), (B, D), (C, F) | ✓ |

**So the correct options for (a), (b) and (c) are (i), (ii) and (ii) respectively.**

**37. A.** Let A, B, C, D, E be P, Q, R, S, T (not in order). Let P, Q, R, S, T have initially the coins of Rs 1, Rs 2, Rs 3, Rs 4 and Rs 5 respectively. Then

| | P | Q | R | S | T |
|---|---|---|---|---|---|
| Initial: | 1 | 2 | 3 | 4 | 5 |
| First Exchange: | 5 | 1 | 2 | 3 | 4 |
| Second Exchange: | 4 | 5 | 1 | 2 | 3 |
| Third Exchange: | 3 | 4 | 5 | 1 | 2 |
| Fourth Exchange: | 2 | 3 | 4 | 5 | 1 |
| Fifth Exchange: | 1 | 2 | 3 | 4 | 5 |

Note that R having Rs 1 after second exchange has Rs 3 initially.
The holding of persons get repeated after five times.
Also the cyclic sequence 1-2-3-4-5-1 follows the cyclic sequence P-Q-R-S-T-P.

**So the correct options for (a), (b) and (c) are (ii), (i) and (i) respectively.**

**B.** In a way similar to as done in part (A), we have

| | P | Q | R | S | T |
|---|---|---|---|---|---|
| Initial: | 1 | 2 | 3 | 4 | 5 |
| First Exchange: | 1 | 5 | 2 | 3 | 4 |
| Second Exchange: | 1 | 4 | 5 | 2 | 3 |
| Third Exchange: | 1 | 3 | 4 | 5 | 2 |
| Fourth Exchange: | 1 | 2 | 3 | 4 | 5 |

From above table the difference between holdings of S and T for first three exchanges is Rs 1 (treating the initial holding also as an exchange as the processes are cyclic)
The difference between their holdings for next successive exchange is Rs 3.
Similarly the difference between holdings of Q and S remains same at Rs 2.

**So the correct options for (a) and (b) are (iii) and (ii) respectively.**

**38.** Note that

| | | | | | |
|---|---|---|---|---|---|
| Initial: | v | w | x | y | z |
| After First Exchange: | z | v | w | x | y |
| After Second Exchange: | y | z | v | w | x |

Noting this sequence, we will have

| | A | B | C | D | E |
|---|---|---|---|---|---|
| Initial: | 1 | 2 | 3 | 4 | 5 |
| After First Exchange: | 2 | 3 | 4 | 5 | 1 |
| After Second Exchange: | 3 | 4 | 5 | 1 | 2 |

$\therefore$ $K_5 = 2$

Note that the cyclic sequences of 1-2-3-4-5-1 as well as z-y-x-w-v-z are maintained.

$\therefore$ when v = 3, x = 1 and
when y =, w = 1

**So the correct options for (a), (b) and (c) are (i).**

**39.** Let

| | Rs 1 | Rs 2 | Rs 3 | |
|---|---|---|---|---|
| A | $x_1$ | $x_2$ | $x_3$ | $= n$ |
| B | $y_1$ | $y_2$ | $y_3$ | $= n$ |
| C | $z_1$ | $z_2$ | $z_3$ | $= n$ |
| | $n$ | $n$ | $n$ | |

$\therefore$ we have

$$\left.\begin{array}{l} x_1 + y_1 + z_1 = n \\ x_2 + y_2 + z_2 = n \\ x_3 + y_3 + z_3 = n \end{array}\right\} \qquad \left.\begin{array}{l} x_1 + x_2 + x_3 = n \\ y_1 + y_2 + y_3 = n \\ z_1 + z_2 + z_3 = n \end{array}\right\}$$

$$\text{and} \left\{\begin{array}{l} x_1 + 2x_2 + 3x_3 = 20 \\ y_1 + 2y_2 + 3y_3 = 30 \\ z_1 + 2z_2 + 3z_3 = 40 \end{array}\right.$$

Adding the third set of equations, we get

$$n + 2n + 3n = 90$$

$\Rightarrow$ $6n = 90 \Rightarrow n = 15.$

Now note that

$$y_1 + 2y_2 + 3y_3 = 30 = 2(y_1 + y_2 + y_3)$$

$\Rightarrow$ $y_1 + 3y_3 = 2y_1 + 2y_3$

$\Rightarrow$ $y_1 = y_3$

Also from $x_1 + x_2 + x_3 = n = 15$ and

$$x_1 + 2x_2 + 3x_3 = 20,$$

$x_1 - x_3 = 15 \times 2 - 20 = 10$

$\Rightarrow x_1 = 10 + x_3$

$\therefore x_1 \geq 10$

**So the correct options for (a), (b) and (c) are (ii), (i) and (iii) respectively.**

**40.** Note that at three times.

$A_1$ ate food of Rs 100, Rs 200, Rs 200;
$A_2$ ate food of Rs 100, Rs 100, Rs 100;
$A_3$ ate food of Rs 200, Rs 200, Rs 200 and
$A_4$ ate food of Rs 100, Rs 100, Rs 200.

$\because$ the bills paid by them are Rs 300, Rs 400, Rs 500 and Rs 600 respectively, we can have

| $A_1$ | $A_2$ | $A_3$ | $A_4$ | Total Bill | |
|---|---|---|---|---|---|
| 100 | 100 | – | 100 | 300 | ($A_1$) |
| 200 | – | 200 | 200 | 600 | ($A_4$) |
| 200 | 100 | 200 | – | 500 | ($A_3$) |
| – | 100 | 200 | 100 | 400 | ($A_2$) |

**So the correct options for (a), (b) and (c) are (iii), (i) and (i) respectively.**

**41.** We can have, after some deliberation,

$$\left.\begin{array}{ccc} n & n+2 & 0 \\ n & 2 & n \\ 2n & 2 & 0 \\ 2n & 0 & 2 \end{array}\right] \text{4 processes}$$

$$\left.\begin{array}{ccc} n-2 & n+2 & 2 \\ n-2 & 4 & n \\ 2n-2 & 4 & 0 \\ 2n-2 & 0 & 4 \end{array}\right] \text{4 processes}$$

(Note that after every 4 processes, C hold 2 litres extra)

$$\begin{array}{ccc} \vdots & \vdots & \vdots \\ n+3 & 0 & n-1 \end{array} \rightarrow \text{upto this, total number of}$$

$$\text{processes} = 4\left(\frac{n-1}{2}\right) = 2(n-1)$$

$$\left.\begin{array}{ccc} 1 & n+2 & n-1 \\ 1 & n+1 & n \\ n+1 & n+1 & 0 \end{array}\right]$$

**So that correct options for (a), (b) and (c) are (ii), (iv) and (iii) respectively.**

**42.** Let us denote

$$\begin{vmatrix} 0 & a & a \\ a & 0 & a \\ a & a & 0 \end{vmatrix} \text{ as } a\begin{vmatrix} 0 & 1 & 1 \\ 1 & 0 & 1 \\ 1 & 1 & 0 \end{vmatrix}$$

Then after first and second processes,

$$a\begin{vmatrix} 0 & 1 & 1 \\ 1 & 0 & 1 \\ 1 & 1 & 0 \end{vmatrix} \to a^2 \begin{vmatrix} -1 & 1 & 1 \\ 1 & -1 & 1 \\ 1 & 1 & -1 \end{vmatrix} \to 2a^4 \begin{vmatrix} 0 & 1 & 1 \\ 1 & 0 & 1 \\ 1 & 1 & 0 \end{vmatrix}$$

$\therefore$ if $a = 1$, then $b = 2$ after two processes.

Also for $a = 1$, $b$ can be equal to 2, 32, ...

Now note that if $x_{n-1}$ and $x_n$ be two values of $b$ after the execution of $2(n-1)$ and $2n$ processes, then

$x_n = 2x_{n-1}^4$ and sequentially

$$x_{n-1} = 2x_{n-2}^4$$

$$\vdots \qquad \vdots$$

$$x_1 = 2a^4$$

$$\therefore x_n = 2\cdot(2)^{41}\cdot(2)^{42} \dots (2)^{4^{n-1}}(a)^{4^n}$$

$$\Rightarrow x_n = 2^{(1+4+4^2+\dots 4^{n-1})}\cdot a^{4^n}$$

$$\Rightarrow x_n = (2)^{(4^n-1)/3}\cdot(a)^{4^n}$$

$$\therefore \text{ for } a = 1, \quad x_n = 2^{\left(\frac{4^n-1}{3}\right)}$$

$$\text{and for } a = 2,\ x_n = 2^{\left(\frac{4^n-1}{3}\right)+4^n} = 2^{\left(\frac{4^{n+1}-1}{3}\right)}$$

**So the correct options for (a), (b), (c) and (d) are (ii), (iv), (i) and (ii) respectively.**

**43.** Let, A, B, C be three such persons. Then we can have three cases:

Case I: A, B, C either all lie or all speak truth.
Case II: A, B lie and C speaks truth.
Case III: A, B speak truth and C lies.

We can construct a table as:

| **Cases** | | $S_1$: Do you both speak truth? | | $S_2$: Do you both lie? | |
|---|---|---|---|---|---|
| I | AB | Yes | Yes | No | No |
| | BC | Yes | Yes | No | No |
| | CA | Yes | Yes | No | No |
| II | AB | Yes | Yes | No | No |
| | BC | Yes | No | Yes | No |
| | CA | No | Yes | No | Yes |
| III | AB | Yes | Yes | No | No |
| | BC | No | Yes | No | Yes |
| | CA | Yes | No | Yes | No |

**So the correct options for (a), (b) and (c) are (iii), (iii) and (iv) respectively.**

**44.** Note that if a particular person speaks truth to two persons, then it implies that he speaks lie to other two persons. We can have four cases:

I. AB, AD speak truth to each other. Then

| Truth | Lie |
|---|---|
| AB, AD, CB, EC, ED | AC, AE, BD, BE, CD |

II. AB, AE speak truth to each other. Then

| Truth | Lie |
|---|---|
| AB, AE, CB, CD, DE | AC, AD, BD, BE, CE |

III. AC, AD speak truth to each other. Then

| Truth | Lie |
|---|---|
| AC, AD, BE, BD, CE | AB, AE, BC, DC, DE |

IV. AC, AE speak truth to each other. Then

| Truth | Lie |
|---|---|
| AC, AE, BD, BE, CD | AD, AB, CB, EC, ED |

**So the correct options for (a), (b), (c) and (d) are (iii), (i), (ii) and (ii) respectively.**

**45.** Let

| | A | B | C | D |
|---|---|---|---|---|
| Initial Amount: | $p$ | $q$ | $r$ | $s$ |

Note that the total amount with them is Rs 180.

Then

$$q + \frac{q\,p}{p+q+r+s} = 45 \text{ and likewise.}$$

$$\therefore \quad \frac{q}{45} = \frac{r}{60} = \frac{s}{75} \Rightarrow \frac{q}{3} = \frac{r}{4} = \frac{s}{5} = x, \text{ say}$$

Then the amount with A, B, C and D will be $12(15 - x)$, $3x$, $4x$ and $5x$ respectively.

Now if B can split his amount likewise, then A, C and D will have respectively

$$12(15 - x) + \frac{12(15-x)3x}{180}, \text{ i.e. } 12(15 - x) + \frac{(15-x)x}{5},$$

$$4x + \frac{3x \cdot 4x}{180}, \quad \text{i.e. } 4x + \frac{x^2}{15} \text{ and}$$

$$5x + \frac{3x \cdot 5x}{180}, \quad \text{i.e. } 5x + \frac{x^2}{12}.$$

Note that $x$ has to be divisible by 2, 3 and 5.

$\because x < 15 \qquad \therefore$ no value of $x$ is possible.

If C can split his money likewise, then

A, B and D will have respectively

$$12(15 - x) + \frac{12(15-x)4x}{180}, \text{ i.e. } 12(15 - x) + \frac{4(15-x)x}{15},$$

$$3x + \frac{3x \cdot 4x}{180}, \text{ i.e. } 3x + \frac{x^2}{15} \text{ and}$$

$$5x + \frac{5x \cdot 4x}{180}, \text{ i.e. } 5x + \frac{x^2}{9}.$$

Note that $x$ must be divisible by 3 and 5. $\because x < 15$.

$\therefore$ this case is rejected.

If D can split his money likewise, then

A, B and C will have respectively

$$12(15 - x) + \frac{12(15-x)5x}{180}, \text{ i.e. } 12(15 - x) + \frac{(15-x)x}{3},$$

$$3x + \frac{3x \cdot 5x}{180}, \text{ i.e. } 3x + \frac{x^2}{12} \text{ and}$$

$$4x + \frac{4x \cdot 5x}{180}, \text{ i.e. } 4x + \frac{x^2}{9}.$$

Note that $x$ must be divisible by 2 and 3.

$\therefore x$ can be equal to 6 or 12 (as $x < 15$)

and the amount with A can be 12·9 or 12·3.

**So the correct options for (a) and (b) are (iv) and (iii) respectively.**

**46.** Let

$$\overset{\text{A}}{\begin{pmatrix} \text{R} \\ \text{B} \end{pmatrix}} \quad \overset{\text{B}}{\begin{pmatrix} \text{B} \\ \text{Y} \end{pmatrix}} \quad \overset{\text{C}}{\begin{pmatrix} \text{Y} \\ \text{G} \end{pmatrix}} \quad \overset{\text{D}}{\begin{pmatrix} \text{G} \\ \text{R} \end{pmatrix}}$$

where R, B, Y, G denote marbles of red, blue, yellow and green colours respectively.

AFTER FIRST ROUND:

$$(\text{A, C}) \equiv \begin{pmatrix} \text{R} & \text{B} \\ \text{G} & , & \text{Y} \end{pmatrix} \text{ or } \begin{pmatrix} \text{R} & \text{G} \\ \text{Y} & , & \text{B} \end{pmatrix} \text{ or } \begin{pmatrix} \text{B} & \text{R} \\ \text{Y} & , & \text{G} \end{pmatrix} \text{ or } \begin{pmatrix} \text{B} & \text{R} \\ \text{G} & , & \text{Y} \end{pmatrix} \text{ and}$$

$$(\text{B, D}) \equiv \begin{pmatrix} \text{B} & \text{Y} \\ \text{G} & , & \text{R} \end{pmatrix} \text{ or } \begin{pmatrix} \text{B} & \text{Y} \\ \text{R} & , & \text{G} \end{pmatrix} \text{ or } \begin{pmatrix} \text{Y} & \text{B} \\ \text{G} & , & \text{R} \end{pmatrix} \text{ or } \begin{pmatrix} \text{Y} & \text{B} \\ \text{R} & , & \text{G} \end{pmatrix}$$

Note that the only possibilities (taking second round in account) will be

$$\begin{array}{lcccc} & A & B & C & D \\ \text{Case I.} & \begin{pmatrix} R \\ Y \end{pmatrix} & \begin{pmatrix} B \\ G \end{pmatrix} & \begin{pmatrix} G \\ B \end{pmatrix} & \begin{pmatrix} Y \\ R \end{pmatrix} \\ \text{Case II.} & \begin{pmatrix} B \\ G \end{pmatrix} & \begin{pmatrix} Y \\ R \end{pmatrix} & \begin{pmatrix} R \\ Y \end{pmatrix} & \begin{pmatrix} B \\ G \end{pmatrix} \end{array}$$

AFTER SECOND ROUND:

Case I: $(A, B) \equiv \begin{pmatrix} R & B \\ Y & G \end{pmatrix}$ or $\begin{pmatrix} R & B \\ G & Y \end{pmatrix}$ or $\begin{pmatrix} Y & R \\ B & G \end{pmatrix}$ or $\begin{pmatrix} Y & R \\ G & B \end{pmatrix}$

$(C, D) \equiv \begin{pmatrix} G & B \\ R & Y \end{pmatrix}$ or $\begin{pmatrix} G & B \\ Y & R \end{pmatrix}$ or $\begin{pmatrix} B & G \\ Y & R \end{pmatrix}$ or $\begin{pmatrix} B & Y \\ R & G \end{pmatrix}$

Taking third round in account, the possibilities can be

$$\begin{array}{ccccl} A & B & C & D & \\ \begin{pmatrix} R \\ G \end{pmatrix} & \begin{pmatrix} B \\ Y \end{pmatrix} & \begin{pmatrix} G \\ R \end{pmatrix} & \begin{pmatrix} B \\ Y \end{pmatrix} & \text{or} \\ \begin{pmatrix} Y \\ B \end{pmatrix} & \begin{pmatrix} R \\ G \end{pmatrix} & \begin{pmatrix} B \\ Y \end{pmatrix} & \begin{pmatrix} R \\ G \end{pmatrix} & \text{or} \\ \begin{pmatrix} Y \\ G \end{pmatrix} & \begin{pmatrix} R \\ B \end{pmatrix} & \begin{pmatrix} G \\ Y \end{pmatrix} & \begin{pmatrix} B \\ R \end{pmatrix} & \end{array}$$

Case II: $(A, B) \equiv \begin{pmatrix} B & G \\ R & Y \end{pmatrix}$ or $\begin{pmatrix} B & G \\ Y & R \end{pmatrix}$ or $\begin{pmatrix} G & B \\ Y & R \end{pmatrix}$ or $\begin{pmatrix} G & B \\ R & Y \end{pmatrix}$

$(C, D) \equiv \begin{pmatrix} R & B \\ G & Y \end{pmatrix}$ or $\begin{pmatrix} R & Y \\ B & G \end{pmatrix}$ or $\begin{pmatrix} Y & R \\ B & G \end{pmatrix}$ or $\begin{pmatrix} Y & R \\ G & B \end{pmatrix}$

Taking third round in account, the possibilities can be

$$\begin{array}{ccccl} A & B & C & D & \\ \begin{pmatrix} B \\ R \end{pmatrix} & \begin{pmatrix} G \\ Y \end{pmatrix} & \begin{pmatrix} R \\ B \end{pmatrix} & \begin{pmatrix} Y \\ G \end{pmatrix} & \text{or} \end{array}$$

$$\begin{pmatrix} B \\ Y \end{pmatrix} \begin{pmatrix} G \\ R \end{pmatrix} \begin{pmatrix} Y \\ B \end{pmatrix} \begin{pmatrix} R \\ G \end{pmatrix} \text{ or}$$

$$\begin{pmatrix} G \\ Y \end{pmatrix} \begin{pmatrix} B \\ R \end{pmatrix} \begin{pmatrix} Y \\ G \end{pmatrix} \begin{pmatrix} R \\ B \end{pmatrix} \text{ or}$$

$$\begin{pmatrix} G \\ R \end{pmatrix} \begin{pmatrix} B \\ Y \end{pmatrix} \begin{pmatrix} R \\ G \end{pmatrix} \begin{pmatrix} B \\ Y \end{pmatrix}$$

The last three possibilities of Case II are mere repetetion of possibilities of Case I. Also note that (A, C) and (B, D) have marbles of same set of colurs.

**So the correct options for (a), (b), (c) and (d) are (i), (iv), (iii) and (iii) respectively.**

**47.** Let $x$ be the cost of a peach be Rs $x$. Then the cost of an orange, an apple and a mango will be Rs $x + 1$, Rs $x + 2$ and Rs $x + 3$ respectively. Then

$4(x + x + 1\ x + 2 + x + 3) = 20 + 22 + 24 + 26 = 4 \times 23$

$\Rightarrow 4x = 17 \qquad \Rightarrow x = 4.25$

Now

A $\rightarrow 4.25 \times 4 + 3 \equiv$ (3P, M); (2P, O, A) or (P, 3O)

B $\rightarrow 5.25 \times 4 + 1 \equiv$ (3O, A); (P, M, 2O); (2A, O, P) or (2P, A, M)

C $\rightarrow 6.25 \times 4 - 1 \equiv$ (3A, O); (2A, M, P); (A, M, 2O) or (2M, O, P)

D $\rightarrow 7.25 \times 4 - 3 \equiv$ (3M, P); (2M, A, O) or (M, 3A)

[P, M, O, A represent a peach, a mango, an orange, an apple repectively]

Note that we need to combine solutions for A, B, C, D such that there are 4P, 4M, 4O and 4A.

Pertaining to part (b), we can have A, B, C, D as buying (P, 3O), (2P, A, M), (2M, O, P) and (M, 3A) respectively.

**So the correct options for (a), (b), (c) and (d) are (ii), (i), (iii) and (iv) respectively.**

**48.** Various possibilities are:

(1)

| | | |
|---|---|---|
| | A | |
| C | B | |
| | | |

Not possible as
D E, H G cannot fit

(2)

| | | |
|---|---|---|
| | | A |
| I | C | B |
| F | | |

(3)

| | | |
|---|---|---|
| | | |
| | A | |
| C | B | |

Not possible as
D E, H G cannot fit

(4)

| | | |
|---|---|---|
| | | |
| | | A |
| | C | B |

Not possible as
D E, H G, I F cannot fit

**So the correct options for (a), (b) and (c) are (iii), (i) and (i) respectively.**

**49. A. (a) The correct option is (iv). EXPLANATION:**

∵ there are three pairs of unique sequences, let them be

| | | |
|---|---|---|
| A | B | C |
| B | C | A |
| C | A | B |

If we interchange first column with second column, then we get

| | | |
|---|---|---|
| B | A | C |
| C | B | A |
| A | C | B |

which has six unique sequences.

**(b) The correct option is (i). EXPLANATION:**
From second figure in part (a), option (i) is clearly evident.

**B. The correct option is (iii). EXPLANATION:**

The only possible arrangement will have same element in any row and one such arrangement will be

| | | |
|---|---|---|
| A | A | A |
| B | B | B |
| C | C | C |

which has four unique sequences, one of them being triple.

50. **The correct option is (iv). EXPLANATION:**
Note that (2, 4), (6, 7) and (3, 8) exchanged their mutual places. Now it is possible that (1, 5) exchanged their places and then 1 exchanged its new place with 9 or (5, 9) exchanged their places and then 5 exchanged its new place with 1.

51. **The correct option is (iii). EXPLANATION:**
Had there been one more member of the board having his choice different from others, then all woud have got the same weightage. ∴ the weightage given to three candidates will be

$$2\times\left(1+\frac{1}{2}+\frac{1}{3}\right)-\frac{1}{3},\ 2\times\left(1+\frac{1}{2}+\frac{1}{3}\right)-\frac{1}{2}\ \text{and}$$

$$2\times\left(1+\frac{1}{2}+\frac{1}{3}\right)-1$$

∴ the required ratio will be $\dfrac{3+1/3}{2+2/3}=\dfrac{10}{8}=\dfrac{5}{4}$

52. From the informations, A is B's only sister and C is unmarried brother in law of B and C, P are brothers, and Z is son of A, we have

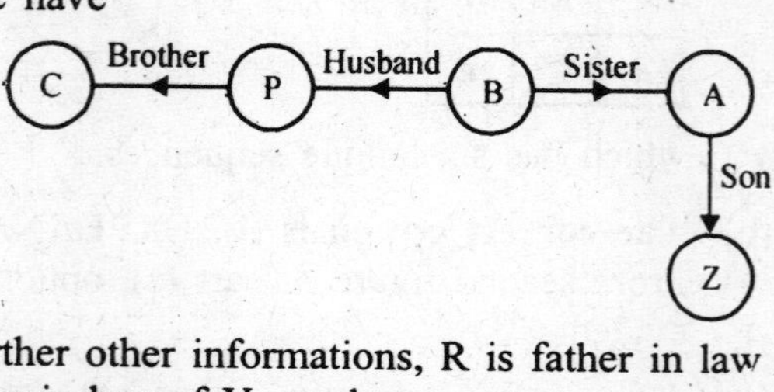


From further other informations, R is father in law of P and X is sister-in-law of Y, we have

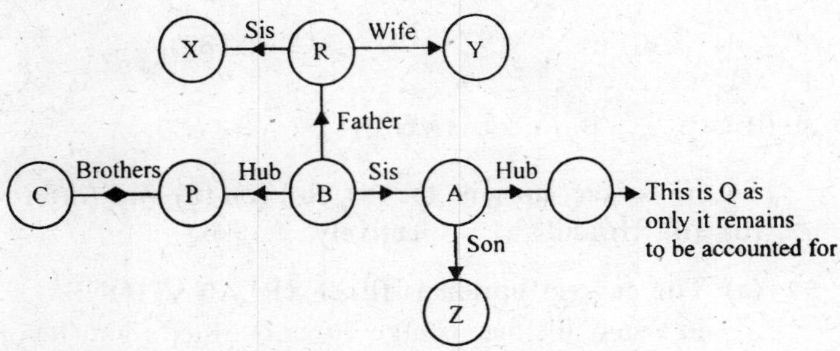


**So the correct options for (a) and (b) are (i).**

**53.** The tournament took $4 \times 3 + 5 = 17$ days to complete. If it started on Jan 15, then there could not have been be any match on Jan 22 and if it started on Jan 14, then there could not have been be any match on Jan 17. Also as it was yet not clear on Jan 20 which teams would to the final, therefore the match could not have started earlier than Jan 13 and it started actually on that day itself. We can have the following arrangement:

13 14 15 17 18 19 21 22 23 25 27 29

(__ __ AC). (BC __ __). (__ AB __). __ . __ . __

↓ ↓ ↓

C B A

(. denotes rest day and down arrow points to winner)

∵ no two teams played in same sequence in any two league matches. ∴ the arrangement will be

(AB BC AC) · (BC AC AB) · (AC AB BC) · — · — · —

↓ ↓ ↓

C B A

(No other possibility exists)

∵ it was not clear on Jan 20 which teams would go to the final ∴ every team won exactly two matches in first two bouts. Also the winner is B or C and it could not have won the highest number of matches. ∴ the actual arrangement will be

| 13 | 14 | 15 | 17 | 18 | 19 | 21 | 22 | 23 | 25 | 27 | 29 |
|---|---|---|---|---|---|---|---|---|---|---|---|
| (AB | BC | AC)·(BC | | AC | AB)· | (AC | AB | BC)· | — · | — · | — |
| ↓ | ↓ | ↓ | ↓ | ↓ | ↓ | ↓ | ↓ | ↓ | | | |
| A | (B or C) | C | B | (A or C) | (A or B) | B | A | (B or C) | | | |

**So the correct options for (a), (b), (c), (d) and (e) are (iv), (ii), (ii), (i) and (ii) respectively.**

**54. (a) The correct option is (ii). EXPLANATION:**

In a step, the man can go either one step right (R) or one up (U). ∴ the number of different ways in which the man can go from A to B will be the number of different ways in which 3R and 3U can be arranged in a line which is equal to

$$\frac{\lfloor 6}{\lfloor 3 \lfloor 3} = \frac{6.5.4}{\lfloor 3} = 20$$

**(b) The correct option is (ii). EXPLANATION:**

For reaching X, there are $\frac{\lfloor 4}{\lfloor 2 \lfloor 2} = 6$ different ways.

For reaching B via X, there are 6 × 2 = 12 different ways.
∴ for reaching B without going to X there are 20 – 12 = 8 ways.

**55. (a) The correct option is (ii). EXPLANATION:**

The actual circuit becomes as shown alongside. There are 3 different ways for signal to reach B without passing through E.

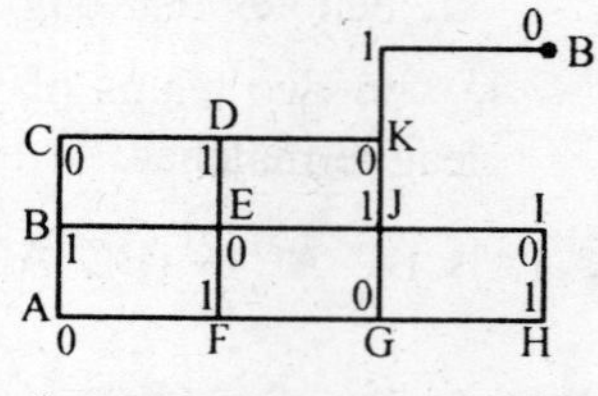


There are 5 different ways of reaching E and total number of ways the signal can further go to B are given as:

(1) ABE + DO, EJO, FGJO, FGHIJO → 4 ways
(2) ABCDE + same as above → 4 ways
(3) AFE + DO, JO, BCDO → 3 ways
(4) AFGJE + DO, BCDO → 2 ways
(5) AFGHIJE + DO, BCDO → 3 ways

∴ the total number of required ways = 3 + 4 + 4 + 3 + 2 + 2

**(b) The correct option is (iv). EXPLANATION:**

The signal cannot pass from A to B as B has to be at 0 state.

**56. (a) The correct option is (iv). EXPLANATION:**

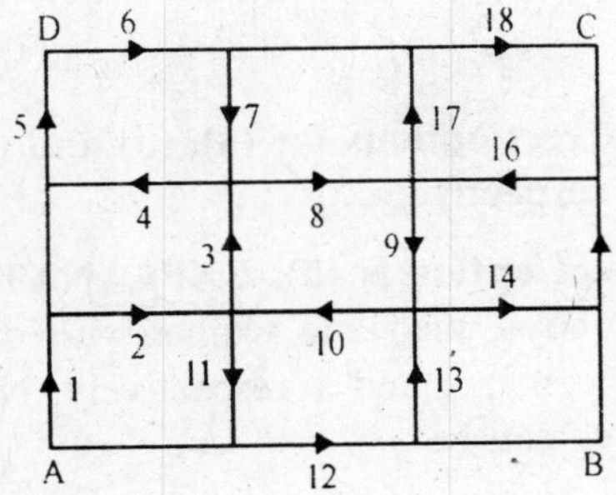


As shown above, he can walk 18 km.

**(b) The correct option is (iii). EXPLANATION:**

Same as above, only the paths 4, 5, 6, 7 has to be counted out. ∴ the man can walk 18 – 4 = 14 km.

**57.** The possible arrangement will be of the form

| 1 | 2 | 3 | 4 | 5 | 6 | 7 | 8 |
|---|---|---|---|---|---|---|---|
| $A_L$ | | | | | | | |

Note that $B_R$, $C_R$, $D_R$ has to be between $A_L$ and $A_R$. Also $C_L$ has to be before $C_R$ while $B_L$, $D_L$ has to be after $B_R$ and $D_R$ respectively. ∴ $A_R$ can be at sixth, seventh or eighth position.

∴ the possible arrangements can be

| | 1 | 2 | 3 | 4 | 5 | 6 | 7 | 8 |
|---|---|---|---|---|---|---|---|---|
| | $A_L$ | $B_R$ | $C_L$ | $D_R$ | $C_R$ | $A_R$ | $B_L/D_L$ | $D_L/B_L$ |
| | $A_L$ | $B_R$ | $D_R$ | $C_L$ | $C_R$ | $A_R$ | $B_L/D_L$ | $D_L/B_L$ |
| | $A_L$ | $C_L$ | $B_R$ | $D_R$ | $C_R$ | $A_R$ | $B_L/D_L$ | $D_L/B_L$ |
| STEPS: | 1 | 5 | 6 | 7 | 8 | 2 | 3 | 4 |

Note that the position of $A_R$ is exchangable with that of seventh or eighth.

**So the correct options for (a), (b) and (c) are (iv), (iii) and (iv) respectively.**

**58.** **A.** The only possibilities are

| | | | | |
|---|---|---|---|---|
| Girls | – | (3, 4) | | (3,4) |
| Boys | – | (1, 8) | | (5,7) |
| Women | – | (5, 6) | or | (2, 8) |
| Men | – | (2, 7) | | (1, 6) |

**So the correct options for (a), (b) and (c) are (iii), (iv) and (iii) respectively.**

**B.** **The correct option is (ii). EXPLANATION:**
Note that boys, men and women will definetly occupy seat numbers 3, 4 and 1 respectively. Now the various possibilities can be

| | | | | | | |
|---|---|---|---|---|---|---|
| Girls | – | (2, 5) | | (2, 8) | | (5, 8) |
| Boys | – | | | (3, 6) | | (3, 6) |
| Men | – | NOT | or | (4, 7) | or | (2, 4) |
| Women | – | POSSIBLE | | (1, 5) | | (1, 7) |

**59.** Consider the table given below wherein the first column denotes the person assumed to be female and second and third columns denote the persons with which the female assumed in first column cannot/can form the triplet of females.

| Persons | Not possible | Possible |
|---|---|---|
| $A_1$ | ($A_2$, $A_6$, $A_8$, $A_5$, $A_7$) | ($A_3$, $A_4$, $A_9$) |
| $A_2$ | (1, 3, 9, 8, 4, 6) | (5, 7) |
| $A_3$ | (2, 4, 5, 8, 7, 6) | (1, 9) |
| $A_4$ | (3, 5, 2, 7, 9) | (1, 6, 8) |
| $A_5$ | (4, 6, 3, 8, 1) | (2, 7, 9) |
| $A_6$ | (5, 7, 1, 2, 3) | (4, 8, 9) |
| $A_7$ | (6, 8, 4, 9, 1, 3) | (2, 5) |
| $A_8$ | (7, 9, 3, 1, 2, 5) | (4, 6) |
| $A_9$ | (8, 7, 2, 4) | (1, 3, 5, 6) |

(For convenience, $A_1$, $A_2$ .... are denoted directly by their subscripts in second and third columns from second row onwards)

From above table, the possible triplets of females are ($A_1$, $A_3$, $A_9$) or ($A_2$, $A_5$, $A_7$) or ($A_4$, $A_6$, $A_8$).

**So the correct options for (a), (b), (c) and (d) are (ii), (iv), (i) and (iii) respectively.**

**60. (a) The correct option is (iii). EXPLANTION:**

Given: C E B and A F D

Now if B is female, then one of C, E has to be female as two males cannot be together $\because$ two females are together $\therefore$ E will be female and consequently F will also be a female while C, A, D will be males.

**(b) The correct option is (iii). EXPLANATION:**

Given: A B and C D

Also we have arrangement of males (M) and females (F) as M F F M F M.

Now if E, F are adjacent to each other, then (A, B) and (C, D) can be first four persons or last four persons or first two and last two persons. In any of these cases, E and F will be of opposite sex.

**61.** A B C D E F G

$\because$ C is a female $\therefore$ either E or F is the unmarried brother.

Case I: Let E be unmarried brother. Then D, F will be males.

A B C D E F G

If B, C are parent, then F is married to A and D is married to G.

If A, B are parent, then C is married to F and D is married to G.

Case II: Let F be unmarried brother. Then E, G will be males.

A B C D E F G

If A, B are parent, then C (female) is married to E and D (female) is married to G;

If B, C are parent, then E is married to A (female) and D is married to G;

If C, D are parent, then (E, G) are married to (A, B) (may not be in that order).

**From above, the correct options for (a), (b), (c), (d) are (iii), (iii), (i) and (ii) respectively.**

**62. A.** Tosses

| | Initial | 1 | 2 | 3 | 4 | 5 | 6 |
|---|---|---|---|---|---|---|---|
| A: | 12 (0) | 3 | 5 | 10 | 2 | 8 | 9 |
| B: | $x$ | $x + 2$ | $x + 5$ | $x + 9$ | $x + 3$ | $x + 4$ | $x + 9$ |
| Difference: | $x$ | $x - 1$ | $x$ | $x - 1$ | $x + 1$ | $x - 4$ | $x$ |

**(a) The correct option is (ii). EXPLANATION:**
They can be at same positions initially and after second and sixth tosses.

**(b) The correct option is (i). SELF EXPLAINED.**

**(c) The correct option is (iv). EXPLANATION:**
$x + 1 = 6 \Rightarrow x = 5$ $\therefore$ they will be closest to each other after fifth toss.

**(d) The correct option is (iv). EXPLANATION:**
The only possibilities are third and fourth tosses, $\therefore$ in fifth toss, the diference in their positions decreases by 5.

**B.** Tosses

| | Initial | 1 | 2 | 3 | 4 | 5 | 6 |
|---|---|---|---|---|---|---|---|
| A: | 0 | 3 | 5 | 10 | 2 | 8 | 9 |
| B: | $x$ | $x - 2$ | $x - 5$ | $x - 9$ | $x - 3$ | $x - 4$ | $x - 9$ |
| Difference: | $x$ | $x - 1$ | $x - 10$ | $x - 7$ | $x - 5$ | $x$ | $x - 6$ |

**(a) The correct option is (ii). SELF EXPLAINED.**

**(b) The correct option is (i) EXPLANATION:**
They can be at same position after first and sixth tosses.

**63. (a) The correct option is (iv). EXPLANATION:**
The movement of the child can be:

| | | | |
|---|---|---|---|
| | 11 | 4 | 15 |
| 3 | 14 | 7 | 10 |
| 12 | 9 | 2 | 5 |
| 1 | 6 | 13 | 8 |

**(b) The correct option is (i). EXPLANATION:**

The movement of child can be:

| | | | |
|---|---|---|---|
| | 3 | | 7 |
| | 6 | | 4 |
| | | 2 | |
| 1 | | 5 | |

**(c) The correct option is (i). EXPLANATION:**

The movements of childrens can be:

| | | | |
|---|---|---|---|
| | $X_2$ | | |
| | | $Y_1$ | |
| $X_3Y_2$ | | $X_1$ | |
| $X_0$ | | | $Y_0$ |

**64. (a) The correct option is (iii). EXPLANTION:**

For them to meet in minimum number of moves, A, B have to move equal number of minimum moves, A up or to the right and B down or to the left. Therefore they are going to meet along diagonal elements as for reaching any diagonal blocks they will have to move 7 blocks each.

**(b) The correct option is (ii). EXPLANATION:**

Note that if a person reaches any one block of a particular diagonal blocks in certain number of moves, then he can equally well reach the other blocks of the same diagonal blocks in the same number of moves. Note that in 9 moves A can move to either central diagonal blocks or diagonal blocks adjacent to diagonal blocks just next to it.

∴ the total number of blocks in which they can meet is $8 + 2 \times 6 = 20$.

**65. (a) The correct option is (i). EXPLANATION:**

| | | |
|---|---|---|
| A | D | H |
| F | E | C |
| B | I | G |

Fig. 1

| | | |
|---|---|---|
| F | H | I |
| G | C | B |
| E | D | A |

Fig. 2

| | | |
|---|---|---|
| I | F | G |
| B | H | A |
| D | C | E |

Fig. 3

Let us start checking from option (i), i.e A.
Fixing A, we get the positions of F and I from fig (2) and fig. (3) respectively. Subsequently the position of others can be similarly known and we get original pattern as

| | | |
|---|---|---|
| A | E | B |
| G | D | I |
| H | C | F |

Since no anomalies are encountered ∴ this solution is retained and there is no need to check other options.

**The correct options for (b) and (c) are (i) as self evident from above figure.**

66. (a) **The correct option is (iv). EXPLANATION:**

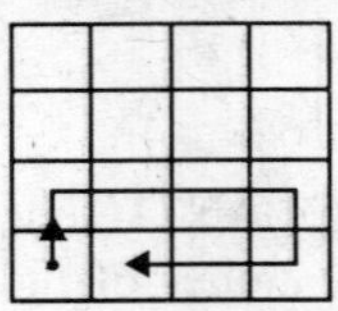

7 moves

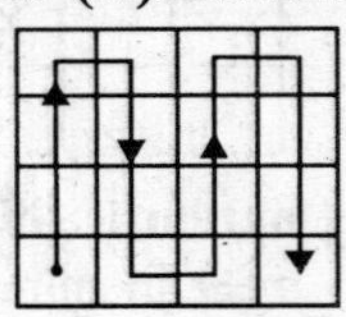

15 moves

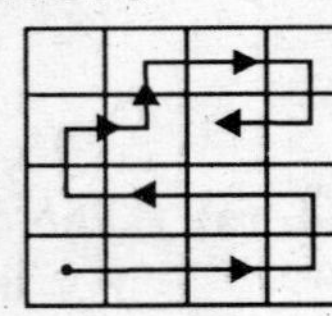

14 moves

There can be minimum of 7 moves and maximum of 15 moves. Figure showing 14 moves is shown so as to prove that there can be even number moves also. ∴ total number of unequal elements of S will be 15 – 7 + 1 = 9.

(c) **The correct option is (i). EXPLANATION:**
Consider the following figure:

| | | | |
|---|---|---|---|
| o | e | o | e |
| e | o | e | o |
| o | e | o | e |
| A | o | e | o |

| | | | |
|---|---|---|---|
| e | o | e | o |
| o | e | o | B |
| e | o | e | o |
| o | e | o | e |

where e denotes position reached after even number of moves and o denotes reached after odd number of moves. ∴ A and B cannot be in a block after equal number of moves.

67. A. (a) **The correct option is (ii). EXPLANATION:**
Exchanging first column with fourth column and second column with fourth column, we get $a = x_{12}$.

(b) **The correct option is (ii). EXPLANATION:**
Note that the property is retained even if two of its columns or rows are exchanged. Here the first and third rows are exchanged, then second and fifth columns are exchanged, then second and fourth rows are exchanged, then first and fourth column are exchanged, then second and fifth rows are exchanged. $\therefore\ a = x_{14}$.

**B.** The blocks can be filled as:

| | | | | | | |
|---|---|---|---|---|---|---|
| 30 | 39 | 48 | 1 | 10 | 19 | 28 |
| 38 | 47 | 7 | 9 | 18 | 27 | 29 |
| 46 | 6 | 8 | 17 | 26 | 35 | 37 |
| 5 | 14 | 16 | 25 | 34 | 36 | 45 |
| 13 | 15 | 24 | 33 | 42 | 44 | 4 |
| 21 | 23 | 32 | 41 | 43 | 3 | 12 |
| 22 | 31 | 40 | 49 | 2 | 11 | 20 |

If we rotate the given block so that 1 comes on the top row, then

| | | | | | | |
|---|---|---|---|---|---|---|
| $y$ | | | 1 | | | |
| | | | | | | |
| | | | | | $x$ | |
| | | | | | | |
| | | | | | | |
| | $z$ | | | | | |
| | | | | 2 | | |

$\therefore\ x = 35,\ y = 30,\ z = 23$

$$\text{and sum of numbers in any row} = \frac{1+2+---49}{7} = \frac{49 \times 50}{2 \times 7} = 175$$

**So the correct options for (a), (b), (c), (d) are (ii), (iii), (iv) and (i) respectively.**

**68. (a) The correct option is (ii). EXPLANATION:**

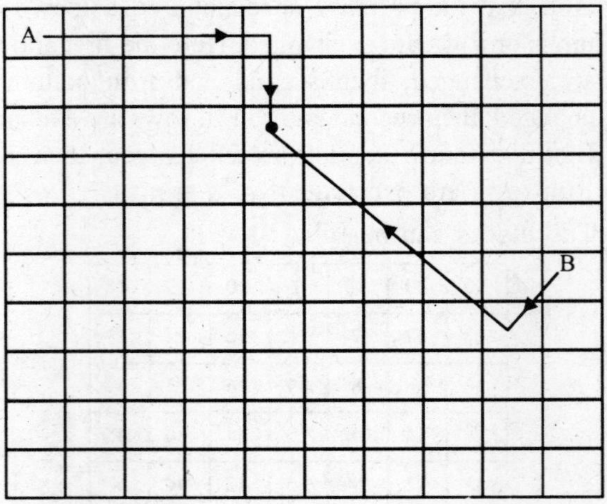


From above figure, minimum sum of moves = 6 (A) + 5(B) = 11

**(b) The correct option is (i). EXPLANATION:**

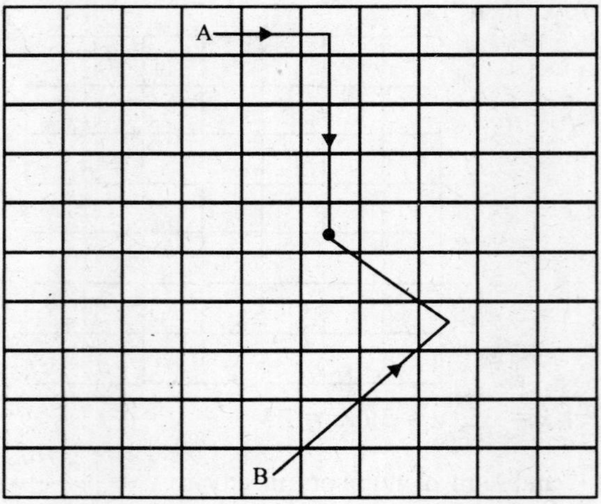


From above figure, minimum sum of moves = 6 (A) + 5 (B) = 11

**69. (a) The correct option is (iii). EXPLANATION:** Note that B, I and J occur twice.

∴ we can construct the blocks as

| | | | |
|---|---|---|---|
| | | N | P |
| | E | J | K |
| O | I | B | M |
| H | D | L | F |

So the letter in third row of last column will be M.

**(b) The correct option is (ii). EXPLANATION:**

Note that $\begin{pmatrix} GL & NG \\ IB & JD \end{pmatrix}$, and $\begin{pmatrix} GL & EH \\ IB & BK \end{pmatrix}$ are not compatiable.

∴ $\begin{pmatrix} G & L \\ I & B \end{pmatrix}$ is rotated and when $\begin{pmatrix} I & O \\ C & M \end{pmatrix}$ is taken into account, then it should be $\begin{pmatrix} L & B \\ G & I \end{pmatrix}$. ∴ the blocks can be constructed as:

| | | | |
|---|---|---|---|
| | | E | H |
| | L | B | K |
| N | G | I | O |
| J | D | C | M |

So the letter in last row and third column will be C.

**70. (a) The correct option is (i). EXPLANATION:**

For the minimum number of distinct pattern, the filling should be most symmetric which can be:

| | | | |
|---|---|---|---|
| R | B | G | Y |
| B | G | Y | R |
| G | Y | R | B |
| Y | R | B | G |

and the number of distinct pattern will be 8.

**(b) The correct option is (iii). EXPLANATION:**

Exchanging third row with fourth row in the figure given in part (a), the arrangement will be

| | | | |
|---|---|---|---|
| R | B | G | Y |
| B | G | Y | R |
| Y | R | B | G |
| G | Y | R | B |

and the number of distinct pattern will be 14.

**(c) The correct option is (iv). EXPLANATION.**
If the arrangement in (b) is changed by exchanging the first row with third row, then the arrangement will be

| | | | |
|---|---|---|---|
| Y | R | B | G |
| B | G | Y | R |
| R | B | G | Y |
| G | Y | R | B |

and the number of distinct pattern will be 16.

**B.**

| | | | |
|---|---|---|---|
| Y | R | B | G |
| | | | |
| | | | |
| | | | |

If we try filling blocks rowise with cyclic sequence YRBG, we get two of the arrangements as:

| | | | |
|---|---|---|---|
| Y | R | B | G |
| B | G | Y | R |
| R | B | G | Y |
| G | Y | R | B |

or

| | | | |
|---|---|---|---|
| Y | R | B | G |
| B | G | Y | R |
| G | Y | R | B |
| R | B | G | Y |

Note that both of them satisfy the given conditions.

∴ the pattern in third and fourth row cannot be uniquely determined and hence

**the correct options for (a) and (b) will be (iv).**

**71.** From both figures, A, B...I can be married to persons as shown below:

A → E, F, I
B → D
C → F, H
D → B, G
E → A
F → C, A
G → I, D
H → C
I → A, G

At least two of the couples must be (B, D), (E, A) or (C, H)

∴ the couples can be

1) (B, D), (E, A), (C, H), (G, I) ... F
2) (B, D) (E, A) (F, C) (G, I) ... H
3) (B, D), (C, H), (F, A), (G, I) ... E

**So the correct options for (a), (b), (c), (d) are (iv), (i), (i) and (ii) respectively.**

**72.** There will be two groups starting from A,
A (in second figure) is in position of I (in first figure)
I (in second figure) is in position of F (in first figure)
F (in second figure) is in position of D (in first figure)
D (in second figure) is in position of A (in first figure)
∴ the two groups are (A, I, F, D) and (B, C, E, G, H)
∵ the number of females is less than that of males ∴ it will be equal to 4.
**So the correct options for (a) and (b) will be (iv).**

**73.**

| | | |
|---|---|---|
| | B | |
| D | E | F |
| | H | I |

None of the above elements are in the row or column they are actually in now.

| | | |
|---|---|---|
| | G | |
| | | A |
| C | | |

Actual arrangement

The position of B can be block numbers 4, 9; D can be 3, 8, 9; E can be 1, 3, 9; F can be 1, 8; H can be 1, 3, 4; I can be 1, 4, 5.

**(a) The correct option is (iii). EXPLANATION:**
Note that I has to be in block number 5 as no other elements can go into it.

**(b) The correct option is (i). EXPlANATION:**
If F is in block number 1, then D has to be in block number 8, and B, E, H can be in block numbers (4, 9), (3, 9) and (3, 4) respectively ie B, E, H can be in block numbers (4, 9, 3) or (9, 3, 4) respectively.

**(c) The correct option is (i). EXPLANATION:**
If D is in block number 3, then F has to be in block number 8 and B, E, H can be in block numbers (4, 9, ~~1~~) or (9, 1, 4) respectively.

**74.** Note that (G, H, Z); (C, F, X); (A, C, Y); (E, H, Y); (E, F, Z) and (A, G, Z) will be in a row/column where
X, Y, Z ≡ B, D, I (may not be in order)

∵ AC is in a row ∴ AG is in a column;
∵ AG is in a column ∴ GH is in a row;
∵ GH is in a row ∴ EH is in a column;
∵ EH is in a column ∴ EF is in a row;
∵ EF is in a row ∴ CF is in a column.

Now the possible arrangements can be:

| | | |
|---|---|---|
| A | | C |
| | E | F |
| G | H | |

or

| | | |
|---|---|---|
| A | C | |
| | F | E |
| G | | H |

**So the correct options for (a), (b) and (c) are (iv), (ii) and (ii) respectively.**

**75.**

| Cell: | 1 | 2 | 3 | 4 | 5 | 6 | 7 | 8 | 9 |
|---|---|---|---|---|---|---|---|---|---|
| | A | C | F | H | D | B | E | G | I |
| | G | I | C | E | A | H | B | D | F |

Note that cells (1, 5, 8) have (A, G), (D, A), (G, D) respectively;
(2, 3, 9) have (C, I), (F, C), (I, F) respectively;
(4, 6, 7) have (E, H), (B, H), (E, B) respectively;

The sequence can be

| | | | | | | | |
|---|---|---|---|---|---|---|---|
| 1 | $x$ | 5 | $y$ | 8 | $z$ | 1 | [where $x$, $y$, $z$ are the number of terms between |
| A | $x$ | D | $y$ | G | $z$ | A | (1, 5), (5, 8) and (8,1) respectively |
| G | $x$ | A | $y$ | D | $z$ | G | Also note that $x + y + z = 6$] |

∴ the space between (A, D) or (A, G) or (G, D) in the cyclic sequence remains constant

∴ $x = y = z = 2$

Now in the cyclic sequence if two letters are separated by two letters, they might as well be separated by five letters.

Similarly cells numbered 2 and 3 in their cyclic sequences must be separated by two cells.

Note that if C, F, I can be as well in cells numbered (1, 5, 8) or (4, 6, 7). ∴ C, F, are in cells numbered 4, 6 then I will be in cell numbered 7.

Now if the sequences are

A B C __ E __ D <u>X</u> __ A and

1 2 4 5 __ 6 __ <u>Y</u> __ 1,

then X = H and Y can be 3 or 9.

**So the correct options for (a), (b), (c) and (d) are (iii), (iii), (ii) and (i) respectively.**

**76.** The columns are (1, 5, $x$); (6, 7, $y$) and (3, 9, z) where $x$, $y$, $z$ = 2, 4 or 8 (may not be in order).

Now (2, 5) or (4, 5) are in a row ∴ $x = 8$. Also as A cannot occupy (1, 5) or (3, 6) ∴ the numbering of cells can be:

| | | |
|---|---|---|
| 8 | 6 | 3 |
| 1 | 7 | 9 |
| 5 | $y$ | $z$ |

∴ position of A will be 8, B will be $y$ (which will be equal to 4 as $z = 2$) and C will be $z$.

**So the correct options for (a), (b) and (c) are (iii), (ii) and (i) respectively.**

**77. (a) The correct option is (i). EXPLANATION:**

Note that the counter can move between two stops as

1 – 2, 2 – 4, 3 – 6, 4 – 8, 5 – 1, 6 – 3, 7 – 5, 8 – 7 and 9 – 9 only.

∴ there can be three different movements of the counter:

1 – 2 – 4 – 8 – 7 – 5 – 1 ( 5 stops)
6 – 3 – 6 (1 stop)
9 – 9 (0 stop)

(b) **The correct option is (iii). EXPLANATION:**
In a similar way as done in part (a), the movements of the counter can be
1– 2 – 4 – 9 – 9, 3 – 6 – 3, 9 – 9,
7 – 5 –1 – 2 – 4 – 9 – 9

(c) **The correct option is (iv). EXPLANATION:**
Checking for
(4, 8), we can have 7 – 5 – 1 – 2 – 8 – 3 – 6 – 3 and for
(8, 7), we can have 5 – 1 – 2 – 4 – 7 – 6 – 3 – 6.

∵ the two options are correct ∴ we need not check the third option.

**78.**

| | | |
|---|---|---|
| A | B | C |
| D | E | F |
| G | H | I |

Note that the unmarried person can be only A, C, G, I or E. When A is the unmarried person, then various set of couples can be {(B, C); (D, E); (G, H); (F, I)} or {(B, C); (D, G); (E, H); (F, I)} or {(B, C); (D, G); (E, F); (H, I)} or {(B, E); (C, F); (D, G); (H, I)}

When E is the unmarried person, then various set of copules can be {(A, B); (C, F); (I, H); (G, D)} or {(A,D); (G, H); (I, F); (C, B)}

∴ total number of possibilities of four set of couples is
4 × 4 + 2 = 18

**So the correct options for (a) and (b) are (iii) and (ii) respectively.**

**79.** (a) **The correct option is (iii). EXPLANATION:**
The only possibilities are:

| | | |
|---|---|---|
| **B** | **C** | **H** |
| **A** | **D** | **G** |
| | **E** | **F** |

or

| | | |
|---|---|---|
| **F** | **G** | **H** |
| **E** | **D** | **C** |
| | **A** | **B** |

**(b) The correct option is (iv). EXPLANATION:**
The arrangements can be:

| | | |
|---|---|---|
| G | F | E |
| B | C | D |
| A | | |

or

| | | |
|---|---|---|
| C | D | G |
| B | E | F |
| A | | |

**(c) The correct option is (i). EXPLANATION:**
If A is at the corner, then all the blanks may be filled

as

| | | |
|---|---|---|
| G | H | I |
| F | E | P |
| A | B | C |

or as

| | | |
|---|---|---|
| | F | G |
| | E | D |
| A | B | C |

If A is at the centre, then all the blanks must be filled

as

| | | |
|---|---|---|
| G | F | E |
| H | A | D |
| I | B | C |

$\therefore m = 1$

If A is the block between two corner blocks, then at least one block must be empty

as

| | | |
|---|---|---|
| F | G | H |
| E | D | C |
| | A | B |

$\therefore n = 4$

**80. (a) The correct option is (iv). EXPLANATION:**
Note that the relative positions of 2, 4, 5, 6, 8 in both the figures are same. ∴ there will be five different positions of A for which four more letters can have the same positions in both the figures.

**(b) The correct option is (iv). EXPLANATION:**
For the positions of 2, 4, 5, 6, 8 there is no need to check. For the positions of four corners, let us check:

| | | | | | |
|---|---|---|---|---|---|
| 1 | 2 | 3 | 1 | 9 | 8 |
| 4 | 5 | 6 | 2 | 3 | 4 |
| 7 | 8 | 9 | 7 | 6 | 5 |

One common pair (1, 7)

| | | | | | |
|---|---|---|---|---|---|
| 8 | 9 | 1 | 3 | 2 | 1 |
| 2 | 3 | 4 | 4 | 5 | 6 |
| 5 | 6 | 7 | 9 | 8 | 7 |

One common pair (1, 7)

| | | | | | |
|---|---|---|---|---|---|
| 4 | 5 | 6 | 4 | 3 | 2 |
| 7 | 8 | 9 | 5 | 6 | 7 |
| 1 | 2 | 3 | 1 | 9 | 8 |

One common pair (1, 4)

| | | | | | |
|---|---|---|---|---|---|
| 2 | 3 | 4 | 6 | 5 | 4 |
| 5 | 6 | 7 | 7 | 8 | 9 |
| 8 | 9 | 1 | 3 | 2 | 1 |

One common pair (1, 4)

So for all nine positions of A, there will be at least one letter having same relative position in both the figure.

**(c) The correct option is (iv). EXPLANATION:**
For (A, D) to have same relative position in both the figures, the difference between their positions denoted by numbers (of given sequence) must be 3. Now note that
$5 - 2 = 3,\ 8 - 5 = 3,\ 4 - 1 = 3,\ 1 + 9 - 7 = 3$
∴ there can be six such positions. [first two correspond to part (a) while latter two correspond to part (b)]

**(d) The correct option is (iv). EXPLANATION:**
For (A, G) to have same relative positions in both the figure, the difference between their positions should be 6 or 3 (as it is a cyclic sequence). Therefore its solution corresponds to that of part (c).

**81. (a) The correct option is (iv). EXPLANATION:**
The two sequences can be written as:

| | | | | | | | | | |
|---|---|---|---|---|---|---|---|---|---|
| First sequence: | A | D | E | F | C | B | G | I | H |
| Second sequence: | A | F | G | H | B | I | D | C | E |

Note that for any such pair, the spacing between them in two sequences must be same. Only (F, I) and (D, G) are found to be such pairs.

**(b) The correct option is (iv). EXPLANATION:**
From part (a), only (F, I) and (D, G) are such pairs,
∴ H is not in any such pairs.

**(c) The correct option is (ii). EXPLANATION:**

The required condition will as well be satisfied if one of the sequences is reversed so that the sequences can be written as:

| | | | | | | | | |
|---|---|---|---|---|---|---|---|---|
| A | D | E | F | C | B | G | I | H |
| A | E | C | D | I | B | H | G | F |

For such pairs, the spacing between two letters must be same. Only (A, B) and (C, H) are found to be such pairs.

**(d) The correct option is (iv). EXPLANTION:**

From part (c), only (A, B) and (C, H) are such pairs.

∴ D is not in any such pairs.

**82.** Given:

| | | |
|---|---|---|
| 5 | *b* | 7 |
| *a* | *c* | 8 |
| 1 | *d* | *e* |

Note that e, c can only be odd numbers while a, b, d can only be even numbers. Few of the possibilities can be:

| | | |
|---|---|---|
| 5 | 2 | 7 |
| 6 | 3 | 8 |
| 1 | 4 | 9 |

and

| | | |
|---|---|---|
| 5 | 4 | 7 |
| 2 | 9 | 8 |
| 1 | 6 | 3 |

**So the correct options for (a) and (b) are (iv).**

**83. Let us number the cells as**

| | | |
|---|---|---|
| 1 | 2 | 3 |
| 4 | 5 | 6 |
| 7 | 8 | 9 |

We can tabulate the cases as:

| Tosses: Cases | I | II | III | IV | V | Cell Numbers of rest | |
|---|---|---|---|---|---|---|---|
| I | 2 | 3 | 4 | – | – | 1, 3, 6, 1 | ⇒ N.P |
| II | 2 | 5 | 4 | – | – | 1, 3, 8, 3 | ⇒ N.P |

| | | | | | | | |
|---|---|---|---|---|---|---|---|
| III | 2 | 6 | 4 | 3 | 5 | 1, 3, 9, 4, 7, 3 | ⇒ N.P |
| IV | 3 | 5 | 4 | – | – | 1, 4, 9, 4 | ⇒ N.P |
| V | 3 | 6 | 4 | – | – | 1, 4, 1 | ⇒ N.P |
| VI | 5 | 6 | 4 | 2 | 3 | 1, 6, 3, 7, 3 | ⇒ N.P |
| VII | 5 | 2 | 4 | 6 | 3 | 1, 6, 8, 3, 6, 3 | ⇒ N.P |

N.P ≡ 'Not possible'.

Note that for first two tosses or for last two tosses in above cases, if $(x, y)$ is not possible, then $(y, x)$ will also not be possible. Also only 2, 3, 5 for the first toss [as asked in part (a)] are checked.

**So the correct options for (a), (b) and (c) are (iv).**

**84. (a) The correct option is (i). EXPLANATION:**

Let the number be in $m$th row and $n$th column of first arrangement. Then the number will be $7(m - 1) + n$. To retain its position, the number in second arrangement will be $10(n - 1) + m$

$\therefore\ 7(m - 1) + n = 10(n - 1) + m$

$\Rightarrow\quad 6m = 9n - 3$

$\Rightarrow\quad 2m = 3n - 1$

$\Rightarrow\quad 2(m - 1) = 3(n - 1)$

The solution of $(m, n)$ can be (4, 3) or (7, 5) and the corresponding numbers can be 24 or 47.

**(b) The correct option is (iii). EXPLANATION:**

As done in part (a),

$25(m - 1) + n = 37(n - 1) + m$ where $m \le 37$ and $n \le 25$

$\Rightarrow\quad 24(m - 1) = 36(n - 1)$

$\Rightarrow\quad 2(m - 1) = 3(n - 1)$

$\Rightarrow\quad m = 3k + 1,\quad k = 0, ...12$ only and correspondingly, $n = 2k + 1$, $k = 0, ... 12$ only.

$\therefore$ there can be 13 such numbers.

**85.** Note that A, C are of same sex and B, D are of same sex and opposite to that of A, C. Now there must be at least one couple in A, B, C, D which can be only A, D. Now if D, E are of opposite sex, then B, E will be another couple as A, D has to be a couple.

**So the correct options for (a) and (b) are (iv) and (iii) respectively.**

**86.** Let $x$ be the number of members with government and $p$ be the % of cross voting. Then $\frac{px}{100}$ should be an integer. Also

$$x - \frac{px}{100} < 50$$

Also as $p < 25$;

$$\therefore \frac{x-50}{x} < \frac{p}{100} \Rightarrow \frac{x-50}{x} < \frac{1}{4}$$

$\Rightarrow 4x - 200 < x$

$\Rightarrow 3x < 200 \quad \Rightarrow x < 66\ 1/3$

From options of part (a), only $x = 60$ is found to be valid

$\therefore x = 60$

Now $\frac{p \cdot 60}{100} = \frac{3p}{5}$ must be an integer.

$\therefore p$ can be 5, 10, 15 or 20. But as

$x - \frac{px}{100} < 50 \quad \therefore p = 20$ will be the only valid option.

Now 48 members with the government voted for the bill

$\therefore$ 2 members from the opposition voted for the bill and % crossvoting occured on the opposition side = $\frac{2}{40} \times 100 = 5\%$

**So the correct options for (a), (b) and (c) are (i), (iv) and (i) respectively.**

**87. (a) The correct option is (ii) EXPLANATION:**

$x_1 + x_2 + x_3 = 1$

$x_2 + x_3 + x_4 = 1/2$

$x_3 + x_4 + x_5 = 1/4$

From first two equations and from last two equations,

$x_1 - x_4 = 1/2$ and $x_2 - x_5 = 1/4$

Similarly $x_3 - x_6 = 1/8$, $x_4 - x_7 = 1/16$,

$x_5 - x_8 = 1/32$ and so on.

$$\therefore\ x_1 - x_4 + x_4 - x_7 + \ldots = \frac{1}{2} + \frac{1}{16} + \ldots$$

$$\Rightarrow x_1 = \frac{1}{2}\left(1+\frac{1}{8}+\frac{1}{8^2}+\cdots\right)$$

$$= \frac{1}{2\,(1-1/8)} = \frac{4}{7}$$

**(b) The correct option is (ii). EXPLANATION:**

$$x_2 - x_5 = \frac{1}{4},\ x_5 - x_8 = \frac{1}{32},\ \ldots.$$

$$\Rightarrow x_2 - x_5 + x_5 - x_8 + \ldots = \frac{1}{4}+\frac{1}{32}+\ldots$$

$$= \frac{1}{4}\left(1+\frac{1}{8}+\frac{1}{8^2}+\ldots\right)$$

$$= \frac{1}{4\,(1-1/8)} = \frac{2}{7}$$

**(c) The correct option is (ii). EXPLANATION:**

$$x_1 + \frac{x_2}{2} + \frac{x_3}{4} = 1$$

$$x_2 + \frac{x_3}{2} + \frac{x_3}{4} = 1\times\frac{1}{2}$$

Subtraction gives

$$x_1 - \frac{x_4}{8} = \frac{1}{2}$$

Similarly, $x_2 - \dfrac{x_5}{8} = \dfrac{1}{2}$

$$x_3 - \frac{x_6}{8} = \frac{1}{2}$$

$$x_4 - \frac{x_7}{8} = \frac{1}{2}$$

$$\therefore x_1 - \frac{x_4}{8} + \frac{1}{8}\left(x_4 - \frac{x_7}{8}\right) + ....$$

$$= \frac{1}{2} + \frac{1}{2}\cdot\frac{1}{8} + \frac{1}{2}\cdot\frac{1}{8^2} + ......$$

$$= \frac{1}{2}\left(1 + \frac{1}{8} + \frac{1}{8^2}...\right)$$

$$= \frac{1}{2}(1 - 1/8) = \frac{4}{7}$$

**88.** The correct responses would be of Question

1. ($M_1$, $M_2$, $M_3$) or ($M_4$, $M_5$)
2. ($M_1$, $M_2$) or ($M_3$ $M_4$, $M_5$)
3. ($M_1$, $M_5$) or ($M_2$, $M_3$, $M_4$)

Note that $M_1$ and $M_4$ always fall in different groups.

$\therefore$ the two students of given qualities are either of these.

$\because$ the number of correct responses is less than that of the wrong responses

$\therefore$ $M_1$ always gave answers correctly,
$M_4$ always gave answers incorrectly and $M_3$ gave correct answer only once.

**So the correct options for (a), (b) and (c) are (i), (iii) and (ii) respectively.**

**89.** Let $n$ be the total number of hours per day for which the computer is used and $x$, the price of computer.

| Persons | Money contributed | Time used |
|---|---|---|
| $M_1$ | $5000 = k\ x$ (say) | $k\ n$ |
| $M_2$ | $x/4$ | $n/4$ |
| $M_3$ | $x/5$ | $n/5$ |
| $M_5$ | $\left(\frac{11}{20} - k\right)x$ | $\left(\frac{11}{20} - k\right)n = 2$ |

Now $k\,x = 5000$ and $\frac{11}{20} - k = \frac{2}{n}$

$$\Rightarrow \quad \frac{11}{20} - \frac{5000}{x} = \frac{2}{n}$$

$$\Rightarrow \quad \frac{5000}{x} = \frac{11}{20} - \frac{2}{n}$$

$$\Rightarrow \quad x = \frac{5000}{\frac{11}{20} - \frac{2}{n}}$$

$$\Rightarrow \quad x = \frac{5000}{\left(\frac{11n - 40}{20n}\right)}$$

$\because$ $x$ is an integer

$\therefore$ $\frac{11n-40}{20n}$ and 5000 should have a common factor.

Checking for $n$ = 10, 11, 12, 13, 14, 15,
we have $11\,n - 40$ = 70, 81, 92, 103, 114, 125 respectively.
Only $n$ = 15 and subsequently $x$ = 12000 is valid.

**(a) The correct option is (ii). EXPLANATION:**

$M_1$ used computer for $k\,n$ hours, i.e.

$$\left(\frac{11}{20} - \frac{2}{n}\right) n = \frac{11}{20} \times 15 - 2$$

$$= \frac{25}{4} = 6 \text{ hours, } 15 \text{ minutes}$$

**(b) The correct option is (ii). EXPLANTION:**

$M_4$ contributed $\left(\frac{11}{20} - k\right) x$, i.e.

$$\frac{2}{n} x = \frac{2}{15} \times 12000 = \text{Rs } 16000.$$

**(c) The correct option is (ii). EXPLANATION:**
Note that the remaining hours = 9

$\therefore$ the money he would have contributed $= \dfrac{9}{24} \times 12000$

$= 4500$

i.e. he would have paid rent for 45 days.

**90.** Let the tickets for A and B bought by betters be $(a_1, b_1)$, $(a_2, b_2)$, $(a_3, b_3)$ and $(a_4, b_4)$ respectively. If 10 unit $p$ be the amount invested by each of them, then

$a_1 + 2b_1 = p \qquad a_2 + 2b_2 = p$

$a_3 + 2b_1 = p \qquad a_4 + 2b_4 = p$

Adding all equations, we get

$(a_1 + a_2 + a_3 + a_4) + 2\,(b_1 + b_2 + b_3 + b_4) = p$

$\because \quad a_1 + a_2 + a_3 + a_4 = b_1 + b_2 + b_3 + b_4$ (given)

$\therefore \quad 3\,(a_1 + a_2 + a_3 + a_4) = 4p$

Now all of $a_i$ and $b_i$ $(i = 1, 2, 3, 4)$ are different and as $a_i + 2\,b_i = p$

$\therefore$ either all $a_i$ are odd or even according as $p$ is odd or even. We can have two cases:

Case I: $p$ is odd. Then checking for minimum values of $a_i$'s, we have

$$3(1 + 3 + 5 + 7) = 4p \rightarrow \text{Not possible}$$
$$3(1 + 3 + 5 + 9) = 4p \rightarrow \text{Not possible}$$
$$3(1 + 3 + 5 + 11) = 4p \rightarrow p = 15, \text{ possible}$$

For $p = 15$, the values of $(a_i, b_i)$ can be

(1, 7), (3, 6), (5, 5) (11, 2) or

(1, 7), (3, 6), (7, 4), (9, 3)

Case III: $p$ is even. Then, similarly

$$3(2 + 4 + 6 + 8) = 4p \rightarrow \text{Not possible}$$
$$3(2 + 4 + 6 + 10) = 4p \rightarrow \text{Not possible}$$
$$3(2 + 4 + 6 + 12) = 4p \rightarrow p = 18$$

But for this value the number of tickets sold is higher than that obtained in case I $\therefore$ this case is not considered.

**So the correct options for (a), (b) and (c) are (iii), (ii) and (ii) respectively.**

**91.** Let the price of an apple and an orange be Rs $x$ and Rs $y$ respectively. Then

A $\to 5x + 2y$ [ '$\to$' denotes 'bought']

B $\to nx + ny$

C $\to 2x + 2ny$

$\because$ each of them spent equal amount

$$\therefore \begin{cases} nx + ny = 2x + 2ny & \text{and} \\ nx + ny = 5x + 2y \end{cases}$$

$$\Rightarrow \begin{cases} (n-2)x = ny & \text{and} \\ (n-5)x = (2-n)y \end{cases}$$

$$\Rightarrow \quad \frac{n-2}{n-5} = \frac{n}{2-n}$$

$\Rightarrow (n - 2)^2 + n\ (n - 5) = 0$

$\Rightarrow 2n^2 - 9n + 4 = 0$

$\Rightarrow (2n - 1)\ (n - 4) = 0$

$\Rightarrow n = 4$ as $n$ is an integer.

$\therefore$ A $\to 5x + 2y = 12y$

B $\to 4x + 4y = 12y$

C $\to 2x + 8y = 12y$

and consequently

D $\to 3x + 6y = 12y$ and

E $\to x + 10y = 12y$

**So the correct options for (a), (b) and (c) are (iii), (iii) and (i) respectively.**

**92.** Let the price of an apple and an orange be Rs $x$ and Rs $y$ respectively. Then three of

$9x + 25y$, $11x + 22y$, $15x + 16y$ and $21x + 8y$ will be equal.

On checking

$9x + 25y = 11x + 22y \Rightarrow 2x = 3y$

$9x + 25y = 15x + 16y \Rightarrow 2x = 3y$

$\therefore$ A, B, C spent equal amount of money.

Now money spent by A $= 15x + 16y = 25\ x + y$ and

the money spent by D $= 21x + 8y = 25x + 2y$

**So the correct options for (a) and (b) are (iv).**

**93.** The reciprocal of given amount of times, in increasing order, are

$$\frac{2}{24}, \frac{4}{24}, \frac{5}{24}, \frac{6}{24}, \frac{8}{24}, \frac{9}{24}, \frac{18}{24}, \frac{20}{24}, \frac{24/x}{24}$$

These nine numbers can be divided into three groups which sum are equal (each sum will correspond to the opening of all the six pipes).

On checking, we get

$$\frac{18}{24}+\frac{9}{24}+\frac{4}{24} = \frac{20}{24}+\frac{6}{24}+\frac{5}{24} = \frac{31}{24} \text{ or}$$

$$\frac{18}{24}+\frac{9}{24}+\frac{5}{24} = \frac{20}{24}+\frac{8}{24}+\frac{4}{24} = \frac{32}{24} \text{ or}$$

$$\frac{18}{24}+\frac{8}{24}+\frac{5}{24} = \frac{20}{24}+\frac{9}{24}+\frac{2}{24} = \frac{31}{24}$$

and corresponding values of $x$ are $\frac{24}{21}, \frac{24}{24}, \frac{24}{21}$ respectively.

**So the correct options for (a), (b), (c) and (d) are (ii), (ii), (i) and (iii) respectively.**

**94. (a) The correct option is (iv). EXPLANATION:**

Let 3 articles be purchased together $m$ times and $n$ articles be purchased $n$ times. Then $4m + 7n = 100 - x$ where $x$ articles are purchased either singly or two at a time.

Let $3m + 5n = 72 - y$ where $y = 0, 2$ or $4$ (as given in options)

From the above two equations, we have

$m = 7(72 - y) - 5(100 - x) = 4 - 7y + 5x$

$n = 3(100 - x) - 4(72 - y) = 12 - 3x + 4y$

$\therefore$ all values of $y$, viz. 0, 2 and 4 are possible for corresponding suitable value of $x$.

**(b) The correct option is (ii). EXPLANATION:**

Let C and S be the cost price and selling price of the article. Then

$(3m + 5n)\text{S} = (1{\cdot}1)100\text{C}$

$$\Rightarrow \qquad \frac{S}{C} = \frac{110}{3m+5n}$$

From given options,

$$\frac{S}{C} = 1.2,\ 1.25,\ 1.4,\ 1.5$$

$\because$ $(3m + 5n)$ is an integer

$\therefore$ only 1.25 will be valid, i.e. $x = 25\%$

**95.** Profit is made on articles which are not used.

For X, CP = 100 – A and SP = 100

$$\therefore \quad \frac{A}{100-A} = \frac{20}{100} \Rightarrow \quad A = \frac{20 \times 100}{120} = \frac{50}{3}$$

For Y, CP = 100 – B and SP = 100

$$\therefore \quad \frac{B}{100-B} = \frac{25}{100} \Rightarrow \quad B = \frac{25 \times 100}{125} = \text{Rs } 20$$

For Z, CP = 100 – C and SP = 100

$$\therefore \quad \frac{C}{100-C} = \frac{50}{100} \Rightarrow \quad C = \frac{50 \times 100}{150} = \text{Rs } \frac{100}{3}$$

Also A + B + C + D = 100 (as X bought them)

$$\Rightarrow \qquad D = 100 - \frac{150}{3} - 20 = \text{Rs } 30$$

**So the correct options for (a), (b) and (c) are (i), (iii) and (iii) respectively.**

**96. A. The correct option is (i). EXPLANATION:**

Let us draw a regular pentagon:

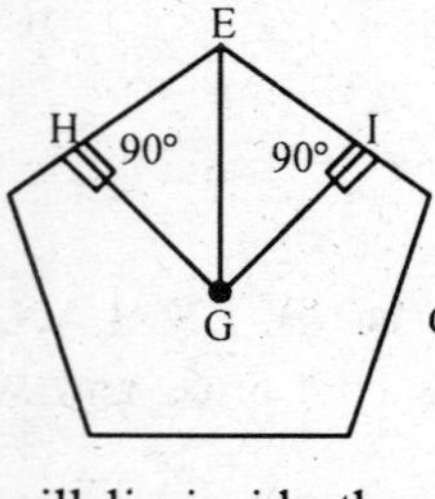


G is the centre of pentagon

Note that O will lie inside the quadrilateral GHEI.

Let O be inside the triangle GHE. Then the naming of vertices will be as

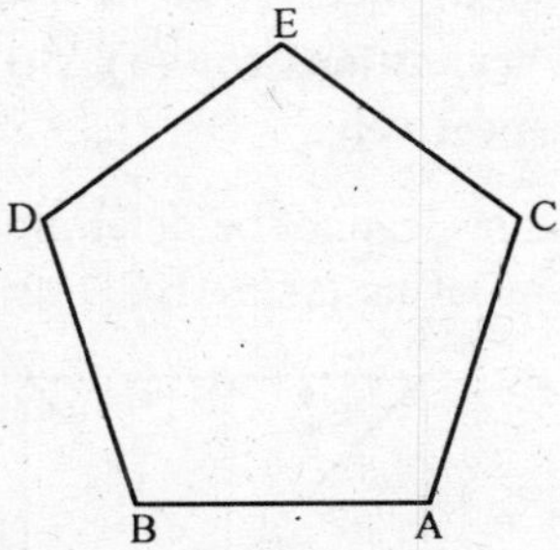


**B.** Let us draw a regular hexagon:

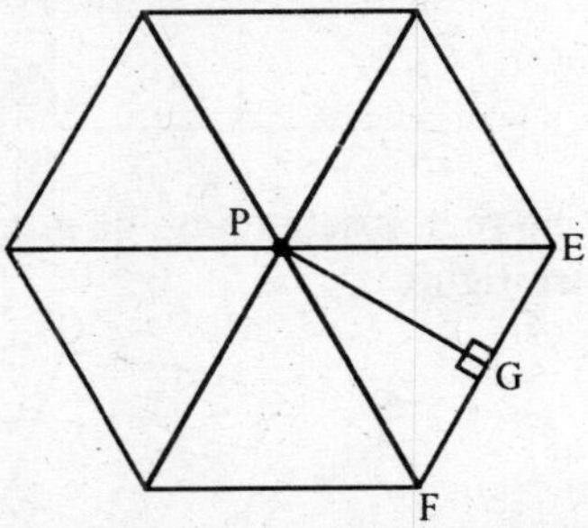


Let P be the centre of the hexagon. Then O will lie inside the triangle which vertices are E, P and F and precisely within triangle PFG where G is the foot of perpendicular dropped from P on EF. The naming of vertices can be done as

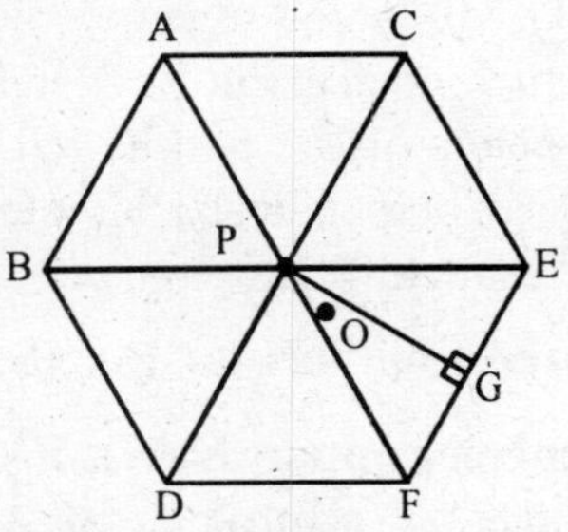


Note that from any point lying on PG, the perpendiculars dropped on PF and PE will be equal. $\because$ O lies inside the triangle PFG $\therefore$ the perpendicular dropped from O on BE will be greater than that on AF. Similarly from any point lying on AF, the perpendiculars dropped on BE or CD

will be same ∵ O lies inside FPE ∴ the perpendicular dropped from O on CD will be longer than that on BE.

**So the correct options for (a), (b) and (c) are (i), (ii) and (iii) respectively.**

**97.** Note that there is no 'cannot be determined' in the options. ∴ for simplification, let us take ABCD as a square:

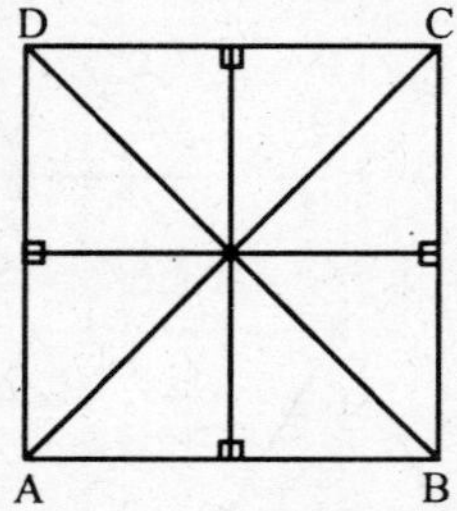


But as there is no region satisfying the given conditions, so let us draw another figure:

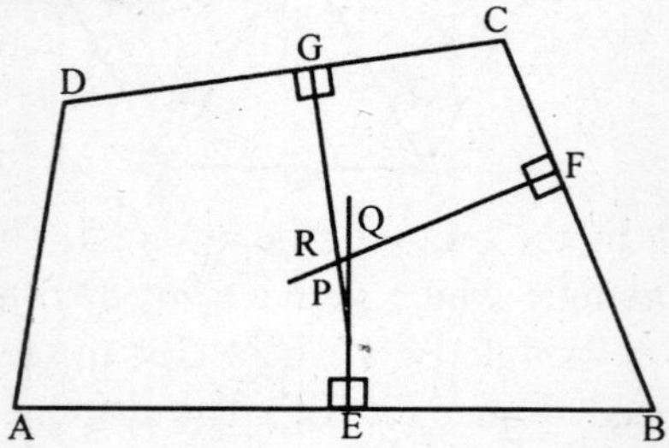


Note that O will lie left to perpendicular bisectors of AB, BC and CA which intersect in P, Q and R. Note that the perpendicular bisectors of DA will lie left to triangle PQR as OD > OA. Similarly perpendicular bisectors of CA and DB will lie left to the triangle PQR.

**So the correct options for (a), (b) and (c) are (iv).**

**98. (a) The correct option is (iv). EXPLANATION:**

Note that the median to longest side is shortest in length and the median to shortest side is longest in length. Now D cannot be on BC. If it is on AC, then one of E,

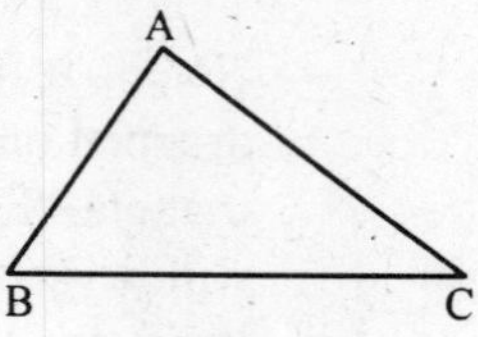

F will lie on BC and AD will be less than BE or CF.

∴ the given case is not possible.

**(b) The correct option is (iv). EXPLANATION:**
Let BC = a, AC = b and AB = c. Note that the length of the medians through vertices A, B and C are

$$\frac{1}{2}\sqrt{2b^2+2c^2-a^2}, \frac{1}{2}\sqrt{2c^2+2a^2-b^2} \text{ and}$$

$$\frac{1}{2}\sqrt{2a^2+2b^2-c^2}$$

If D is on BC, then E and F can be on AC and AB respectively satisfying the given condition.
If D is on AC, then E can be on BC satisfying the given condition as

$$\frac{1}{2}\sqrt{2c^2+2a^2-b^2} > \frac{a}{2}$$

$$\Rightarrow 2c^2 + 2a^2 - b^2 > a^2$$

$\Rightarrow 2c^2 + a^2 > b^2$, which is true

So D can lie on BC or AC.

**99.**

| | | | |
|---|---|---|---|
| | | $A_4$ | |
| | $B_2$ | | |
| $C_1$ | | | |
| | | | $D_3$ |

Note that the block just below $A_4$ can be filled by $B_1$ or $B_3$ and the arrangements can be

| | | | |
|---|---|---|---|
| $A_2$ | $A_3$ | $A_4$ | $A_1$ |
| $B_3$ | $B_2$ | $B_1$ | $B_4$ |
| $C_1$ | $C_4$ | $C_3$ | $C_2$ |
| $D_4$ | $D_1$ | $D_2$ | $D_3$ |

| | | | |
|---|---|---|---|
| $A_3$ | $A_1$ | $A_4$ | $A_2$ |
| $B_4$ | $B_2$ | $B_3$ | $B_1$ |
| $C_1$ | $C_3$ | $C_2$ | $C_4$ |
| $D_2$ | $D_4$ | $D_1$ | $D_3$ |

**So the correct options for (a), (b), (c) and (d) will be (ii), (i), (iii) and (iv) respectively.**

**100. (a) The correct option is (iii). EXPLANATION:**

If D wins all his games, then, in whichever order they bet, he will get half the worth of each of the amounts others have directly or indirectly. ∴ his final amount will be

$$8+\frac{8+8+8}{2} = \text{Rs } 20.$$

**(b) The correct option is (iii). EXPLANATION:**

If D wins all his bets and A loses all his bets, then the amount they will have respectively will be Rs 20 and Rs 1. Suppose B won the bet with only A. Then the money he will have will be Rs 3 and consequently the amount with C will be

$4 \times 8 - (20 + 1 + 3) = \text{Rs } 8$

∴ the difference in the amount of B and C will be Rs 5.

**101. (a) The current option is (iii). EXPLANATION:**

The various possibilities can be:

```
   1                  1                    1
○     2     or     ○     ○     or     ○     ○
 ○  ○                  ○  2                2  ○
```

which on further probing give

```
   1                  1                  1
5     2     or     3     4     or     4     3
 4  3                  2  4               3  1
  (I)                  (II)              (III)
```

**(b) The correct option is (iii). EXPLANATION:**

For (I), the shifting process can be repeated three times as

```
   1             3              2              4
5     2  →  5       1  →  5       4  →  5       3
 4  3         2  4          3  1          1  2
```

Note that (I) changes to (II) and (III) after first and second shifting process. ∴ the minimum number of process corresponds to (I) which is 3.

**(c) The correct option is (ii). EXPLANATION:**
Checking for (I), (II) and (III), only (II) and (III) are found to satisfy the condition.

**102.** Note that the coins they can have will be given as:

| A | B | C | D | E | F |
|---|---|---|---|---|---|
| 1 | (2 – 3) | (4 – 9) | (8 – 27) | (16 –81) | (32 – 100) |

(A = 2 is not possible as minimum coins with D, E, F will be 16, 32, 64 which sum is more than 100)

**(a) The correct option is (i). EXPLANATION:**
The maximum number of coins with F sums up to be
$(100 - (1 + 2 + 4 + 8 + 16) = 69$
but note that 69 is more than thrice of 16.
$\therefore$ the minimum number of coins will be
$100 - (1 + 2 + 4 + 8 + x) = 85 - x$ where
$85 - x \leq 3x$
$\Rightarrow x \geq 22$
$\therefore$ the minimum number of coins = 85 – 22 = 63

**(b) The correct option is (ii). EXPLANATION:**
Let the coins with children be roughly as:

| A | B | C | D | E | F |
|---|---|---|---|---|---|
| 1 | (2,3) | $x$ | $2x$ | $4x$ | $8x$ + few extra coins |

$\therefore 15x \leq 97$ or $96 \Rightarrow x \leq 6$
For $x = 6$, let the distribution be as:

| A | B | C | D | E | F |
|---|---|---|---|---|---|
| 1 | 2 | 6 | 12 | 24 | 48 + 7 extra coins |

Now extra two coins can be distributed as:
D gets one coin, E gets 2 coins and F gets 4 coins or
E gets 2 coins, F gets 4 coins and B gets 1 coin
$\therefore$ the minimum number of coins F will get is
48 + 4 = 52

**(c) The correct option is (iv). EXPLANATION:**
If D gets 13 coins, then E and F must get minimum of 26 and 52 coins while C, B, A must get minimum of 5, 2 and 1 coin respectively so that total coins sums up to be 99. One extra coin may be received by C or F.

**103.** The distribution of marks can be

Maths: 7 × 4, A > B > C > D → Doing it third, 10 > 8 > 6 > 4
Physics: 8 × 4, B > D > C > A → Doing it last, 10 > 9 > 8 > 5
Chemistry: 6 × 4, C > A > D > B → Doing it first, 9 > 6 > 5 > 4
Biology: 8 × 4, D > B > A > C → Doing it second, 10 > 9 > 7 > 6
or 10 > 9 > 8 > 5

This is rejected after maths is done

**So the correct options for (a), (b) and (c) are (iv), (iv) and (i) respectively.**

**104. A.** Note that 1 + 2 = 3, 1 + 3 = 4, 1 + 5 = 6, 1 + 6 = 7,
2 + 3 = 5, 2 + 4 = 6, 2 + 5 = 7 and 3 + 4 = 7

∵ nine sets are given ∴ the number of marbles will be 1, 2, 3, 4, 5, 6 and 7.

In the above set,

| | | | |
|---|---|---|---|
| 1 | → | 5 times | ∵ F is used five times ∴ F = 1 |
| 2 | → | 4 times | C, D → 3 times. Note that 6 is used twice with F ∴ C = 7, D = 6 |
| 3 | → | 4 times | ∵ F + B = D ∴ B = 5 |
| 5 | → | 4 times | ∵ A + B = C ∴ A = 2 |
| 6 | → | 3 times | Now A + F = G ∴ G = 3 and as only |
| 7 | → | 3 times | E is left, it is equal to 4. |

['→' denotes 'is found']

**So the correct options for (a), (b), (c), (d) and (e) are (iii), (ii), (iv), (i) and (ii) respectively.**

**B.** Note that only four such sets are possible if and only if the number of marbles are 3, 4, 5, 6, 7, 8 and 9 so that 3 + 4 = 7, 3 + 5 = 8, 3 + 6 = 9 and 4 + 5 = 9.

∵ 3 is used thrice ∴ D = 3

∵ 4, 5, 9 are used twice ∴ A, B = 4, 5 and F = 9

Consequently G = 6 and C, E = 7, 8 or 8, 7 according as A, B = 4, 5 or 5, 4.

**So the correct options for (a), (b) and (c) are (iii), (ii) and (iv) respectively.**

**105.** Note that when

$P \to A$, then $Q \to (C, D)$ and $S \to (B, C)$. Also when $R \to C$, $S \to (A, B)$ ['$\to$' denotes 'over']

$\therefore$ we can have four cases:

| Cases | P | Q | R | S |
|---|---|---|---|---|
| I | A | D | B | C |
| II | A | D | C | B |
| III | A | C | D | B |

Now we can have three cases according as P is against Q, R or S. Also we have to verify

$Q \to B$, $R \to (A, D)$;
$R \to C$, $S \to (A, B)$ and
$S \to D$, $P \to (B, C)$

Case I: P is against Q.

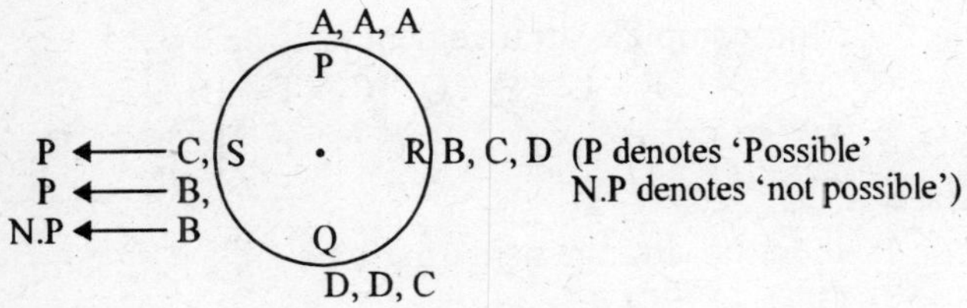


Case II: P is against R.

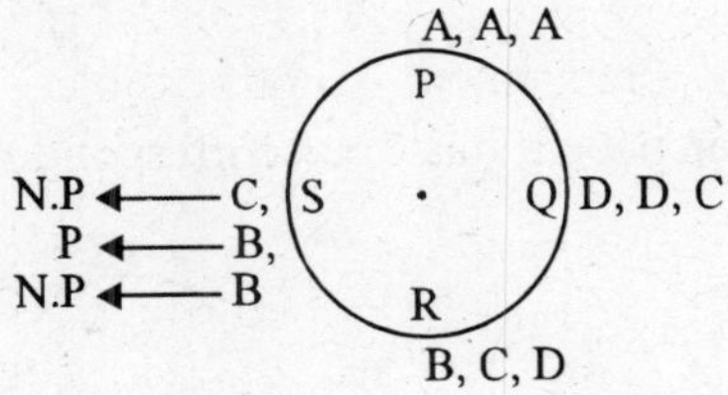


Case III: P is against S.

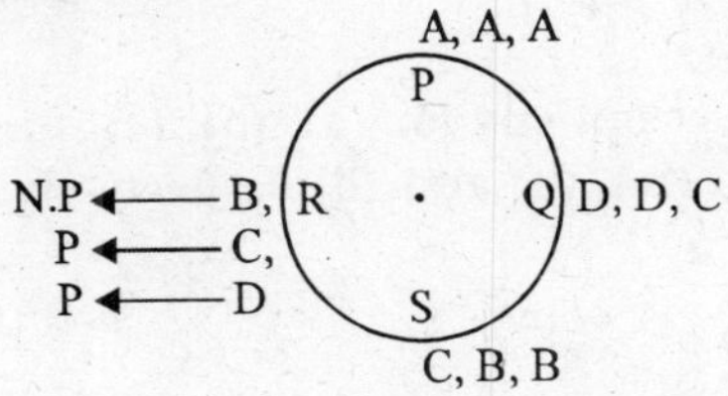


**So the correct options for (a), (b), (c), (d) and (e) are (iii), (ii), (i), (i) and (iv) respectively.**

**106.** Note that (A, F), (B, E) and (C, D) are together. Also (Q, T) and (P, S, U) are together. Now all the letters can be arranged cyclically in a line with alternate positions being occupied by letters of any one paper. Now the arrangement can be for three statements as

APF and QDT;
BRF and SFU; (order of triplets insignificant)
CQD and PAS

We can have the arrangement as

P A S __ U __ __ __ __ __ __ __

where F can be at an alternate position just preceding or just following A.

Case I: P A S F U __ __ __ __ __ __ __

Other sub arrangements must be

DQCT/TCQD or BRE/ERB

∴ the complete arrangement will be

P A S F U D Q C T B R E
E B

Case II: P A S __ U __ __ __ __ __ __ __ F

Other sub arrangements must be

CQDT or TDQC and

R __ __ B __ E or B __ E __ __ R
E B E B

The complete arrangement is not possible.

∴ the circular papers must be (corresponding to case I)

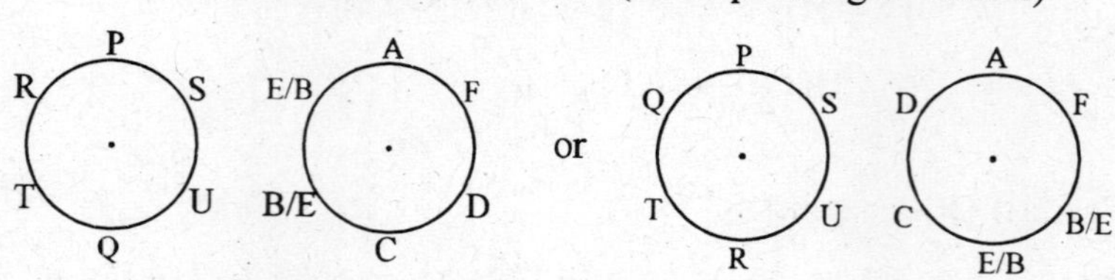


**So the correct options for (a), (b), (c), (d), (e) and (f) are (iii), (iii), (i), (iv), (ii) and (ii) respectively.**

**107.** Let

| A | B | C | |
|---|---|---|---|
| $a$ | $b$ | $c$ | $\rightarrow +1$ |
| $a'$ | $a'$ | $c'$ | $\rightarrow -1$ |

where ($a$, $b$, $c$, $a'$, $b'$, $c'$) are numbers through 1 to 6 and A gets +1 or –1 according as $a$ or $a'$ is turned up and likewise.

Now,

| | A | B | C | |
|---|---|---|---|---|
| First Round | 5 | 4 | 6 | $\rightarrow -1, 1, 1$ |
| Second Round | 2 | 3 | 4 | $\rightarrow -1, 1, 1$ |
| Third Round | b′ | c | a | $\rightarrow 1, -1, 1$ |

Note that turning up of 4 cannot give anybody –1 as 5, 6, 2, 3 will, then, give +1 which is not possible $\therefore$ turning up of 4 gives 1 and

$5, 6 \rightarrow -1, 1$ (each accorded to different persons)
$2, 3 \rightarrow -1, 1$ (each accorded to different persons but same pair as above)

$\therefore$ turning up of 1 gives –1 and is accorded to same person to whom 4 accorded.

Now $b'$ can be equal to 1, 3 and 6 only;
$c$ can be equal to 2, 5 and 6 only;
$a$ can be equal to 2, 3 and 5 only

$\therefore$ $a$, $c$ cannot be equal to 4 $\therefore$ $b$ has to be equal to 4 and $b'$ equal to 1. And for others, we can have

$$\left.\begin{matrix} c = 2, \ a = 5 \\ c' = 6, a' = 3 \end{matrix}\right\} \text{ or } \left.\begin{matrix} c = 5, \ \ a = 2, 3 \\ c' = 3, 2 \ a' = 6 \end{matrix}\right\} \text{ or } \left.\begin{matrix} c = 6, \ \ a = 2, 3 \\ c = 3, 2 \ a' = 5 \end{matrix}\right\}$$

**So the correct options for (a), (b), (c) and (d) are (i) (ii), (ii) and (iv) respectively.**

**108.** Note that eight childrens can be born in minimum 7 years and six months, which leaves extra six months to be adjusted according to given dates. We can draw a chart as:

| Case | Extra Months | Jan +1 | Feb +2 | Apr +2 | Jun +3 | Sep +2 | Nov +2 |
|---|---|---|---|---|---|---|---|
| I | > 6 | First | – | Third | Fifth | Second | Fourth |
| II | 5 | Sixth | First | Third | Fifth | Second | Fourth |
| III | > 6 | Fourth | – | First | Third | Fifth | Second |
| IV | > 6 | Second | – | Fourth | First | Third | Fifth |
| V | > 6 | – | – | Second | Fourth | First | Third |
| VI | > 6 | Third | – | – | Second | Fourth | First |

$\therefore$ only case II is found to be valid, the order of age of children (youngest to eldest) will be A, D, F, C, E, B.

**So the correct options for (a), (b), (c), (d) and (e) are (i), (ii), (ii), (iii), and (i) respectively.**

**109.** We can draw a chart as:

| | Maths | Phy | Chem | Bio |
|---|---|---|---|---|
| Rose | A | ③ | ⑤ | C |
| Monica | ① | C | B | ⑦ |
| Lily | C | ④ | A | ⑧ |
| Tina | ② | B | ⑥ | B |
| To Be Filled By: | (A, B) | (A, B) | (A, B) | (A, C) |

Note that ⑧ cannot be B ∴ ④ has to be B.

Now stepwise, we have

④ → B

③ → A

⑤ → B

⑥ → A

⑧ → C (∵ Rose and Lily will have different ranks)

⑦ → A

① → B (∵ Rose and Monica will have different ranks)

② → A

Now weightage given to Rose, Monica, Lily and Tina will be A + A + A/2 + A/3, A + A/2 + A/2 + A/3, A + A/2 + A/3 + A/3 and A + A + A/2 + A/2 respectively.

**So the correct options for (a), (b), (c) and (d) are (iv), (iii), (iii) and (iii) respectively.**

**110.** We need to form four rows and four columns, each row belonging to one student and each column belonging to one subject so that no row or column has any number repeated. We can have six cases for position of 11 and 12 in the following chart:

| | | | | |
|---|---|---|---|---|
| A | 8 | 9 | 10 | 11 |
| B | | | | |
| C | | | | |
| D | | | | |

11 will be in third row and any of first three columns while 12 will be in second and fourth rows and can be in any column not occupied by 11.

Case I

| | | | | |
|---|---|---|---|---|
| A | 8 | 9 | 10 | 11 |
| B | $7_9$ | $12_2$ | $9\}$ | $8_7$ |
| C | $11_1$ | $7\}$ | $8\}_4$ | $10_6$ |
| D | $10_{10}$ | $8\}_5$ | $12_3$ | $9_8$ |

where the subscripts show the sequence of steps in which the filling is done.

Case II

| | | | | |
|---|---|---|---|---|
| A | 8 | 9 | 10 | 11 |
| B | $7_7$ | $8_8$ | $12_3$ | $9_{10}$ |
| C | $11_1$ | $7_9$ | $8\}$ | $10_{11}$ |
| D | $10_6$ | $12_2$ | $9\}_4$ | $8_5$ |

Case III

| | | | | |
|---|---|---|---|---|
| A | 8 | 9 | 10 | 11 |
| B | $12_2$ | $8_9$ | $9\}$ | $7_{10}$ |
| C | $7\}$ | $11_1$ | $8\}_4$ | $10_6$ |
| D | $9\}_5$ | $10_7$ | $12_3$ | $8_8$ |

Case IV

| | | | | |
|---|---|---|---|---|
| A | 8 | 9 | 10 | 11 |
| B | $9\}$ | $8_9$ | $12_3$ | $7_{10}$ |
| C | $7\}_5$ | $11_1$ | $8\}$ | $10_6$ |
| D | $12_2$ | $10_7$ | $9\}_4$ | $8_8$ |

Other cases need not be examined as all the questions can be answered by these four cases only.

**So the correct options for (a), (b), (c), (d), (e) and (f) are (iv), (i), (iv), (iv), (i) and (ii) respectively.**

**111.** Given:

| | | | |
|---|---|---|---|
| $P \rightarrow A$ | A | B | C; |
| $Q \rightarrow A$ | B | C | C; |
| $R \rightarrow A$ | B | C | C; |
| $S \rightarrow A$ | B | B | C |

Note that they should be arranged as four rows and four columns such that four columns correspond to four subjects and there must be (A, A, B, C); (A, B, B, C) (A, B, C, C) and (A, B, C, C) in columns as well as rows. We can, for a start, have an initial arrangement as

| | | | |
|---|---|---|---|
| A | A | B | C |
| B | – | – | – |
| – | B | – | – |
| – | – | – | B |

Note that each row and each column must have at least one A. Also 2A can only be in first row and second column and ∵ these columns are symmiterical ∴ let us assume that 2A is in first column. Then the arrangement can be

| | | | |
|---|---|---|---|
| A | A | B | C |
| B | — | — | A |
| A | B | — | — |
| C | — | A | B |

or

| | | | |
|---|---|---|---|
| A | A | B | C |
| B | — | A | — |
| C | B | — | A |
| A | — | — | B |

or

| | | | |
|---|---|---|---|
| A | A | B | C |
| B | — | — | A |
| C | B | A | — |
| A | — | — | B |

Now in all the above blanks, one of them will be occupied by B and all others by C. Also B can occupy any of the blanks in any arrangement.

Note that P definetly gets A in maths and by same analogy (since A, B are symmeterical in the conditions given in the problem), S definetly gets B in Physics.

From additional information provided for (c), (d) and (e), first second, thrid and fourth column belongs to Maths, X, Y, Z respectively while first, second, third and fourth row belongs to P, L, M/N, N/M respectively (Note that M got A in Maths)

**So the correct options for (a), (b), (c), (d) and (e) are (i), (iii), (ii), (iv) and (iii) respectively.**

**112.** The table can be drawn as:

| | Maths | Phy | Chem | Bio |
|---|---|---|---|---|
| P | 8, 9 | 6, 7 | 4, 5 | 6, 7 |
| Q | 4, 5 | 6, 7 | 6, 7 | 8, 9 |
| R | 6, 7 | 4, 5 | 8, 9 | 4, 5 |
| S | 4, 5 | 8, 9 | 6, 7 | 6, 7 |

∵ no students got same marks in any of the two subjects
∴ sum of marks obtained by
P in Phy and Bio is 13;
Q in Phy and Chem is 13;
R in Phy and Bio is 9;
S in Chem and Bio is 13.
Also P, Q, S got total marks in the range of 25 – 27 while R got total marks in the range of 23 – 25.
Similarly the number of marks obtained in Maths is in the range of 23 – 25 while the marks obtained in
Phy, Chem and Bio are in the range of 25 – 27.
∵ the total marks obtained in all subjects are different
∴ the marks obtained in Maths will be 23 or 24.
As marks obtained by R in Maths is 7 so the marks obtained in Maths will be 24. Consequently, marks obtained by R will also be equal to 24. Also the marks obtained by P in Maths and R in Chemistry will be 8. Now there can be four cases (two pertaining to Q getting 4 in maths and another two to him getting 5 in maths):

| | Maths | Phy | Chem | Bio | Total |
|---|---|---|---|---|---|
| P | 8 | | 5/4 | | 26/25 |
| Q | 4 | | | 8/9 | 25/26 |
| R | 7 | 5/4 | 8 | 4/5 | 24 |
| S | 5 | 9 | | | 27 |
| Total | 24 | 27/26 | 26/25 | 25/27 | |

(Note that either all numbers before slash or after slash are chosen together)

| | Maths | Phy | Chem | Bio | Total |
|---|---|---|---|---|---|
| P | 8 | | 5/4 | | 26/25 |
| Q | 5 | | | 9 | 27 |
| R | 7 | 4/5 | 8 | 5/4 | 24 |
| S | 4 | 8/9 | | | 25/26 |
| Total | 24 | 25/27 | 26/25 | 27/26 | |

**So the correct options for (a), (b), (c), (d) and (e) are (ii), (ii), (i), (ii) and (iv) respectively.**

**113.** Note that either the numbers of fruits with (A and B) or (C and D) are equal or differ by one. So we can have two cases, either the difference in cost of an apple and an orange is Rs 1 or else the cost of an orange is Rs 1.

Case I: Cost of an orange = Rs 1

The distribution of fruits will be as:

| A | B | C | D |
|---|---|---|---|
| 2 apples | 2 apples | 1 apple | 1 apple |
| 2 oranges | 1 orange | 2 oranges | 1 orange |

The cost of an apple = Amount received by D – that received by B
= Rs 8

Case II: Cost of an (apple – orange) = Rs 1

The distribution of fruits can be

| | A | B | C | D |
|---|---|---|---|---|
| | 3 apples | 2 apples | 1 apple | – |
| a. | 2 oranges | 3 oranges | – | 1 orange |
| b. | 1 orange | 2 oranges | 1 orange | 2 oranges |
| c. | – | 1 orange | 2 oranges | 3 oranges |

For a., cost of 2 (apples + oranges) = Rs 8

⇒ cost of an apple and an orange = Rs 3 and Rs 2

For b., cost of 2 apples = Rs 8

⇒ cost of an apple and an orange = Rs 4 and Rs 3

For c., cost of 2 (apples – oranges) = Rs 8 ⇒ not possible

**So the correct options for (a), (b), (c) and (d) are (iii), (iv), (iii) and (iv) respectively.**

**114.** The distribution of marbles pairwise can be
(B, G), (B, R), (G, G), (R, R) or
(B, B), (G, R), (G, G), (R, R) only

The distribution of marbles among persons can be

| | A | B | C | D |
|---|---|---|---|---|
| a. When R is most expensive, G is least | B<br>R | B<br>G | G<br>G | R<br>R |
| b. When R is most expensive, B is least | B<br>R | G<br>G | B<br>G | R<br>R |

(A and B columns of b.: uncertain ∴ rejected)

| | | | | |
|---|---|---|---|---|
| c. When R is most expensive, B is least | G | G | B | R |
| | R | G | B | R |
| d. When G is most expensive, R is least | B | B | R | G |
| | R | G | R | G |
| e. When G is most expensive, B is least | R | B | B | G |
| | R | G | R | G |

(first two columns: uncertain ∵ rejected)

| | | | | |
|---|---|---|---|---|
| f. When G is most expensive, B is least | R | G | B | G |
| | R | R | B | G |
| g. When B is most expensive, G is least | R | B | G | B |
| | R | G | G | R |

(first two columns: uncertain ∴ rejected)

| | | | | |
|---|---|---|---|---|
| h. When B is most expensive, G is least | R | G | G | B |
| | R | R | G | B |

**So the correct options for (a), (b), (c) and (d) are (iii), (ii), (i) and (iii) respectively**

**115. (a) The correct option is (iv). EXPLANATION:**

Let A, B got $2m$ and $2n$ marbles respectively. Then the marbles received by C and D will be $(m + n)$ and $(m + n + x)$ respectively and

$$2m + 2n + m + n + m + n + x = 20$$

$$\Rightarrow \quad x = 20 - 4(m + n) = 4\{5 - (m + n)\}$$

$\because m, n > 0$ and $(m + n)$ is odd

$$\therefore \quad m + n = 3 \text{ and } x = 8$$

**(b) The correct option is (ii). EXPLANATION:**

Note that D will get an odd number of marbles. Let the marbles received by A, B, C and D be $2m$, $2n$, $2k + 1$ and $2k + 9$ respectively. Then

$$2m + 2n + 2k + 1 + 2k + 9 = 20$$

$$\Rightarrow \quad m + n + 2k + 5 = 10$$

Now one of $2m$, $2n$ has to be 2, let us say $2m = 2$.

Then $\quad n + 2k = 4$

Now $n$ has to be 2 and $\because$ $k$ is a positive integer
$\therefore$ $k = 1$ and number of marbles D got is 11.

**116.** The amount of milk received by P, Q, R and S will be

| P | Q | R | S |
|---|---|---|---|
| $\frac{n}{2}$ | $\frac{n+2}{4}$ | $\frac{n+6}{8}$ | $\frac{n+14}{16}$ |

$\because$ S got the integeral number of litres

$\therefore$ let $\frac{n+14}{16} = m$, an integer.

$\Rightarrow$ $n = 16(m - 1) + 2$

$\because$ $n$ is a multiple of 10 less than 100

$\therefore$ $m = 4$ and $n = 50$

So the amounts of milk received are

| Initial | P | Q | R | S | Remaining |
|---|---|---|---|---|---|
| 50 | 25 | 13 | 7 | 4 | 4 |

The amount of water in the remaining milk

$= \cdot 9 \times 4 = 3 \cdot 6\ell$

The amount of dehydrated pure milk $= \cdot 4\ell$

The amount of pure milk $= \frac{\cdot 4\ \ell}{1/5} = 2\ell$

The content of pure milk remains same for the amount of milk with S and that of the remaining milk. The amount of milk with R has one litre of water less than 8 litres of milk with S and the remaining amount. $\therefore$ the amount of pure milk with R is $4\ell$. Similarly the amount of pure milk with $Q$ is $8\ell$, with P is $16\ell$ and in initial amount in can is $32\ell$. $\therefore$ the percent dilution in amount of milk with P, Q, R and S are $\frac{9}{25} \times 100$ $= 36\%$, $\frac{5}{13} \times 100 \simeq 38\%$, $\frac{3}{7} \times 100 \simeq 43\%$ and $\frac{2}{4} \times 100 \simeq$ 50% respectively.

**So the correct options for (a), (b), (c) and (d) are (iii), (ii), (ii) and (iv) respectively.**

**117.** Note that from
1st, 2nd and 4th group, A will be one of (I, K) and from 1st, 3rd and 4th group A will be one of (J, F).
Now we can have four cases regarding A:

Case I: A ≡ I and J. The given groups get reduced to triplets: (C, D, E) ; (C, K, L); (D, F, H), (G, H, L) and (B, G, K). So we can have

| (I) | | | (II) | | | (III) | | |
|---|---|---|---|---|---|---|---|---|
| C | D | E | C | D | E | C | D | E |
| C | K | L | C | L | K | C | L | K |
| H | D | F | F | D | H | H | D | F |
| H | G | L | G | L | H | H | L | G |
| Not possible as G, K are distinct | | | G | B | K | Not possible as G, K are distinct | | |

Case II: A ≡ I and F. This is not possible as fifth group will not have A.

Case III: A ≡ K and J. This is not possible as fifth group will have A twice.

Case IV: A ≡ K and F. The given groups get reduced to triplets: (C, D, E); (C, I, L) ; (D, H, J); (G, H, L) and (B, G, J). So we can have

| | | | | | | | | |
|---|---|---|---|---|---|---|---|---|
| C | D | E | C | D | E | C | D | E |
| C | I | L | C | L | I | C | L | I |
| H | D | J | J | D | H | H | D | J |
| H | G | L | G | L | H | H | L | G |
| B | G | J | Not possiple as G, J are distinct. | | | Not possible as E, I, J, G can't be same person. | | |

∴ we have two possible cases:

| | | | | | | | | |
|---|---|---|---|---|---|---|---|---|
| A | C | D | E | | A | C | D | E |
| I | F | L | K | or | K | H | I | L |
| J | G | B | H | | F | B | G | J |

**So the correct options for (a), (b), (c) and (d) are (ii), (ii), (iv) and (iii) respectively.**

**118.** Consider the ranks of A, B, C and D which can be 1, 2, 3 or 4. Now if $x$ be the rank of A in a subject, then the ranks of

$(4 - x)$ students will be behind him. Therefore if $x_1, x_2, x_3, x_4$ be the ranks of A in four subjects, then

$$\overline{4 - x_1} + \overline{4 - x_2} + \overline{4 - x_3} + \overline{4 - x_2} = 6$$

(as out of 16 possible ranks, 6 will be behind A's ranks)

$$\Rightarrow \quad 16 - (x_1 + x_2 + x_3 + x_4) = 6$$

$$\Rightarrow \quad x_1 + x_2 + x_3 + x_4 = 10$$

i.e. the sum of ranks of A will be 10.

Similarly the sum of ranks of B, C and D will also be 10. Now the ranks of the students (may not be in order) can be

| Case I | Case II | Case III |
|---|---|---|
| (1, 1, 4, 4) | (1, 1, 4, 4) | (1, 2, 3, 4) |
| (2, 2, 2, 4) | (2, 2, 3, 3) | (1, 2, 3, 4) |
| (1, 3, 3, 3) | (1, 2, 3, 4) | (1, 2, 3, 4) |
| (1, 2, 3, 4) | (1, 2, 3, 4) | (1, 2, 3, 4) |

where the order of ranks within a bracket may not be in order of the given subjects.

**(a) The correct option is (i). EXPLANATION:**
From case I, the result is obvious.

**(b) The correct option is (ii). EXPLANATION:**
From case I, $m = 3$, $n = 2$ and $p = 2$

**(c) The correct option is (iii). EXPLANATION:**
we have,

| Ranks | : | 1 | 2 | 3 | 4 |
|---|---|---|---|---|---|
| Maths | : | A | C | — | — |
| Physics | : | A | B | — | — |
| Chemistry | : | B | — | — | A |
| Biology | : | C | — | — | A |

[Note that ranks of A has to be last in chemistry and Biology as sum of the ranks of A in four subjects is 10]

Note that the above case corresponds to the case II where the ranks of D are (2, 2, 3, 3). From above table, D must get rank 2 in Chemistry and Biology and rank 3 in Maths and Physics.

**(d) The correct option is (iii). EXPLANATION**

∵ A got second highest marks in three of the subjects ∴ this case will correspond to the case I. Now, we have,

A → ( 2 , 2 , 2 , 4 )
B → ( 1 , 1 , 4 , 4 )
(Maths) , (Physics)
C → ( 1 , 2 , 3 , 4 )
(Chem)
D → ( 1 , 3 , 3 , 3 )

From above table, C cannot get second lowest mark (i.e. rank 3) in Chemistry. ∴ D must have got second lowest marks in Chemistry.

**(e) The correct option is (iv) . EXPLANATION:**

∵ A got rank 2 in two subjects and B got rank 4 also in two subjects ∴ this case corresponds to case II. Now, we have

A → ( 2 (Maths) , 2 (Phy) , 3 (Chem) , 3 (Bio) )
B → ( 1 (Maths) , 1 (Phy) , 4 (Chem) , 4 (Bio) )

From above table, none of the first three given options seems feasible.

**119.** Consider two tables:

| Student | Given Ranks (For two subjects) |
|---|---|
| A | 1, 4 |
| B | 1, 3 |
| C | 2, 3 |
| D | 2, 4 |

and

| Subject | Ranks Left (For two students) | Students who occupy these ranks |
|---|---|---|
| Maths | 2, 4 | C, D |
| Physics | 3, 4 | A, C |
| Chemistry | 1, 2 | B, D |
| Biology | 1, 3 | A, B |

(a) **The correct option is (iii). EXPLANATION**
From second table the ranks of A can be chosen in 2 × 2, i.e. 4 ways and that of D can also be chosen in 2 × 2, i.e. 4 ways. [Note that the ranks for B and C will be the remainging ones]. ∴ total number of possibilities = 4 × 4 = 16

(b) **The correct option is (iv). EXPLANATION:**
The sum of ranks for
A can be 5 (From first table) + (4, 5, 6 or 7) (From second table)
D can be 6 (From first table) + (3, 4, 5 or 6) (From second table)
Now the sum of ranks for both A and D can be 9, 10, 11 or 12.
∴ four required possibilities exist.

(c) **The correct option is (iv). EXPLANATION:**
Note that the maximum value of sum of ranks of B will be 4 (from first table) + 5 (from second table) = 9
while the minimum value of sum of ranks of C and D are respectively
5 (from first table) + 5 (from second table) = 10 and
6 (from first table) + 3 (from second table) = 9
As the sum of ranks of B or C can be both 9
∴ the conclusion cannot be made about which of them will get the least marks.

**120.** Let us convert the grades into relative marks by assuming that grade D in both systems correspond to 3 marks. Then the relative marks for the grades will be as:

| | A | B | C | D |
|---|---|---|---|---|
| System I : | 12 | 6 | 4 | 3 |
| System II: | 12 | 9 | 6 | 3 |

Note that the relative marks in system II are multiples of 3.
∵ by the evaluation of system II, the ranks of P and S are

three and one respectively ∴ if $n$ be the marks obtained by P, then the marks obtained by S should be at least $(n + 6)$

Now the decrements of marks from system II to system I are 0, 3, 2, 0 for the grades A, B, C and D respectively. ∵ by the evaluation of system I, the marks obtained by S is less than that of P and P got grade C in one of the subjects ∴ the decrements of marks from system II to system I for P and S should be 2 and 9 respectively. So that their marks became $(n - 2)$ and $(n - 3)$ respectively. As the decrement of marks for S is 9 ∴ S must have got grade B in all the three subjects and consequently $(X - 3)$ must be equal to $6 \times 3$, i.e. $n$ must be equal to 21.

Now the relative marks obtained by students can be tabulated as:

| | System I | System II |
|---|---|---|
| P | 19 | 21 |
| Q | – | – |
| R | – | – |
| S | 18 | 27 |

∵ by evaluation of system II, relative marks obtained by Q and R are equal and between that of P and S

∴ it must be 24 (as the relative marks for system II are multiples of 3).

Now $24 = 12 + 9 + 3$ or $12 + 6 + 6$ or $9 + 9 + 6$

∴ the grades obtained by Q, R can be (A, B, D) or (A, C, C) or (B, B, C)

∵ by the evaluation of system I, R got the highest rank and Q, the lowest ∴ the grades obtained by R can be (A, B, D) or (A, C, C) and those obtained by Q will be (B, B, C)

Also the grades obtained by P will be (A, C, D) as it is the only possibility. We can tabulate the results as:

| | Grades |
|---|---|
| P → | (A, C, D) |
| Q → | (B, B, C) |
| R → | (A, B, D) or (A, C, C) |
| S → | (B, B, B) |

**So the correct options for (a), (b), (c), (d) and (e) are (iii), (iii), (i), (i) and (i) respectively.**

**121.** Ball could have been passed among three persons in four different ways: $\overline{ABC}, \overline{ABD}, \overline{ACD}$ or $\overline{BCD}$ and let the number of times it was passed among them be $a$, $b$, $c$ and $d$ respectively. Then

| A | B | C | D |
|---|---|---|---|
| $a$ | $a$ | $a$ | – |
| $b$ | $b$ | – | $b$ |
| $c$ | – | $c$ | $c$ |
| – | $d$ | $d$ | $d$ |

**A.** There will be 14 sequences (triplets) as the total number of times the ball held by them was 16. If we note down the sequence in which the ball is passed then it will start from AC and end in DA.

$\therefore\ a + b + c = 3 \times 3 + 2 \times 1 = 11$ (sequence involving A)

$a + b + d = 3 \times 3 = 9$ (sequence involving B),

$a + c + d = 3 \times 3 + 1 \times 2 = 11$ (sequence involving C),

$b + c + d = 3 \times 3 + 1 \times 2 = 11$ (sequence involving D).

Also

$a + b + c + d = 14.$

$\therefore\ a = 3,\ b = 3,\ c = 5$ and $d = 3$.

**So the correct options for (a), (b) and (c) are (i), (iii) and (i) respectively.**

**B.** Note that if we note down the sequence in which ball is passed, then we will have six different pairs (written consecutively), viz. (A, B), (A, C), (A, D), (B, C), (B, D) and (C, D). Also A, B, C and D can form 8, 6, 8, 8 pairs respectively.

**(a) The correct option is (ii). EXPLANATION:**

The question only implies that total numbers of all pairs involving A, B or C only must be added which will be

equal to $\dfrac{8 + 6 + 8 - 8}{2} = 7$

**(b) The correct option is (ii). EXPLANATION:**

As done in part (a), it will be equal to

$$\frac{8+6+8-8}{2} = 9$$

**122.** (D, G, E, H) will be in middle or lowest shelf.

Note that any book of one subject can be absent from only one shelf.

$\because$ B and chemistry book are not on one shelf

$\therefore$ B is on top shelf.

Similarly F and H are on middle and lowest shelves respectively.

$\because$ E and biology books are not on one shelf and E is in middle or lowest shelf $\therefore$ one of these shelves will also not have biology book and that shelf will only have two books.

$\therefore$ we can have two different arrangements:

$$\begin{array}{lcl} \text{Books} & & \text{Subjects} \\ \left\{\begin{array}{l} \text{A, B, C} \\ \text{F, D, G} \\ \text{H, E} \end{array}\right. & \begin{array}{c} \longrightarrow \\ \longrightarrow \\ \longrightarrow \end{array} & \begin{array}{c} \text{M, P, B} \\ \text{C, P, B} \\ \text{M, C} \end{array} \end{array}$$

$$\text{or} \left\{\begin{array}{l} \text{A, B, C} \\ \text{F, E} \\ \text{H, D G} \end{array}\right. \begin{array}{c} \longrightarrow \\ \longrightarrow \\ \longrightarrow \end{array} \begin{array}{c} \text{M, P, B} \\ \text{P, C} \\ \text{B, M, C} \end{array}$$

**So the correct options for (a), (b), (c), (d) are (iii), (iv) (iii) and (iv) respectively.**

**123.** Let P be the initial amount the man has. Then

$$5A + B + x = P$$
$$4B + 2C + y = P \text{ and}$$
$$3C + 3A + z = P$$

where $0 < x, y, z < A, B, C$

Note that $A = B = C$ and $x = y = z$ is also a possibility

$\therefore$ the relative price of A, B and C cannot be determined.

**So the correct options for (a) and (b) are (iv).**

**124.** Taking first, third and fifth rows together, the money spent on each article are same and equal to $(x + y + z)$.

Same are the cases for second, fourth and sixth rows.

$\therefore\ 28 + 31 + 31 = 29 + k + k'$

$\Rightarrow \qquad k + k' = 61$

Now let $x/A = p$, $y/A = \alpha p$, $z/A = \beta p$

(Note that $p$, $\alpha p$, $\beta p$ are integers)

Similarly, let $x/B = q$, $y/B = \alpha q$, $z/B = \beta q$

and $x/c = r$, $y/c = \alpha r$, $z/c = \beta r$

Now, we have

$$\left.\begin{array}{ccccccc} p & + & \alpha q & + & \beta r & = & 28 \\ p & + & \beta q & + & \alpha r & = & 29 \\ \alpha p & + & \beta q & + & r & = & 31 \\ \alpha p & + & q & + & \beta r & = & k \\ \beta p & + & q & + & \alpha r & = & 31 \end{array}\right\}$$

$$\Rightarrow \left\{\begin{array}{lccc} (\alpha-\beta) & (q-r) & = & -1 \\ (\beta-1) & (q-r) & = & 31-k \\ (1-\alpha) & (p-r) & = & -2 \\ (\alpha-\beta) & (p-r) & = & k-31 \end{array}\right.$$

From first two equations, we have $(\alpha - 1)(q - r) = 30 - k$

$$\therefore\ \frac{k-31}{2} = \frac{-1}{30-k}$$

$\Rightarrow (k - 31)(k - 30) = 2$

$k = 32$ or $28$

$\because\ k < 32$, given

$\therefore\ k = 28$. Subsequently $k' = 61 - k = 33$

Now $(\alpha - \beta)(q - r) = -1$

$(\alpha - \beta)(p - r) = k - 31 = -3$

$$\therefore\ \frac{q-r}{p-r} = \frac{1}{3}$$

$\Rightarrow 3q - 3r = p - r \Rightarrow 3q = p + 2r$

Again $(\alpha - \beta)(q - r) = -1$

$(\beta - 1)(q - r) = 31 - k = 3$

$$\therefore \quad \frac{\alpha - \beta}{\beta - 1} = -\frac{1}{3}$$

$\Rightarrow 3\alpha - 3\beta = 1 - \beta$

$\Rightarrow 3\alpha = 1 + 2\beta$

$\because \alpha = y/x$ and $\beta = z/x$

$\therefore \quad 3y = x + 2z$

**So the correct options for (a), (b), (c) and (d) are (i), (iv), (iv) and (ii) respectively.**

**125.** Three articles comprises of 2A + B, 2B + A, 2A + C, A + B + C or A + 2C. For successive articles, we can have following cases:

| Cases | Three articles | Four articles | Five articles | Six and Seven articles |
|---|---|---|---|---|
| I. | 2A + B | A = 2B or B = 2C or A = B + C | Two of the conditions of fourarticles must be satisfied and it must not give B = C | (i) A = 2B and B = 2C. Six articles will be A + B + 4C while the seven articles will be A + 6C.<br>(ii) B = 2C and A = B + C. Six articles will be A + 5C while the seven articles will be B + 6C. |
| II. | 2B + A | A = 2B or B = 2C or A = B + C | | (i) A = 2B and B = 2C. Six articles will be 2B + 4C and seven articles will be B + 6C.<br>(ii) B = 2C and A = B + C. Six articles will be B + 5C and seven articles will 7C. |
| III. | 2A + C | A = 2B or A = B + C | Not possible as B = C | |
| IV. | A + 2C | A = 2B or A = B + C | Not possible as B = C | |
| V. | A + B + C | | A = 2B or B = 2C or A = B + C | (i) A = 2B and B = 2C. Six articles will be B + 5C and seven ar'icles will be 7C.<br>(ii) B = 2C and A = B + C. Not possible as seven articles is not possible. |

**So the correct options for (a), (b), (c), (d) and (e) are (iv), (i), (iv), (i) and (i) respectively.**

**126.** Let $x$, $y$, $z$ be the prices of A, B and C respectively. Then
$4x + y = 240$
There can be three cases for second condition, viz.
$2(x + y) = 240$ or $2(x + z) = 240$ or $2(y + z) = 240$

Case I: $2(x + y) = 240$ and $4x + y = 240$
$\Rightarrow 2x = y$ $\Rightarrow x = 40, y = 80$
Now $x + y + 3z$, $x + z + 3y$ or $y + z + 3x$ is equal to 240
which give $z = 40$; not possible; 40 respectively.
$\because$ $x, y, z$ are different $\therefore$ this case is rejected.

Case II : $2(x + z) = 240$ and $4x + y = 240$
Now $x + y + 3z$, $x + z + 3y$ or $y + z + 3x$ is equal to 240.
which give $x = z$; $y = 40$, $x = 50$ and $z = 70$; $x = 60$, $y = 0$.
$\therefore$ only the case $x + z + 3y = 240$ is acceptable where $x = 50$, $y = 40$ and $z = 70$.

Case III: $2(y + z) = 240$ and $4x + y = 240$
Now $x + y + 3z$, $x + z + 3y$ or $y + z + 3x$ is equal to 240.

which give $x = z$; $x = \frac{360}{7}, y = \frac{240}{7}$ and $z = \frac{600}{7}$; $x = z$.

$\therefore$ only the case $x + z + 3y = 240$ is acceptable

where $x = \frac{360}{7}, y = \frac{240}{7}$ and $z = \frac{600}{7}$.

**So the correct options for (a), (b), (c) and (d) are (iii), (ii), (iv) and (ii) respectively.**

**127.** Note that the least expensive article will be less than or equal to $\frac{180}{6} = 30$.

From part (d), either this is 25 or 30. Also note that

$\frac{210}{7} = 30$.

$\therefore$ let us start with putting least expensive articles as Rs 30. Then
$160 = 30 \times 4 + 40 \times 1$, $40 \times 4$, $30 \times 2 + 50 \times 2$

[no other possibilities occurs due to constraint on least expensive and most expensive articles from part (d) and (e)]

Also $180 = 30 \times 6, 30 \times 3 + 50 \times 1 + 40 \times 1,$
$50 \times 2 + 40 \times 2$

$\therefore$ the cost of articles as Rs 30, Rs 40 and Rs 50 is most probable and these are also verified by

$210 = 30 \times 7, 30 \times 4 + 50 \times 1 + 40 \times 1, 50 \times 1 + 40 \times 4$

Now P can buy articles in following four ways only:

$30 \times 2 + 50 \times 2$; $40 \times 4$; $30 \times 4 + 40 \times 1$,
$2 \times 40 + 30 \times 1 + 50 \times 1$

Q can buy articles in following five ways only:

$50 \times 3 + 30 \times 1$; $40 \times 3 + 30 \times 2$;
$30 \times 3 + 40 \times 1 + 50 \times 1$; $40 \times 2 + 50 \times 2$; $30 \times 6$.

R can buy articles in following six ways only:

$30 \times 3 + 40 \times 3$; $30 \times 2 + 50 \times 3$; $4 \times 40 + 50 \times 1$; $30 \times 4 + 40 \times 1 + 50 \times 1$; $40 \times 2 + 30 \times 1 + 50 \times 2$; $30 \times 7$

**So the correct options for (a), (b), (c), (d) and (e) are (iii), (iii), (iv), (ii) and (ii) respectively.**

**128. (a) The correct option is (i). EXPLANATION:**

Consider six consecutive integers say 0, 1, 2, 3, 4 and 5. The minimum such sum will be 3 and maximum such sum will be 12. $\therefore$ minimum of 10 such sums are possible.

**(b) The correct option is (iv). EXPLANATION:**

All we need to find the number of distinct sums of part (a), for which there exits at least three distinct solutions. Note that

$6 = 0 + 2 + 4 = 0 + 1 + 5 = 1 + 2 + 3$
$7 = 0 + 2 + 5 = 0 + 3 + 4 = 1 + 2 + 4$
$8 = 0 + 3 + 5 = 1 + 2 + 5 = 1 + 3 + 4$
$9 = 0 + 4 + 5 = 1 + 3 + 5 = 2 + 3 + 4$

$\therefore$ there exist four such triplets.

**129.** Given that

I. three of (A B, C, D) $\rightarrow$ Maths ($\rightarrow$ denotes 'teaches')
II. three of (B, D, E, F) $\rightarrow$ Physics
III. three of (A, C, E, F) $\rightarrow$ Chemistry
IV. one of (B, E); (C, D); (A, F) $\rightarrow$ Biology

These can be three cases for A, viz.

A → (Maths, Bio) or (Chem, Bio) or (Maths, Chem).

Case I: A → Maths, Bio

∵ A does not teach Chem ∴ C, E, F teach Chem (Statement I).

∵ A teaches Bio ∴ F does not teach Bio but Phy (IV and III).

∴ F → Chem, Phy

Now C, E teach Chem and one of C, E has to teach Maths and another Bio. ∵ only E can teach Maths

∵ C → Chem, Maths and

E → Chem, Bio

Now E teaches Bio ∴ B cannot teach it (IV).

Only (Maths, Phy) and (Bio, Phy) are left

∴ B → Maths, Phy and

D → Bio, Phy

Case II: A → Chem, Bio

∵ A does not teach Maths ∴ B, C, D teach it (I).

∵ A teaches Bio ∴ F cannot teach Bio (IV) and consequently

F → Phy, Chem (II and III)

One teacher has to teach (Maths, Chem) and it can only be C (I and III)

∴ C → Maths, Chem

∵ C does not teach Bio ∴ D teaches it (IV).

∴ D → Maths, Bio

Now only (Maths, Phy) and (Phy, Bio) are left

∴ B → Maths, Phy and

E → Phy, Bio

Case III: A → Maths, Chem

∵ A does not teach Bio ∴ F teaches it IV.

Also as C cannot teach (Maths, Chem) ∴ C has to teach Bio and consequently

D → Maths, Phy (I and II)

∵ B cannot teach (Maths, Phy) together ∴ B has to teach Bio and consequently

E → Phy, Chem

Now B → Bio, Maths/Phy

C → Bio, Chem/Maths

F → Bio, Phy/Chem

We can tabulate the results of three cases as:

| Case I | Case II | Case III |
|---|---|---|
| A → Maths, Bio | A → Chem, Bio | A → Maths, Chem |
| B → Maths, Phy | B → Maths, Phy | B → Bio, Maths/Phy |
| C → Maths, Chem | C → Maths, Chem | C → Bio, Chem/Maths |
| D → Phy, Bio | D → Maths, Bio | D → Maths, Phy |
| E → Chem, Bio | E → Phy, Bio | E → Phy, Chem |
| F → Phy, Chem | F → Phy, Chem | F → Bio, Phy/Chem |

**So the correct options for (a), (b), (c), (d) and are (iii), (iv), (iii), (iii) and (ii) respectively.**

**130.** Note that E, F, G, H, I, J will be supervisors. Now

E → A and B (→ denotes 'report to')
I → C and D
F → (A and B) or (A and D) or (B and D)
G → (B and C) or (B and D) or (C and D)
H → (A and C) or (A and D) or (C and D)
J → (A and B) or (A and C) or (B and C).

Now each supervisor report to two persons only and each manager (three of A, B, C, D) reports to the director only. ∴ the total number of instances of a person reporting to another person must be 15. ∵ A, B, D each gets report from four persons ∴ C must get report from three persons. Also A, B, C, D each gets report form at least one supervisor ∴ the director must get report from four persons (three managers and a supervisor). As C gets report from three persons only ∴ C cannot be the director and must get reports from two of (G, H, J).

Now, we can have three cases:

Case I: A is the director. Then

F → B and D
H → C and D
G → B and D
J → B and C

Case II: B is the director. Then

F → A and D
G → C and D

H → A and D
J → A and C

Case III: D is the director. Then
F → A and B
G → B and C
H → A and C
J → A and B

**So the correct options for (a), (b) and (c) are (ii), (iv) and (ii) respectively.**

**131.** Note that

| | | |
|---|---|---|
| Maths | → | C, E, F, G only |
| Physics | → | A, B, C, D only |
| Chemistry | → | A, E, G, H only |
| Biology | → | B, D, F, H only |

Note that A has to be physics or chemistry. We can have two cases:

Case I: A → Physics

| A | B | C | D | E | F | G | H |
|---|---|---|---|---|---|---|---|
| Phy | Bio | Maths | Phy | Maths | Bio | Chem | Chem |
| 1 | 2 | 5 | 6 | 7 | 8 | 3 | 4 |

where numbers denote the sequence of the steps in which A, B...H are assigned subjects

Case II: A → Chemistry

| A | B | C | D | E | F | G | H |
|---|---|---|---|---|---|---|---|
| Chem | Phy | Phy | Bio | Chem | Maths | Maths | Bio |
| 1 | 2 | 8 | 7 | 5 | 6 | 4 | 3 |

**So the correct options for (a), (b), (c) and (d) are (iv), (i), (iii) and (iv) respectively.**

**132.** Note that there will be three gold, three silver and three bronze medals.

∴ $X_1$ → B, G, G (S, S is not possible)
$X_2$ → G, S
$X_3$ → B, S
$X_4$ → S
$X_5$ → B

We can for a table as:

| Event | $X_1$ | $X_2$ | | | | | $X_3$ $X_4$ $X_5$ | | | | | | |
|---|---|---|---|---|---|---|---|---|---|---|---|---|---|
| 1 | G | S | B | — | — | | B | — | — | | B | — | — |
| 2 | G | — | S | — | B | or | — | S | B | or | B | S | — |
| 3 | B | G | — | S | — | | S | — | — | | S | — | — |

**So the correct options for (a), (b) and (c) are (i), (iii) and (iv) respevtively.**

**133.** Note that the total calorie needed = the total calorie bought [as 1600 + 1800 + 2200 + 2400 = 4 × (400 + 450 + 500 + 650)]

Now

A → 1600 → 4P or Q + R + S

B → 1800 → 2S + R (∵ B preferred to have only three packets)

C → 2200 → 2Q + 2S or 3P + 2R or 2S + P + R or 2Q + 2P +R

∴ the distribution to A, B, C, D can be respectively

(4P, 2S + R, 2Q + 2S, 3R + 2Q) or

(Q + R + S, 2S + R, 3P + 2R, S + 3Q + P) or

(Q + R + S, 2S + R, 2Q + 2P + R, S + R + Q + 2P)

**So the correct options for (a), (b), (c) and (d) are (ii), (i), (iii) and (iv) respectively.**

**134.** Let the cost of articles be $c$, $c + x$, $c + y$ $(y > x)$ where $c$, $x$, $y$ are positive integers. Then we need to verify if there exist integers $m$, $n$ $(0 < m + n < 4)$ such that

$m(c + x) + n(c + y) + (4 - m - n)c = 23, 24, 25, 26$

$\Rightarrow mx + ny + 4c = 23, 24, 25, 26$ ...(i)

Let us put $c = 5$. Then

$mx + ny = 3, 4, 5, 6$

For $x = 1$, $y = 2$, there can be values of $(m, n)$ satisfying $m + 2n = 3, 4, 5, 6$

For $x = 1$, $y = 3$, there can still be values of $(m, n)$ satisfying $m + 3n = 3, 4, 5, 6$

For $x = 2$, $y = 3$, there can still be values of $(m, n)$ satisfying $2m + 3n = 3, 4, 5, 6$

∴ the cost of articles which are expensive with respect to third articles cannot be determined.

Now if we put $c = 4$ in (i), we will have
$mx + ny = 7, 8, 9$ or 10
For $x = 3$ and $y = 4$, there can be values of $(m, n)$ satisfying $3m + 4n = 7, 8, 9$ or 10
$\therefore$ the cost of even cheapest article cannot be determined.

**So the correct options for (a), (b) and (c) are (iv).**

**135.** For all these cases, the sum of surplus amount over Rs 80 for each article bought (when the lower number of articles are bought) must be $\geq$ Rs 80 and < 160
Now
P can have Rs 240 $\rightarrow$ 120 + 120 or 80 + 80 + 80;
Q can have $\rightarrow$ 120 + 120 + $n$ or 80 + 80 + 80 + $n$ where $n$ = 80, 90, 100 or 120

For minimum value, $n = 80$ and for maximum value, $n = 120$
$\therefore Q_{min}$ = Rs 320 and $Q_{max}$ = Rs 360.
R can have $\rightarrow 120 + 120 + n_1 + n_2$ where
$(n_1 - 80) + (n_2 - 80) \leq 80$
$\therefore R_{min}$ = Rs 400 and $R_{max}$ = Rs 460
S can have $\rightarrow 120 + 120 + n_1 + n_2 + n_3$ where
$(n_1 - 80) + (n_2 - 80) + (n_3 - 80) < 80$
$\therefore S_{min}$ = Rs 480 and $S_{max}$ = Rs 550

**So the correct options for (a), (b), (c), (d) and (e) are (iii), (ii), (ii), (ii) and (ii) respectively.**

**136.** From statement I, A is between C and D and from statement II, C is between B and D. $\therefore$ we have B < C < A < D and D – A = A – C = C – B = $x$, say.
Now $R$ = 5B = 150 (from statements III and IV)
$\because$ R can buy at least three articles $\therefore$ R can buy any three articles from cheapest combination (2B + C) to costliest combination 3D and their price can vary from $90 + x + 90 + 9x$ which must be equal to 150, i.e. $x$ to $9x = 60$
$\because$ $x$ have only integral solution
$\therefore x$ = 60, 30, 20 15, 12 or 10.
We can have following cases:

| $x$ | B | C | A | D | |
|---|---|---|---|---|---|
| 10 | 30 | 40 | 50 | 60 | |
| 12 | 30 | 42 | 54 | 66 | |
| 15 | 30 | 45 | 60 | 75 | → Rejected |
| 20 | 30 | 50 | 70 | 90 | |
| 30 | 30 | 60 | 90 | 120 | → Rejected |
| 60 | 30 | 90 | 150 | 210 | → Rejected |

Note that for $x = 60$, 30 or 15, the lowest number of articles R can buy will be one (1A), two (C + A) or two (2D) respectively. ∴ these cases are rejected.

Pertaining to part (e), R can buy four articles only if $x = 10$ and he can buy (3B, D) or (3C, B) or (2B, C, A)

**So the correct options for (a), (b), (c), (d) and (e) are (iii), (iv), (iii), (iv) and (iv) respectively.**

**137.** Let L be the lowest amount and H be the highest amount possessed by the persons. Then we can have a chart as:

| | A | B | C | D | E |
|---|---|---|---|---|---|
| Initial Amount | L + 20 | H – 40 | | | |
| Ist Enchange | L + 20 | H | 70 | L | 50 |
| IInd Exchange | H | H – 40 | H – 30 | $x$ | $x - 10$ |

We can have four cases corresponding to
$H - 40 = 70$, $H - 30 = 70$, $x = 70$ and $x - 10 = 70$

Case I: H = 110
Amounts in IInd exchange are 110, 70, 80, $x$, $x - 10$
Now L < 50 ∴ $x = 50$, $L = x - 10 = 40$
But L + 20 is not accounted for. ⇒ REJECTED

Case II: H = 100
Amounts in IInd exchange are 100, 60, 70, $x$, $x - 10$. Now L < 50 ∴ $x = 50$, $L = x - 10 = 40$.
But H – 40 and L + 20 cannot be equal ⇒ REJECTED

Case III: $x = 70$
Amounts in IInd exchange are 70, 60, H, H – 40 and H – 30. Now one of them has to be 50 and one less than

50 ∴ H – 30 = 50, H – 40 = 40 ⇒ H = 80

**RETAINED**

Case IV: $x - 10 = 70$

Amounts in IInd exchange are 70, 80, H, H – 40 and H – 30. Now one of them has to be 50 and one less than 50. ∴ H – 30 = 50 ⇒ H = 80 which is not possible as $x = 80$ ⇒

**REJECTED**

∴ from case III, we have

| | A | B | C | D | E |
|---|---|---|---|---|---|
| Initial Amount: | 60 | 40 | 80 | 50 | 70 |
| Ist Exchange: | 60 | 80 | 70 | 40 | 50 |
| IInd Exchange: | 80 | 40 | 50 | 70 | 60 |

**So the correct options for (a), (b), (c), (d) and (e) are (ii),(i), (iii), (i) and (ii) respectively.**

**138.** We can draw a table as:

| | A | B | C | D |
|---|---|---|---|---|
| Initial | 100 | 200 | 300 | 400 |
| 1st Exchange | | | | |
| 2nd Exchange | | | | |
| 3rd Exchange | 200 | 300 | 400 | 100 |
| 4th Exchange | | | | |
| 5th Exchange | | | | |
| 6th Exchange | 100 | 200 | 300 | 400 |

Note that the amount A had initially is with D after third exchange: A → D

Similarly B → A

C → B

D → C

We can have the order of first three selections as

(A, B) → (B, C) → (C, D) – 1
(A, B) → (B, D) → (B, C) – 2
(A, B) → (C, D) → (B, D) – 3

[These dencte equation numbers]

(A, C) → (A, B) → (C, D) – 4
(A, C) → (C, D) → (A, B) – 5

(A, D) → (A, C) → (A, B) – 6
(A, D) → (B, C) → (A, C) – 7
(A, D) → (A, B) → (B, C) – 8

(B, C) → (C, D) → (D, A) – 9
(B, C) → (C, A) → (C, D) – 10
(B, C) → (A, D) → (A, C) – 11

(B, D) → (A, D) → (B, C) – 12
(B, D) → (B, C) → (A, D) – 13

(C, D) → (D, B) → (D, A) – 14
(C, D) → (D, A) → (A, B) – 15
(C, D) → (A, B) → (B, D) – 16

Now the reverse order of the last three selections will be same as above. We need to combine two such triplets such that all six exclusive pairs are chosen. The possible sequences are from the combination of (3, 7); (3, 11) [Now we should ignore 1,2, 3]; (4, 12); (4, 13); (5, 12); (5, 13); (7, 16) and (11, 16).

**So the correct options for (a), (b), (c), (d), (e) and (f) are (i), (iii), (i), (i), (ii) and (iii) respectively.**

**139.** We can draw a table as:

| | A | B | C | D | | |
|---|---|---|---|---|---|---|
| Initial | 40 – x | 32 | 48 | 40 + $x$ | → | ⑥ |
| 1st Selection | 40 | 32 | 48 | 40 | → | ⑤ |
| 2nd Selection | 36 | 36 | 48 | 40 | → | ④ |
| 3rd Selection | 36 | 42 | 42 | 40 | → | ① |
| 4th Selection | | | ✓ | ✓ | | |
| 5th Selection | 39 | 41 | 39/41 | 41/39 | → | ③ |
| 6th Selection | 39 | 41 | 40 | 40 | → | ② |

where encircled number denotes the sequence of steps in which the filling is done. Let A, B, C, D also represent the amount possessed by the persons represented by them. Now the explanation for each steps are:

① (B, C) are selected.

② (C, D) are selected.

③ Note that C, D will have amount equal to one of 39, 41. Also in 3rd and 5th selections, no person has the same amount. ∴ in 4th and 5th selections, two exclusive pairs are chosen. And the only possible exclusive pairs are (A, C) and (B, D). ∵ one of the selected pair is (A, C) ∴ C = 39 although the order of selections of (A, C) and (B, D) cannot be known.

④ Now the pairs (A, C); (B, D); (C, D) and (B, C) are exhausted. ∴ the remaining pairs are (A, B) and (A, D). Now (A, D) couldnot have been selected as amounts with them are distinct. ∴ (A, B) were selected. ∴ B = 36 and C = 48.

⑤ (A, D) are selected and A = D = 39.

⑥ Initially A, D have 40 – $x$ and 40 + $x$ where $x$ is any arbitrary integer less than 40.

**So the correct options for (a), (b), (c), (d) and (e) are (i), (iv), (iv), (iii) and (iii) respectively.**

**140.** Let A, B, C, D be the amount possessed by the persons represented by them. Let A + B + C + D = $x$. Then

$$\frac{A+C}{B+D} = \frac{35}{45} = \frac{7}{9}$$

$$\Rightarrow A + C = \frac{14}{32}x \text{ and } B + D = \frac{18}{32}x$$

$$\text{Similarly } A + B = \frac{13}{32}x \text{ and } C + D = \frac{19}{32}x$$

$$A + D = \frac{85}{85+n}x \text{ and } B + C = \frac{n}{85+n}x$$

Let $p$, $q$, $r$ be the cost of a mango, an orange and an apple respectively. Then

$x = (35 + 45)\,p = 80p = 128q = (85 + n)r$

For $x$ to be multiple of 10 ($\leq$ 4000) and $qo$ to be an integer, $x = 128 \times (5, 10, 15, 20, 25 \text{ or } 30)$

For $r$ to be an integer and $50 < n < 100$, we can have $85 + n = 160$ and $x = 160 \times (4, 8, 12, 16, 20 \text{ or } 24)$ [Note that no other values of $n$ is possible]

Now from $B + D = \frac{18}{32}x$, $C + D = \frac{19}{32}x$ and $B + C = \frac{15}{32}x$,

we have $B + D + C = \frac{26x}{32}$ and consequently

$B = \frac{7x}{32}$, $C = \frac{8x}{32}$ $D = \frac{11x}{32}$ and $A = \frac{6x}{32}$.

**So the correct options for (a), (b), (c) and (d) are (ii), (i), (iii) and (ii) respectively.**

**141.** Let A, B, C, D be the cost of articles they represent while *a*, *b*, *c*, *d* be their respective weights. Then

| | |
|---|---|
| $B + C = 130$ | $a + c = 4$ |
| $A + D = 140$ | $b + d = 6$ |
| $B + D = 150$ | $c + d = 7$ |
| $\Rightarrow A + C = 130 + 140 - 150$ | $\Rightarrow a + b = 4 + 6 - 7$ |
| $= 120$ | $= 3$ |
| | Now a, b, cannot be 3kg (as another will be zero) |
| | $\therefore$ one of c, d is 3kg |

Case I: Let c = 3 kg. Then
a = 1 kg, b = 2 kg; c = 80, B = 50, A = 40
and D = 100

Case II: Let d = 3 kg. Then
c = 4 kg, b = 3 kg which canno t be possible

**So the correct options for (a), (b) and (c) are (i), (ii) and (i) respectively.**

**142.** Let

| Fruit | kg per dozen | cost per dozen |
|---|---|---|
| Orange | $x$ | Rs $p$ |
| Apple | $y$ | Rs $q$ |
| Mango | $z$ | Rs $r$ |

where $(x, y, z) \in (1, 2, 3)$
Now

$$p = 1{\cdot}5\ (r/z)$$
$$q = p/x + 2 \text{ and}$$
$$r = 3\ (q/y) + 12$$

$$\Rightarrow \qquad p = \frac{1.5}{z}\left\{\frac{3}{y}\left(\frac{p}{x}+2\right)+12\right\}$$

$\Rightarrow$ $p\,xyz = 4.5\ (p + 2x + 4xy)$

$\Rightarrow$ $6p = 4.5\ (p + 2x + 4xy)$ $(\because xyz = 6)$

$\Rightarrow$ $p = 6x\ (1 + 2y)$ and subsequently

$q = 4\ (2 + 3y)$ and

$r = 4\ (12 + xz)$

$\because q/y$ is an integer $\therefore y \neq 3$

$\because p/x < 30 \therefore y \neq 2$

So $y = 1$ and

$q = 20, r = 72$ and $\because r/z < 30$ $\therefore z = 3$

$\Rightarrow$ $x = 2$ and $p = 36$

**So the correct options for (a), (b) and (c) are (ii), (ii) and (iii) respectively.**

**143.** Let the cost of an apple, a mango and an orange be Rs $x$, Rs $y$, and Rs $z$ respectively, Then

A $\rightarrow$ $11x, 10y, 13z$

B $\rightarrow$ $12x, 11y, 15z$

C $\rightarrow$ $10x, 9y, 12z$

D $\rightarrow$ $14x, 12y, 16z$

where '$\rightarrow$' implies the amount possessed by them roughly. Then

$11x \le A < 12x$
$10y \le A < 11y$
$13z \le A < 14z$

$10x \le B < 13x$
$11y \le B < 12y$
$15z \le B < 16z$

$10x \le C < 11x$
$9y \le C < 10y$
$12z \le C < 13z$

$14x \le D < 15x$
$12y \le D < 13y$
$16z \le D < 17z$

From these equations, we get
$(11/13)\ y < x < (13/14)y$,
$(12/11)z < x < (17/14)z$ and
$(15/12)z < y < (14/10)\ z$

Note that for $y = 7, x = 6$ but no value of $z$ is possible.
For $y = 8, x = 7$ and $z = 6$ which are the least values.

Now for these values,
$80 \le A < 84$
$\because$ A is a multiple of 5
$\therefore A = 80$.

**So the correct options for (a), (b), (c) and (d) are (iii), (iv), (ii) and (iii) respectively.**

**144.** Let $A, B, C, D, E, F$ also denote the amount possessed by the persons they denote. Then

$D + E + F = A + B + C$ and

$A + C + D = B + D + F$

Addition gives $E + D = 2B$.

$\therefore$ there can be three cases, viz.

I. $B = 600$ and $D, E = 450, 750$

II. $B = 500$ and $D, E = 400, 600$

III. $B = 450$ and $D, E = 400, 500$

Now from $B + F = A + C$, only I and II hold as

$600 + 500 = 400 + 700$ (i.e. $F = 500$; $A, C = 400, 700$) and

$500 + 700 = 450 + 750$ (i.e. $F = 700$; $A, C = 450, 750$)

$\because$ $Z$ can be bought by $(A, C, F)$ only

$\therefore$ $Z = 1600$ or $1900$

But for $Z = 1600$, $Z$ can be bought by $D$, $E$ and one of $A$, $C$ as well $(450 + 750 + 400)$. $\therefore$ the case I is rejected and only case II holds good.

$\therefore$ $X = A + C + B = 1200 + 500 = 1700$,

$Y = A + C + D =$ cannot be determined,

$Z = 1900$ as already obtained

**So the correct options for (a), (b), (c) and (d) are (i), (iv), (iii) and (ii) respectively.**

**145.** Let $a$, $2b$, $5c$, $d$ and $e$ be the number of fruits in 1 kg of mango, guava, orange, apple and peach respectively. Then

$$d = b + 5c \quad \text{...(i)}$$

$$2a = b + 4c \quad \text{...(ii)}$$

$$2b = e + a - 2 \quad \text{...(iii)}$$

$$2e = 3 + d \quad \text{...(iv)}$$

From (i), (ii) and (iv), we have

$$2\,(2b - a + 2) = 3 + b + 5c$$

$$\Rightarrow \quad 4b - 2a + 4 = 3 + b + 5c$$

$$\Rightarrow \quad 3b - 2a + 1 = 5c$$

From (ii), we get

$$3b - b - 4c + 1 = 5c$$

$\Rightarrow \quad 2b + 1 = 9c$

Now $\quad c = 1$ or 3 only

For $c = 3$, $\quad b = 13$ but a is not an integer

$\therefore$ $c = 1$ is the only possibility and consequently $b = 4$, $a = 4$, $d = 9$ and $e = 6$.

**So the correct options for (a), (b) and (c) are (iii), (ii) and (ii) respectively.**

**146.** Let R be the radius of the circle. Then

$$\frac{2\pi R}{V_A - V_B} = \frac{4\pi R}{V_A} \text{ if } V_A > V_B \text{ and}$$

$$\frac{2\pi R}{V_B - V_A} = \frac{4\pi R}{V_B} \text{ if } V_A < V_B$$

$$\therefore \quad V_A = 2V_B \text{ if } V_A > V_B$$
$$= 2/3\ V_B \text{ if } V_A < V_B$$

Similarly,

$$\frac{2\pi B}{V_B - V_C} = \pm \frac{6\pi R}{V_B} \text{ according as } V_B \gtrless V_C$$

$$\Rightarrow \quad V_B = 3/2\ V_C \text{ if } V_B > V_C$$
$$= 3/4\ V_C \text{ if } V_B < V_C.$$

And $$\frac{2\pi R}{V_C - V_D} = \frac{8\pi R}{V_C} \text{ according as } V_C \gtrless V_D$$

$$\Rightarrow \quad V_C = 4/3\ V_D \text{ if } V_C > V_D$$
$$= 4/5\ V_D \text{ if } V_C < V_D$$

For part (a), $\quad V_A = 3V_C$ or $\frac{3}{2} V_C$

$$\Rightarrow \quad \frac{V_A}{V_A - V_C} = \frac{3}{2} \text{ or } 3$$

i.e. $$\frac{2\pi R}{V_A - V_C} = (3/2)\ \frac{2\pi R}{V_A} \text{ or } 3 \cdot \frac{2\pi\ R}{V_A}$$

i.e. A would have met C after it made 3/2 or 3 revolutions. Similarly part (b) and (c) can be done.

For part (d), note that

$$V_A = \left(2 \text{ or } \frac{2}{3}\right) \times \left(\frac{3}{2} \text{ or } \frac{3}{4}\right) \times \left(\frac{4}{3} \text{ or } \frac{4}{5}\right) V_D .$$

**So the correct options for (a), (b), (c) and (d) are (i), (iii), (iii) and (iii) respectively.**

**147.** **(a) The correct is (iv). EXPLANATION:**

Let the correct description of stick be long, thick and light. Then none of them would be speaking truth or lie about all the qualities.

**(b) The correct option is (ii). EXPLANATION:**

Note that exactly one exclusive description by A, B and C match with that given by D. If any of these are right and other two wrong, then the one speaking the truth about all the descriptions can be known. If any of these are wrong and other two right, then the case will not be possible. However the case that D speaks truth only is possible.

**148.** Note that

$$\left.\begin{array}{lll} A & \longrightarrow & (B, C) \text{ and } (D, E) \\ B & \longrightarrow & (C, E) \text{ and } (A, D) \\ C & \longrightarrow & (B, D) \text{ and } (A, E) \\ D & \longrightarrow & (A, E) \text{ and } (B, C) \\ E & \longrightarrow & (A, D) \text{ and } (B, C) \end{array}\right\}$$

[Here '⟶' denotes 'speaks truth to one each of ']

Also note all the pairs chosen on R.H.S must have each persons twice.

**(a) The correct option is (ii). EXPLANATION:**

We have

$A \to D$

$B \to A, C$

$C \to E, D$

$D \to E$

$E \to A$

**(b) The correct option (iii). EXPLANATION:**

We have

$A \to E$

$B \to D, E$

C → A, B
D → A
E → D

**(c) The correct option is (iii). EXPLANATION:**
We have
A → E
B → E, D
C → A, B
D → A
E → D

**149.** From three statement, we have

| Statement → | I | | | II | | | III | | |
|---|---|---|---|---|---|---|---|---|---|
| Floors | | | | | | | | | |
| Top | B | | A | D | | B | — | | E |
| 3 | B | | A | D | | — | C | | — |
| 2 | — | or | B | B | or | B | E | or | C |
| 1 | A | | — | — | | B | E | | C |
| Ground | B | | A | D | | D | E. | | C |

where all the possibilities of occupation by (A, B), (B, D) and (C, E) according to three statements are given. Note that A, C cannot occupy second and top floors respectively.

**So the correct options for (a) and (b) are (i) and (iii) respectively.**

**150.** Let

| | Australia | India | Pakistan |
|---|---|---|---|
| A | $a_1$ | $a_2$ | $a_3$ |
| B | $b_1$ | $b_2$ | $b_3$ |
| C | $c_1$ | $c_2$ | $c_3$ |

where $a_1$, $a_2 ... c_3$ denote the amount invested. Similarly their respective gains can be tabulated as:

| | Australia | India | Pakistan |
|---|---|---|---|
| A | $a_1 - (a_2 + a_3)$ | $2a_2 - (a_1 + a_3)$ | $3a_3 - (a_1 + a_2)$ |
| B | $b_1 - (b_2 + b_3)$ | $2b_2 - (b_1 + b_3)$ | $3b_3 - (b_1 + b_2)$ |
| C | $c_1 - (c_2 + c_3)$ | $2c_2 - (c_1 + c_3)$ | $3c_3 - (c_1 + c_2)$ |

Adding the columns, we get

$\Sigma a_1 - \Sigma a_2 - \Sigma a_3 = -1900$ ...given

$2\Sigma a_2 - \Sigma a_1 - \Sigma a_3 = -600$ ...given

$3\Sigma a_3 - \Sigma a_1 - \Sigma a_2 = +3100$ ...given

Solving, we get

$\Sigma a_1 = 1300, \Sigma a_2 = 1300, \Sigma a_3 = 1900$

**So the correct options for (a), (b) and (c) are (ii), (i) and (iv) respectively.**

**151.** We have

| | | | |
|---|---|---|---|
| | B > D, A > C | or | B < D, A < C |
| | C > F, E > D | or | C < F, E < D |
| 1 | E > A, B < F | or | ② E < A, B > F |

From first two informations, we have

| | | | |
|---|---|---|---|
| (I.) | B > D<br>E > D | , | A > C > F |
| (II.) | B > D > E | , | A > C<br>F > C |
| (III) | B < D < E | , | A < C<br>F < C |
| (IV) | B < D<br>E < D | , | A < C < F |

Now we can have eight cases:

① + (I) ⇒ E > A > C > F > B > D

① + (II) ⇒ F > B > D > E > A > C

① + (III) ⇒ no unique solution

① + (IV) ⇒ no unique solution

② + (I) ⇒ no unique solution

② + (II) ⇒ no unique solution

② + (III) ⇒ C > A > E > D > B > F

② + (IV) ⇒ D > B > F > C > A > E

**So the correct options for (a), (b), (c), (d) and (e) are (iii), (iv), (iv), (iii) and (i) respectively.**

**152.** Note that from first four statements, professor, artist, lawyer, doctor do not live in blue, green, red and yellow houses respectively. From last two options, we can have two possible cases:

I. Professor → red house , Doctor → green house
Artist → blue house , Lawyer → yellow house

II. Artist → yellow house , Lawyer → blue house
Professor → green house , Doctor → red house

Note that when A is not a professor, then he lives in blue house and can be an artist or a lawyer.
Similarly when B is not an artist, then he lives in green house and can be a doctor or a professor.
Also C can be a lawyer and when he is not a lawyer, he lives in red house and can be a professor or a doctor.
Similarly D can be a doctor and when he is not a doctor, he lives in yellow house and can be a lawyer or an artist.

**So the correct options for (a), (b), (c) and (d) are (i), (iii), (ii) and (i) respectively.**

**153.** There can be six cases pertaining to first statements:

Case I: A → Professor, B → Doctor ('→' implies 'is')
Let us find Professor, doctor pair in other statements. We find them in IIrd statement. On inspection, this case is ruled out.

Case II: B → Doctor, C → Lawyer
On inspection of statement IV, this case is ruled out.

Case III: C → Lawyer, E → Accountant
On inspection of statement II, this case is ruled out.

Case IV: A → Professor, C → Lawyer
On inspection of statement II, though this case seems feasible, it is rejected on further inspection of statement III.

Case V: A → Professor, E → Accountant
On inspection of other statements, this case is found to be valid and
C → Doctor (using statements I and II)
B → Chemist
D → Lawyer
F → Actor
{ using statements II: E is not professor, F is not accountant }

Case VI: B $\rightarrow$ Doctor, E $\rightarrow$ Accountant
This case need not be examined as case V is already established but for those who does this case prior to Case V, from statement II, though the case seems feasible, on further inspection of statement III, this is rejected.

**So the correct options for (a), (b), (c) and (d) are (i), (iii), (i) and (iii) respectively.**

**154.** Note that only one of them is female and youngest.
There can be five cases:

| | | | |
|---|---|---|---|
| Case I: | A is female , | $E < A$ | ...Rejected. |
| Case II: | B is female , | $B > C$ | ...Rejected. |
| Case III: | C is female , | $B > C$ | ...Retained. |
| Case IV: | D is female , | $A < D$ | ... Rejected. |
| Case V: | E is female , | $E < A, C < E$ | .. Rejected. |

$\therefore$ only valid case is that of case III:
C is female and $B > C$, $A > E$, $D > A$, $E > C$, $B > D$
$\therefore$ $A > E > D > C$ and
$B > D$

**So the correct options for (a), (b) and (c) are (iv), (iv) and (ii) respectively.**

**155.** Note that (A, B) and (G, H) are of opposite sex while (C, D), (E, F), (B, F), (C, G) are of same sex.
When there are six males in the group, then the females have to be A and H.
Similarly when there are six females in the group, then the males have to be A and H.
When there are four males and four females in the group, then (C, D, G, A) have to be of one sex and (B, E, F, H) have to be of another sex. $\therefore$ when A is male, then H will be female.

**So the correct options for (a), (b) and (c) are (iv), (i) and (iv) respectively.**

**156.** Let A like green. Then we will have only one valid possibility:

| A | B | C | D | E |
|---|---|---|---|---|
| green | yellow | black | red | blue |

Let B like blue. Again we will have only one valid possibility:

| A | B | C | D | E |
|---|---|---|---|---|
| yellow | blue | red | green | black |

**So the correct options for (a), (b) and (c) are (iii), (iii) and (ii) respectively.**

**157.** There can be four cases for pair of males, viz. (A, B), (A, D), (B, C) or (C, D) and corresponding choice of colours can be tabulated as

| Cases: | I | II | III | IV |
|---|---|---|---|---|
| Males: | (A, B) | (A, D) | (B, C) | (C, D) |
| | A → yellow | A → yellow | A → red | A → green |
| | B → blue | B → red | B → yellow | B → red |
| | C → green | C → blue | C → green | C → yellow |
| | D → red | D → green | D → blue | D → blue |

**So the correct options for (a), (b), (c) and (d) are (iii), (iv), (iv) and (i) respectively.**

**158.** Only one of (A, G), (B, D) or (D, E) will be a couple. Let (A, G) be one of the couple. Then others will be (B, E), (C, H) and (D, F).
Let (B, D) be one of the couple. Then two of the other couples can be (C, E), (A, F) but the fourth couple cannot be possible.
Let (D, E) be one of the couple. Then others will be (B, H), (A, F) and (C, G).

**So the correct options for (a) and (b) are (iv).**

**159.** Note that in statements, A, F; D, E; C, H; and B, G are exclusive couples. If A, B are males, then B, G will be one of the couple and two of the couples in other statements will be as given (∵ there are four females) while the third couple will not be as given which is not possible. ∴ A, B cannot be males and have to be females. Now one of the other given pairs must also be female.
If G, E are females, then C, H will be a couple which is not possible as C, H are males.
If F, H are females, then D, E will be a couple which is also not possible as D, E are males.

If C, D are females, then A, F will be a couple and other couples can be
B, E; C, G; D, H or B, H; C, E; D, G

**So the correct options for (a), (b) and (c) are (i).**

**160.** In the given statements, we replace 1, 3, 4 by males and 2, 5 by females. Then in each of the following pairs, one is wrong, one is correct:

$$\begin{pmatrix} A \rightarrow M \\ E \rightarrow M \end{pmatrix}, \quad \begin{pmatrix} D \rightarrow M \\ A \rightarrow M \end{pmatrix} \quad \text{and} \quad \begin{pmatrix} E \rightarrow M \\ B \rightarrow F \end{pmatrix}$$

where M, F denote male and female respectively.

We can have two cases:

| | | | | | | | | | | | | |
|---|---|---|---|---|---|---|---|---|---|---|---|---|
| M | M | M | F | F | F | | M | M | M | F | F | F |
| A | C | F | E | B | D | or | E | D | B | A | C | F |
| 3 | 1 | 4 | | 2 | | | 4 | | | | | 5 |

**So the correct options for (a), (b), (c) and (d) are (i), (ii), (iv) and (iv) respectively.**

**161.** Given statement can be written as:

| | | | | |
|---|---|---|---|---|
| I. | A = 2 | and | C > D | |
| II. | B = 1 | and | A > E | |
| III. | C = 4 | and | F > E | (Do not confuse: |
| IV. | D = 5 | and | A > B | the highest rank is 1 |
| V. | E = 3 | and | F > C | and the lowest, 6) |
| VI. | F = 6 | and | D > B | |

Let B = 1. Then A > B and D > B will be incorrect and
∴ D = 5 and F = 6. Now F > E cannot be correct
∴ C = 4. But only three of the first part of statements are correct. ∴ our assumption B = 1 cannot be valid. ∴B ≠ 1 and A > E.

Now let F = 6. Then F > E and F > C will be incorrect and
∴ C = 4 and E = 3 and consequently,
A ≠ 2, B ≠ 1 and D ≠ 5. Also C < D, A > E, A > B and D < B. ∴ D has to be 1 or 2 (∵ C < D), and
∴ D < B < A. ∴ B has to be 2, D = 5 and A = 1 which cannot be possible. ∴ F ≠ 6.

Now we have B ≠ 1, F ≠ 6 and D > B, A > E

If we let D = 5, then A < B. For D > B, B has to be equal to 6 but A < B will not be valid.

$\therefore$ D $\neq$ 5.

So, we finally have

A = 2, C = 4, E = 3, F = 5 ($\because$ F < C and F $\neq$ 6),

D = 1 ($\because$ D > C) and B = 6.

**So the correct options for (a), (b), (c) and (d) are (i), (iii), (iii) and (ii) respectively.**

**162. (a) The correct option is (iii). EXPLANATION:**

There can be four cases:

Case I: AB, DE, BE, CF are together

$\because$ DEB are together $\therefore$ E cannot be at the other end.

$\because$ there is no 'none of these' options $\therefore$ other cases should be ignored as E will be the only valid option.

**(b) The correct option is (iv). EXPLANATION:**

We can have five cases: one case pertaining to A being at an end with E beside him [which is rejected from the result of part (a)] or A is flanked on both sides wherein only one of the statements containing A will be correct. If

EAB are together, then DEB are also together $\Rightarrow$ Rejected;

EAC are together, then BEF are also together $\Rightarrow$ Rejected;

EAF are together, then DEF are also together $\Rightarrow$ Rejected;

EAD are together, then DEF are also together $\Rightarrow$ Rejected;

So the given case is not possible.

**(c) The correct option is (ii). EXPLANATION:**

There can be five cases:

E is adjacent to A $\rightarrow$ Rejected by part (b)

E is adjacent of F $\rightarrow$ CAFE $\rightarrow$ Rejected as further arrangement not possible.

E is adjacent to D $\rightarrow$ CFABDE $\rightarrow$ POSSIBLE CASE

E is adjacent to B $\rightarrow$ EBACFD $\rightarrow$ POSSIBLE CASE

E is adjacent to C $\rightarrow$ Rejected as A cannot be adjacent to three persons.

So when E is at one end, then C or D will be at the other end.

**(d) The correct option is (ii). EXPLANATION:**

There can be five cases:

F is adjacent to A → Rejected as A cannot be adjacent toand B at the same time.

F is adjacent to B → Rejected as B cannot be adjacent to A and E at the same time.

F is adjacent to C → ABEDCF → Possible Case.

F is adjacent to D → Rejected as A will be adjacent to B and D and none of the statements of second given information will becorrect.

F is adjacent to E → FEB (CAD/DAC) → Possible case

So when F is at a end, B cannot be at the other end.

**(e) The correct option is (iv). EXPLANATION:**

From the first case of part (d), F cannot be adjacent to A when it is at the end. ∴ X cannot be F.

**163.** From first two statements:

$$\begin{Bmatrix} \text{CAD} & & \text{FBE} \\ \text{DAC} & \text{and} & \text{EFB} \end{Bmatrix} \quad \text{or} \quad \begin{Bmatrix} \text{ADC} & & \text{BEF} \\ \text{CDA} & \text{and} & \text{FEB} \end{Bmatrix}$$

From third statement:

Let C be between A and E, then the arrangement will be DACEBF but fourth statement is not satisfied. ∴ this case is rejected.

Let F be between B and D, then the arrangement will be CADFBE, the fourth statement is also verified.

**So the correct options for (a) and (b) are (i) and (ii) respectively.**

**164. (a) The correct option is (iv). EXPLANATION:**

Note that the wrong statements correspond to the persons at the ends. Now if I and IV are wrong, then the arrangement will be A E C B F D. If I and V are wrong, then the arrangement will be A F B C D E and if I and VI are wrong, then the arrangement will A E D C B F.

Note that the forward or reverse arrangements do not matter.

**(b) The correct option is (i). EXPLANATION:**
If II and IV are wrong, then the arrangement can be
B E C A F D or B E A C F D
There is no need to check the other two options.

**(c) The correct option is (iv). EXPLANATION:**
If III and IV are wrong, then the arrangement will be
C B E A F D
If III and V are wrong, then the arrangement will be
C B A F D E
And if III and VI are wrong, then the arrangement will be
C D A E B F

**165.** From first statement, we have four cases:

$$\begin{pmatrix} E & D \\ \downarrow & \downarrow \\ A & G \end{pmatrix} \text{ or } \begin{pmatrix} D & D \\ \downarrow & \downarrow \\ B & G \end{pmatrix} \text{ or } \begin{pmatrix} E & F \\ \downarrow & \downarrow \\ A & C \end{pmatrix} \text{ or } \begin{pmatrix} D & F \\ \downarrow & \downarrow \\ B & C \end{pmatrix}$$

Where $\begin{matrix} x \\ \downarrow \\ y \end{matrix}$ denotes 'y is son of x'.

From last two statements, we have other three cases:

$$\begin{pmatrix} A & \rightarrow & F \\ D & \rightarrow & E \end{pmatrix} \text{ or } \begin{pmatrix} B & \rightarrow & G \\ D & \rightarrow & E \end{pmatrix} \text{ or } \begin{pmatrix} B & \rightarrow & G \\ C & \rightarrow & A \end{pmatrix}$$

where $x \rightarrow y$ denotes 'x is brother of y'.
Also we have the family tree of the form

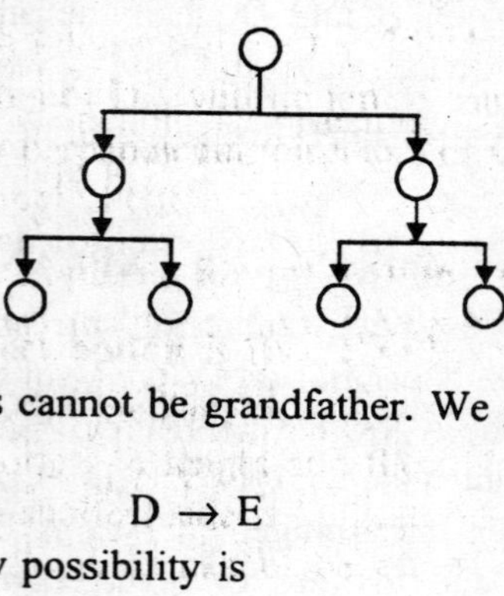

Now brothers cannot be grandfather. We can have following cases:

Case I: $A \rightarrow F$, $D \rightarrow E$
The only possibility is

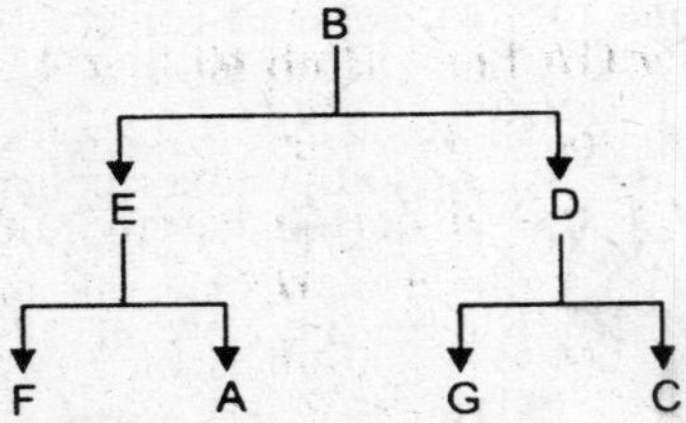


Case II: B → G, D → E

The only possibility is

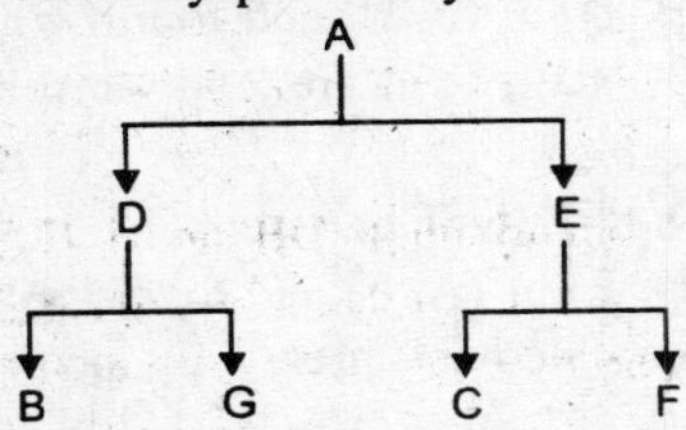


From part (a), D, E has to be a brother. ∴ the case B → G, C → A need not be checked as D, E cannot be brothers (statement IV).

**So the correct options for (a), (b), (c), (d) and (e) are (iii), (iv), (i), (i) and (i) respectively.**

**166.** Note that at least one of each pairs (I, II); (I, III); (I, IV); (I, V); (II, VI), (III, VI); (IV, VI) and (V, VI) is incorrect. If either of I or VI is correct, then II, III, IV and V must be incorrect. But only three statements are incorrect. ∴ I and VI must be incorrect. We can have four cases, viz.

Case I: II, III, IV correct.

Case II: II, III, V correct.

Case III: II, IV, V correct.

Case IV: III, IV, V correct.

And the arrangements can be tabulated as:

| | yellow | Green | Black | White | Pink | Blue | Red | Orange |
|---|---|---|---|---|---|---|---|---|
| Case I: | F | H | E | G | B | D | C | A |
| Case II: | F | H | E | G | D | B | A | C |
| Case III: | F | H | G | E | B | D | C | A |
| Case IV: | H | F | E | G | B | D | C | A |

**So the correct options for (a), (b) and (c) are (i), (iv) and (iv) respectively.**

**167.** Let I be correct. Then IV will be totally incorrect and the third couple can be (C, E) or (C, G). ∴ the couples can be

(A, F) , (B, D) , (C, E) , (G, H) or
(A, F) , (B, D) , (C, G) , (E, H)

Let II be correct. Then III will be totally incorrect and the third couple can be (B, D) or (F, H) and fourth will be (F, H) or (B, D). ∵ two of the statements are totally incorrect ∴ this case is rejected.

Let III be correct. Then II will be totally incorrect and the third couple can be (D, E) or (A, F) and fourth will be (A, F) or (D, E). ∵ two of the statements are totally incorrect. ∴ this case is also rejected.

Let IV be correct. Then I will be totally incorrect.
The third couple can be (A, G) or (C, G) and the fourth couple can be (C, B) or (A, B). ∴ the couples can be

(D, E) , (F, H) , (A, G) , (C, B) or
(D, E) , (F, H) , (C, G) , (A, B)

**So the correct options for (a), (b), (c) and (d) are (ii), (ii), (iii) and (i) respectively.**

**168.** There can be eight cases from first three statements:

Case I: $\left.\begin{aligned} a+b&=5 \\ a+c&=4 \\ a+d&=7 \end{aligned}\right\}$ Then $d-c \neq 2$ ∴ $b=3, a=2, c=2 \rightarrow$ Rejected

Case II: $\left.\begin{aligned} a+b&=5 \\ a+c&=4 \\ b+c&=8 \end{aligned}\right\} \rightarrow$ Not possible as $a$ is an integer

Case III: $\left.\begin{aligned} a+b&=5 \\ b+d&=9 \\ a+d&=7 \end{aligned}\right\} \rightarrow$ Not possible as $a$ is an integer

Case IV: $\left.\begin{array}{r} c+d=10 \\ a+c=4 \\ a+d=7 \end{array}\right\} \rightarrow$ Not possible as $a$ is an integer

Case V: $\left.\begin{array}{r} a+b=5 \\ b+d=9 \\ b+c=8 \end{array}\right\}$ Then $d-c \neq 2 \therefore b-a=1$ $\Rightarrow b=3, a=2, c=5, d=6$

A solution

Case VI: $\left.\begin{array}{l} c+d=10 \\ b+d=4 \\ a+d=8 \end{array}\right\}$ Then $b-a \neq 1 \because d-c=2$ $\Rightarrow d=6, c=4, a=0 \rightarrow$ Rejected

Case VII: $\left.\begin{array}{r} c+d=10 \\ b+d=9 \\ a+d=7 \end{array}\right\}$ $\Rightarrow b-a \neq 1 \quad \therefore d-c=2$ $\Rightarrow d=6, c=4, b=3, a=1$

A solution

Case VIII: $\left.\begin{array}{r} c+d=10 \\ b+d=9 \\ b+c=8 \end{array}\right\} \rightarrow$ Not possible as $b$ is an integer

**So the correct options for (a), (b), (c) and (d) are (iv), (ii), (iv) and (iii) respectively.**

**169. (a) The correct option is (ii). EXPLANATION:**

If $C$ is the least number, then

$A < B$, $B > D$ and $A < D$

$\therefore$ the greatest number is $B$.

**(b) The correct option is (i). EXPLANATION:**

From first two statements, we can have four cases:

Case I: $A < B$, $C < D$, $A > C$, $B > D$

$\Rightarrow C < D < B < A \rightarrow$ Rejected

Case II: $A < B$, $C < D$, $A < C$, $B < D$

$\Rightarrow A < B < C < D \rightarrow$ Rejected

Case III: $A > B$, $C > D$, $A > C$, $B > D$

$\Rightarrow A > B > C > D \rightarrow$ Rejected

Case IV: $A > B$, $C > D$, $A < C$, $B < D$

$\Rightarrow B < A < C$

From third option,
$B < D < A < C$
$\therefore$ the extreme terms are B, C.

**170.** There can be eight cases:

Case I: $\left.\begin{array}{l} A+B=2F \\ C+D=2E \\ A+F=2C \end{array}\right\} \Rightarrow A\,C\,F\,E\,B\,D$

Case II: $\left.\begin{array}{l} A+B=2F \\ C+D=2E \\ E+C=2A \end{array}\right\} \Rightarrow C\,A\,E\,F\,D\,B$

Case III: $\left.\begin{array}{l} A+B=2F \\ E+F=2B \\ A+F=2C \end{array}\right\} \Rightarrow$ Not possible

Case IV: $\left.\begin{array}{l} A+B=2F \\ E+F=2B \\ E+C=2A \end{array}\right\} \Rightarrow$ Not possible

Case V: $\left.\begin{array}{l} B+C=2D \\ C+D=2E \\ A+F=2C \end{array}\right\} \Rightarrow$ Not possible

Case VI: $\left.\begin{array}{l} B+C=2D \\ C+D=2E \\ E+C=2A \end{array}\right\} \Rightarrow$ Not possible

Case VII: $\left.\begin{array}{l} B+C=2D \\ E+F=2B \\ A+F=2C \end{array}\right\} \Rightarrow$ Not possible

Case VIII: $\left.\begin{array}{l} B+C=2D \\ E+F=2B \\ E+C=2A \end{array}\right\} \Rightarrow$ Not possible

**So the correct options for (a), (b), (c), (d) and (e) are (iii), (iii), (i), (iv) and (iv) respectively.**

**171.** We have

$$\left.\begin{aligned} a-b+c &= 0 \text{ or } -1 \\ c &= -2 \text{ or } -1 \\ a+b+c &= -2 \text{ or } 1 \\ 4a+2b+c &= 0 \text{ or } 1 \end{aligned}\right\}$$

Case I: $c = -2$

Then $a - b = (0 \text{ or } -1) + 2$ ...(i)

$a + b = (-2 \text{ or } 1) + 2$ ...(ii)

$4a + 2b = (0 \text{ or } 1) + 2$ ...(iii)

Now (i) + 3 × (ii) gives $4a + 2b = (0 \text{ or } -1) + 3(-2 \text{ or } 1) + 8$

From (iii), $4a + 2b = 2$ or $3$

$\therefore$ only possibility is $a - b = 2$ and $a + b = 0$.

$\Rightarrow$ $a = 1$ and $b = -1$

Case II: $c = -1$

Then $a - b = (0 \text{ or } -1) + 1$ ...(i)

$a + b = (-2 \text{ or } 1) + 1$ ...(ii)

$4a + 2b = (0 \text{ or } 1) + 1$ ...(iii)

(i) + 2 × (ii) gives $4a + 2b = (0 \text{ or } -1) + 3 \times (-2 \text{ or } 1) + 4$ which cannot be equal to the R.H.S. of (iii).

$\therefore$ this case is rejected.

**So the correct options for (a), (b) and (c) are (iii), (i) and (i) respectively.**

**172.** (a) **The correct option is (i). EXPLANATION:**

The given pair of numbers can be treated as points of which three lie on a line and fourth not. Now slope of the lines joining the points

(1, 2) and (–3, 1) will be $\dfrac{2-1}{1+3} = \dfrac{1}{4}$

(1, 2) and (2, –1) will be $\dfrac{2+1}{1-2} = -3$

(1, 2) and (4, 3) will be $\dfrac{3-2}{4-1} = \dfrac{1}{3}$

i.e. (1, 2) cannot lie on a line with any two of the other points. $\therefore$ (1, 2) cannot satisfy the given relation.

(b) **The correct option is (ii). EXPLANATION:**
The given values of $(x, y)$ can be treated as points which are to lie on a circle. Note that the points $(-3, -1)$, $(0, 2)$ and $(1, 3)$ lie on a line $y = x + 2$ and $\because$ no three collinear points can lie on a circle. $\therefore$ $(1, -1)$ must be included with two of the above three points to lie on a circle.

**173.** Given:
A – (5, 6, 1)
B – (6, 1, 2)
C – (1, 2, 3) (Notice the symmetry of triplets)
D – (2, 3, 4)
E – (3, 4, 5)
F – (4, 5, 6)

$\because$ in option (b) and (c), A = 1 is used $\therefore$ let us start our solution with assumption of A = 1. We can have following cases:

| A | B | C | D | E | F | |
|---|---|---|---|---|---|---|
| 1 | 2 | 3 | 4 | 5 | 6 | |
| → | → | ← | ← | ← | ← | ...(sequence of filling for first case) |
| 1 | 6 | 2 | 3 | 4/5 | 5/4 | |
| 1 | 6 | 2 | 4 | 3 | 5 | |
| 1 | 6 | 2 | 2 | 4/5 | 5/4 | |

Similarly there will be six cases for A = 5 and A = 6 each.

**So the correct options for (a), (b) and (c) are (iii), (iv) and (ii) respectively.**

**174.** Note that

$A = 2B \pm 1$
$B = 2C \pm 2 \quad \times 2$
$C = 2D \pm 4 \quad \times 4$
$D = 2A \pm 3 \quad \times 8$

Adding, we get

$15A = -(\pm 1 \pm 4 \pm 16 \pm 24)$

$\because$ $A$ is an integer

$\therefore$ $15A = -(1 + 4 + 16 + 24)$ or $1 + 4 + 16 + 24$

$\Rightarrow A = -3$ or 3 and correspondingly
$B = -2$ or 2
$C = -2$ or 2 and
$D = -3$ or 3

**So the correct options for (a) and (b) are (ii).**

**175.** Let us tabulate the given conditions roughly as:

| | A | B | C | D |
|---|---|---|---|---|
| | 4 | 4 | 4 | 4 |
| | 4 | 4 | 4 | 4 |
| | 2 | 0 | 3 | 2 |
| Total | 10 | 8 | 11 | 10 |

Note that for third round (a round consists of four questions), questions asked first to A would not be answered, while to B would be answered by C or D, and to C would be answered by A while to D would not be answered. Again for fourth round, questions asked to A would not be answered while to B would be answered by one of C, D who did not answer in third round. Note that two questions asked to A, one question to D would not be answered. For minimum questions to be asked, B should not have given answer to any questions he was asked first but rather he should have given answer to questions asked to A (twice) and D. The rounds can be tabulated as:

| A | B | C | D |
|---|---|---|---|
| 4 | 0 | 4+3 | 4 |
| 4 | 0 | 4 | 4+2 |
| 2 | 3+2 | 0 | 0 |
| 0 | 3 | | |

(Note that to complete all the questions asked by the third round itself is not possible).

**So the correct options for (a), (b) and (c) are (ii).**

**176.** Consider the number of block in $m$th row and $n$th column. Then by
first numbering, its number will be

$$\left.\begin{array}{r} 10(m-1)+n \text{ if } m \text{ is odd} \\ 10(m-1)+11-n \text{ if } m \text{ is even} \end{array}\right\}, 1 \le n \le 10;$$

Second numbering, its number will be

$$\left.\begin{array}{r} 10(n-1)+m \text{ if } n \text{ is odd} \\ 10(n-1)+11-m \text{ if } n \text{ is even} \end{array}\right\}, 1 \le m \le 10;$$

(a) **The correct option is (ii). EXPLANATION:**
If $m$, $n$ are both odd, then
$10(m - 1) + n = 10(n - 1) + m$
$\Rightarrow m = n$ which comprises of 5 cases, viz.
(1, 1), (3, 3), (5, 5), (7, 7) and (9, 9)

If $m$, $n$ are both even, then also
$m = n$ which will also comprise of 5 cases, viz.
(2, 2), (4, 4), (6, 6), (8, 8) and (10, 10).

If $m$ is even and $n$ is odd, then
$10(m - 1) + 11 - n = 10(n - 1) + m$
$\Rightarrow 9m = 11(n - 1)$ which cannot be possible.
Similarly $n$ being even and $m$ being odd will also be not possible.

(b) **The correct option is (i). EXPLANATION:**
If $m$, $n$ are both odd, then
$\{10(m - 1) + n\} - \{10(n - 1) + m\} = 9$
$\Rightarrow 9(m - n) = 9$
$\Rightarrow m - n = 1$ which cannot be possible
$\because m, n$ are both odd.
Similarly $m$, $n$ both being even will also be not possible.
Now let $m$ be odd and $n$ even, then
$\{10(m - 1) + n\} - \{10(n - 1) + (11 - m)\} = 9$
$\Rightarrow 11m - 9n - 11 = 9$
$\Rightarrow 11(m - 1) = 9(n + 1)$
No value of $(m, n)$ is possible.
For even $m$ and odd $n$,

$\{10(m-1)+11-n\}-\{10(n-1)+m\}=9$
$9m+11-11n=9$
$\Rightarrow 9(m-1)=11(n+1).$
No value of $(m, n)$ is possible.

(c) **The correct option is (iii). EXPLANATION:**
We have for $(m, n) \equiv$ (even, even) or (odd, odd)
$9(m-n)=18$
$\Rightarrow m=n+2$ which can be satisfied by 8 values of $(m, n)$
For $(m, n) \equiv$ (odd, even), we have
$11m-9n-11=18 \quad \Rightarrow 11(m-1)=9(n+2)$
No value of $(m, n)$ is possible.
For $(m, n) \equiv$ (even, odd)
$9m+11-11n=18 \quad \Rightarrow 9(m-2)=11(n-1)$
Again no values of $(m, n)$ is possible.

**177.** As the man returns to his initial point,
$\therefore$ the total distances covered in eastward and westward directions or northward and southward directions are equal. So from the given relations,
$A_0A_1, A_2A_3 \rightarrow$ eastward direction
$A_4A_5, A_6A_7, A_8A_9 \rightarrow$ westward direction
$A_1A_2, A_5A_6, A_8A_9 \rightarrow$ northward direction (assumed)
$A_3A_4, A_7A_8 \rightarrow$ southward direction
$\because$ there are two exclusive pairs of roads which intersect each other $\therefore$ we can draw the roads as:

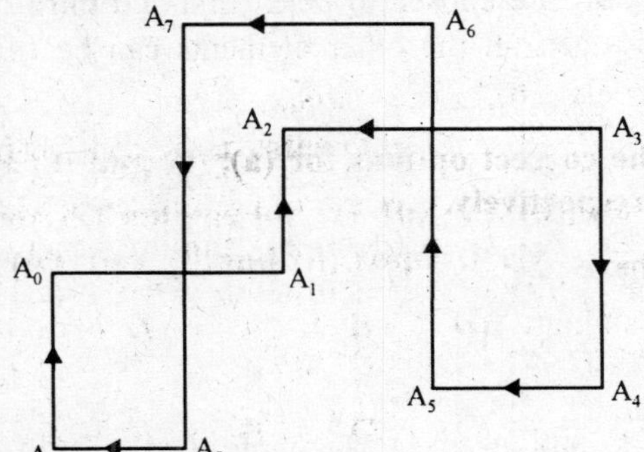


**So the correct options for (a), (b) and (c) are (iii), (i) and (i) respectively.**

**178.** We can have the possibilities of arrangement as:

| | | | | | | |
|---|---|---|---|---|---|---|
| | | $A_1$ | | $A_2$ | | Given |
| | | | $B_2$ | | $B_3$ | |
| Possibilities for | $C_4$ | | | $C_5$ | | |
| $A_3$ | $A_3$ | | $A_3$ | | | 3 ways |
| $A_4$ | | | $A_4$ | | $A_4$ | |
| $A_5$ | $A_5$ | | $A_5$ | | $A_5$ | |
| $B_1$ | $B_1$ | | | $B_1$ | | 2 ways |
| $B_4$ | | $B_4$ | | $B_4$ | | |
| $B_5$ | $B_5$ | $B_5$ | | | | |
| $C_1$ | | | $C_1$ | | $C_1$ | 2 ways |
| $C_2$ | | $C_2$ | | | $C_2$ | |
| $C_3$ | | $C_3$ | $C_3$ | | | |

Note that if $A_5$ is in first column and $A_3$ is in third column, then there will be only one way of filling. If only one of these is in corresponding column, then the number of ways will be four and when none of these are in corresponding columns then there will be two ways. So total number of ways of filling = 1 + 4 + 2 = 7

Also third column can be filled in maximum number of different ways (= 5).

If $A_3$, $A_5$ are chosen to be in first and third columns respectively, then all the other elements can be filled in a unique way.

**So the correct options for (a), (b) and (c) are (i), (iii) and (iv) respectively.**

**179.** We have

B ___sibling___ H
(+)

D ___sibling___ ( ) ___couple___ G ('+' denotes male
(+) '–' denotes female)

C sibling ( ) couple J
(–)

Also from given statements, we can construct the family tree as:

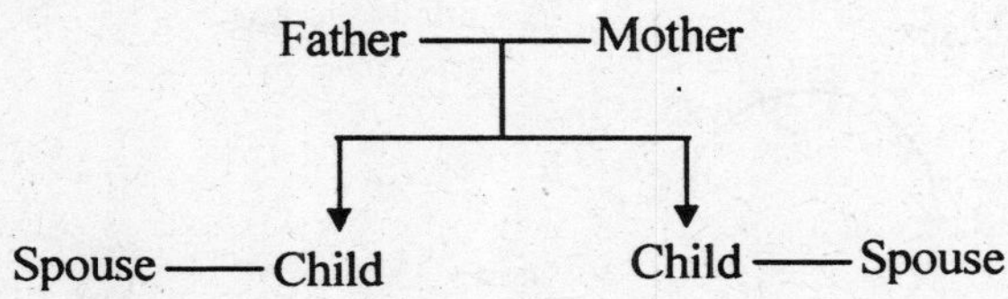


So we will have

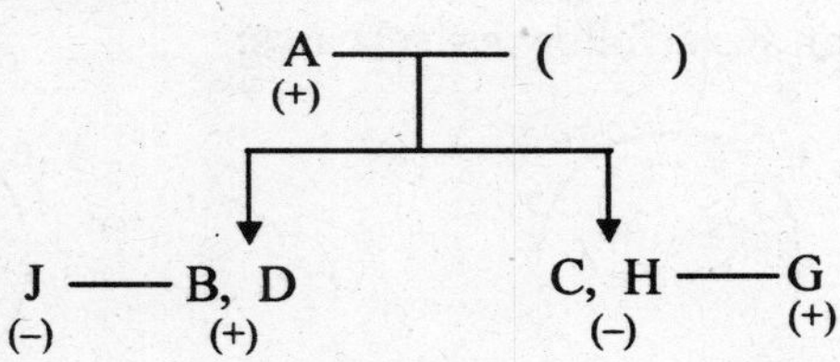


∵ K is son in law of I
∴ K, G are same persons and I is the mother.
∵ E is husband of L
∴ (A, E) and (I, L) are same persons and consequently (F, J) are the same persons.
∴ we have the family tree as

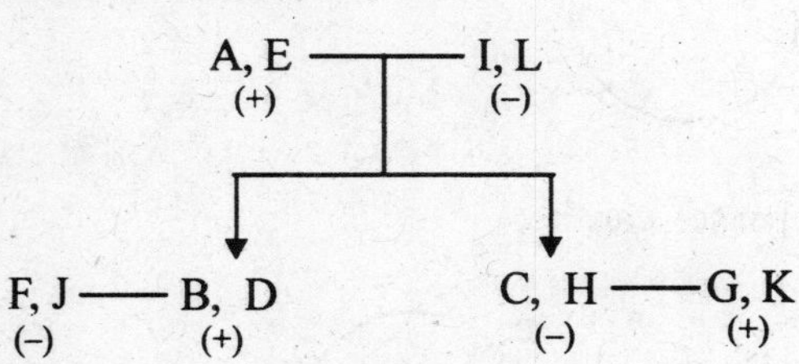


**So the correct options for (a), (b) and (c) are (i), (ii) and (ii) respectively.**

**180.** Note that the distance between any two vertices of a regular heptagon can have only three values which correspond to the number of vertices (0, 1 or 2) they have in between them.

Now the number of vertices between

(A, B); (D, F); (C, G) and (D, E) $\rightarrow$ 2 or 3

(D, G); (B, E); (B, F) and (A, C) $\rightarrow$ 1 or 2

Let us start naming the vertices with D. There can be following cases:

Case I:

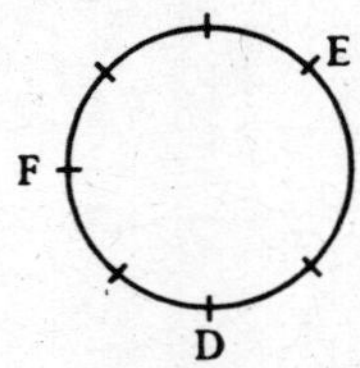


We can have following subcases:

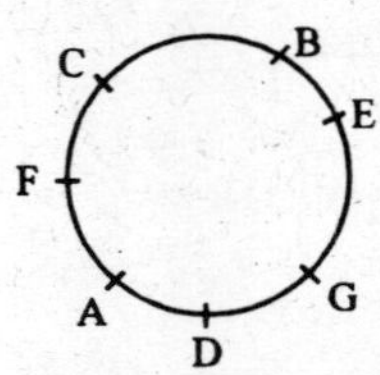


and

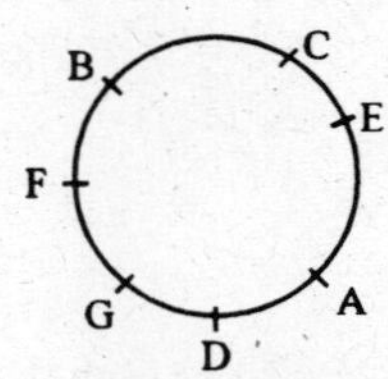


Rejected as DE > AC is not satisfied

Rejected as DF > BE is not satisfied

Case II:

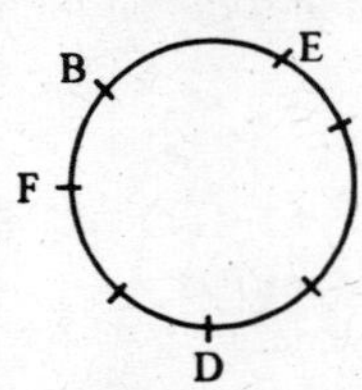


The subcases can be:

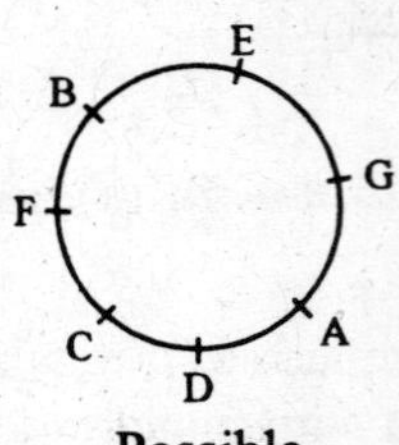


Possible

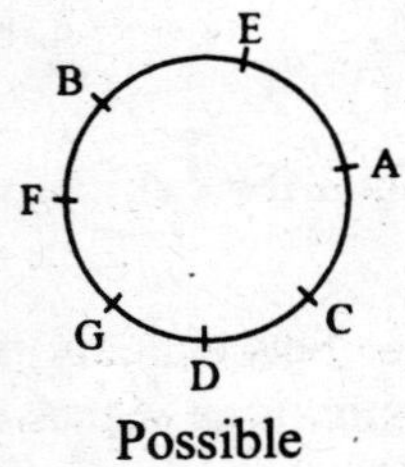


Possible

and

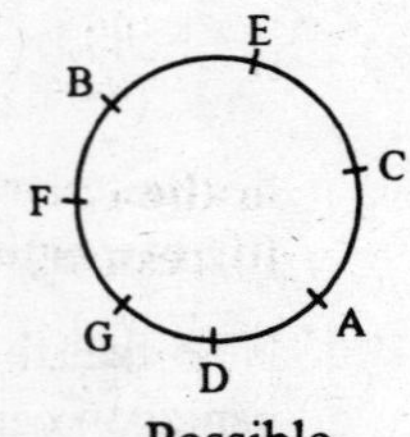


Possible

Case III:

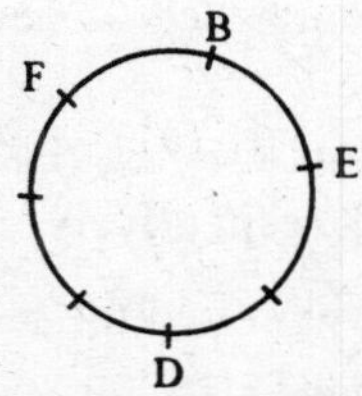


For DE > AC, A, C should be adjacent vertices

∴ the naming can be:

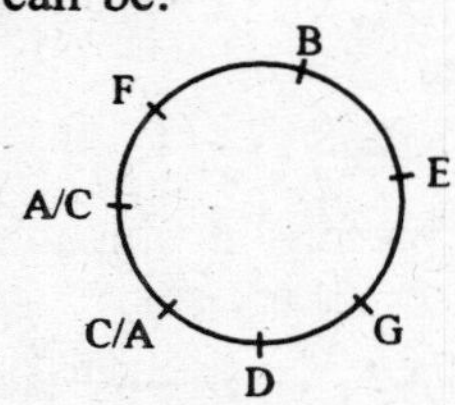


Possible

Case IV:

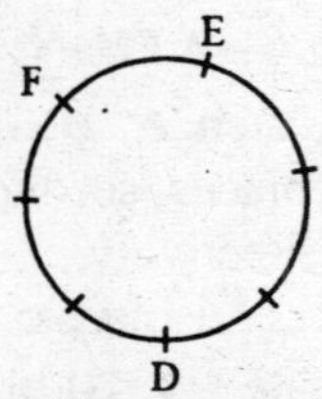


The subcases can be:

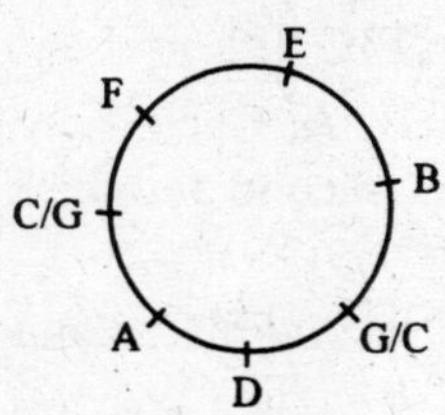


,

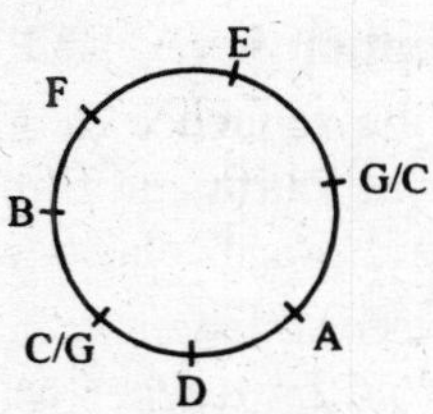


and

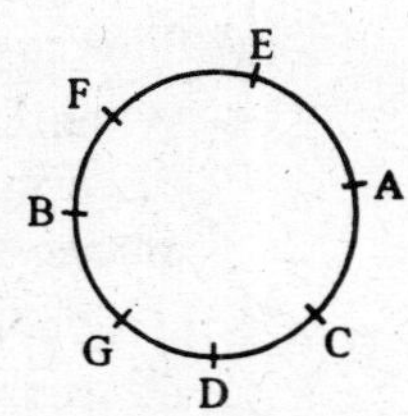


Possible Possible Possible

**So the correct options for (a), (b), (c), (d) and (e) are (iv).**

**181.** Only two cases are possible, viz.

| | Q | S | R | P |
|---|---|---|---|---|
| B | X | $B_1$ | | $P_2$ |
| C | $C_7$ | X | $R_4$ | |
| D | | $S_3$ | $D_8$ | X |
| A | | | X | $A_6$ |

or

| | Q | S | R | P |
|---|---|---|---|---|
| B | X | $S_2$ | | $B_1$ |
| C | $Q_7$ | X | $C_5$ | |
| D | | $D_6$ | $R_4$ | X |
| A | $A_3$ | | X | $P_8$ |

where subscripts of alphabets denote the priorities in which they filled the blocks.

**So the correct options for (a), (b), (c), (d) and (e) are (ii), (iii), (ii), (i) and (ii) respectively.**

**182.** Note that the student who told the sequence to another student directly will have places of only two of the letters in his sequence different from what the second student tells to next person. Now

| A | B | C | D |
|---|---|---|---|
| Q R P T S | Q P R T S | Q R T P S | Q P R S T |

Now the sequence of persons in which the letters are told will be either

Teacher → C → A → B → D → Teacher or
Teacher → D → B → A → C → Teacher

(a) **The correct option is (i). EXPLANATION:**

When A told the sequence to B, then A, B, D got confused in letters at third and fourth places, second and third places, fourth and fifth places respectively.
∴ C got confused in first and second places.

(b) **The correct option is (iii). SELF EVIDENT FROM ABOVE ANALYSIS.**

(c) **The correct option is (i). EXPLANATION:**

When B told the sequence to A, then B, A, C got confused in letters at fourth and fifth places, second and third places, third and fourth places respectively.

∴ D got confused in letters at first and second places and the sequence told by teacher was P Q R S T.

**183.** Note that the sequence can be only
1, 0, 2, 0, 2 or 1, 2, 0, 2, 0

Case I: Sequence is 1, 0, 2, 0, 2. Then

$$k_1 + k_2 + k_3 = 0$$
$$k_3 = 2 \quad \text{and}$$
$$4k_1 + 2k_2 + k_3 = 0$$

which gives $k_1 = 1, k_2 = -3, k_3 = 2$

Case II: Sequence is 1, 2, 0, 2, 0. Then

$$k_1 + k_2 + k_3 = 2$$
$$4k_1 + 2k_2 + k_3 = 0 \text{ and}$$

$$k_3 = 2$$

which gives $k_1 = -1$, $k_2 = 1$ and $k_3 = 2$.

**So the correct options for (a), (b), (c) and (d) are (i), (iii), (iii) and (iii) respectively.**

**184.** **(a) The correct option is (iii). EXPLANATION:**
Note that the cyclic sequence ABCDE is never broken, only it gets clockwise or anticlockwise. Only DEABC satisfies this condition.

(b) **The correct option is (ii). EXPLANATION:**

$$\underbrace{\text{ABC}}\ \underbrace{\text{DE}} \longrightarrow \underbrace{\text{CBAE}}\ \underbrace{\text{D}} \longrightarrow \text{EABCD}$$

(b) **The correct option is (ii). EXPLANATION:**

$$\underbrace{\text{ABCD}}\ \underbrace{\text{E}} \longrightarrow \underbrace{\text{DCB}}\ \underbrace{\text{AE}} \longrightarrow \underbrace{\text{BC}}\ \underbrace{\text{DEA}}$$

$$\longrightarrow \underbrace{\text{CBA}}\ \underbrace{\text{ED}} \longrightarrow \text{ABCDE}$$

**185.** There can be three cases:

Case I: $G_1$ $G_2$

$(A_1, A_3, \_\_, \_\_)$ $(A_5, A_7, \_\_, \_\_)$

$\because 1 + 7 = 3 + 5 = 2 \cdot 4$ $\therefore$ they cannot form pairs.

Let $(A_1, A_5)$ form pair. The next pair will be $(A_3, A_7)$. And the third pair will be $(A_5, ...)$ which is not possible. $\therefore$ this case is rejected and $A_1$, $A_3$ can't be in a group.

Case II: $G_1$ $G_2$

$(A_1, A_5, \_\_, \_\_)$ $(A_3, A_7, \_\_, \_\_)$

$\because 1 + 7 = 3 + 5 = 2.4$ $\therefore$ they can't form pairs.

Let $(A_1, A_3)$ form pair. The next pair will be $(A_2, A_6)$ or $(A_2, A_8)$. If we consider $(A_2, A_6)$, then the next pair will be $(A_4, A_8)$ and the last pair will be $(A_6, \_\_)$ which is not possible. Now if $(A_2, A_8)$ is the second pair, then the third pair will be $(A_5, A_7)$ and the fourth pair will be $(A_6, A_4)$.

$\therefore G_1 \equiv (A_1, A_5, A_2, A_6)$ and $G_2 \equiv (A_3, A_7, A_8, A_4)$ and formation of pairs is sequentially

$(A_1, A_3) \rightarrow (A_2, A_8) \rightarrow (A_5, A_7) \rightarrow (A_6, A_4)$

Although we need not examine case III, but it is given here in case it is done before case II.

Case III: $G_1$ $(A_1, A_7, \_\_, \_\_)$ $G_2$ $(A_3, A_5, \_\_, \_\_)$

If the first pair is $(A_1, A_3)$, then the second pair can be $(A_2, A_6)$ or $(A_2, A_8)$.

If the second pair is $(A_2, A_6)$, then the third pair is $(A_4, A_8)$ but $4 + 8 = 2{\cdot}6$. $\therefore$ this is rejected.

If the second pair is $(A_2, A_8)$, then $A_5$ should be in $G_1$, $\therefore$ this is rejected.

If the first pair is $(A_1, A_5)$, then $A_3$ should be in $G_1$, $\therefore$ this is also rejected.

**So the correct options for (a), (b) and (c) are (iii), (ii) and (iv) respectively.**

**186.** Note that one of (A, B), (B, C) and (C, D) has to be adjacent and (C, D) can't be adjacent. Also when (B, C) is adjacent, then (A, B) has to be adjacent; $\therefore$ (A, B) has to be adjacent in any case. There will be two cases

$D \ ^1\ A \ ^1\ B \ ^3\ C$ or $C \ ^2\ A \ ^1\ B \ ^2\ D$

**So the correct options for (a) and (b) are (iv).**

**187. The correct option is (i). EXPLANATION:**

We must divide 100 coins into two groups, say A and B. The minimum number of measurements used to separate the fake coin from group A must be equal to or at least close to its corresponding values for B. Also from a group of three coins (out of which one is fake), the fake coin can be separated by single measurement (on weighing two coins, the fake coin will weigh lighter and if both coins are of same weight, then the third coin will be fake)

$\therefore$ coins upto $3^4$ (= 81) can be checked for fake coins by using the balance just five times (by dividing them first into three groups of 27 coins and using balance twice to check if there is a fake coin or not and if it is there, then it can be separated by using the balance thrice as done for three coins explained above). If there is no fake coin in 81 coins, then the fake coin can be separated from 19 coins using the balance thrice (by first dividing them into two groups of 9 coins each and a third group of single coin and then weighing the coins of first two groups and ...). In any case, the minimum number of measurement is 5.

(b) **The correct option is (i). EXPLANATION:**

As explained in part (a), if one coin is fake in 9 coins, then it can be separated in two measurements. We divide the coins into four groups of 9 coins each and take three measurements to ascertain which group (or groups) contain fake coin. ∴ minimum number of measurements taken if two groups have fake coin = $3 + 2 \times 2 = 7$.

If one group has two fake coins, then we divide them into three groups of 3 coins each and take two measurements to ascertain which groups have fake coins. If two groups have fake coins, then minimum measurements = $3 + 2 + 2 = 7$. If one group has fake coins, then total measurements = $3 + 2 + 1 = 6$. So we need to have minimum of 7 measurements to separate fake coins.

**188.** For minimum number of such weights, they should be of values 1, 3, 9, 27 and 81 kg. Also they can weigh upto $1 + 3 + 9 + 27 + 81 = 121$ kg.

**So the correct options for (a) and (b) are (i).**

**189.** (a) **The correct option is (iv). EXPLANATION:**

Note that $(m + n)\, y = m\, x + n\, z, \quad m, n, x, y, z > 0$ implies that $y$ is between $x$ and $z$.

∴ A is between B and C; and

B is between C and D

So we can have the order of A, B, C, D (in increasing or decreasing order of their prices) as D B A C.

(b) **The correct option is (i). EXPLANATION:**

We will have corresponding order as E D B A C where B is between A and E.

**190.** Note that in all ratios, the money spent by C is most and that by A is least. ∴ the number of articles bought by A, B and C can be (1, 1, 3) or (1, 2, 2). Also let the price of Y be greater than that of X. Then

for A, B, C ≡ (1, 1, 3)

A = X, B = Y, C = 2X + Y or 2Y + X

$\therefore$ C = 2A + B or 2B + A ...(i)

for A, B, C ≡ (1, 2, 2),

A = X, or Y, B = 2X, C = 2Y

$\therefore$ B or C = 2A. ...(ii)

So one of conditions of (i) or (ii) must be satisfied.

**So the correct options for (a) and (b) are (iv).**

**191. (a) The correct option is (iii). EXPLANATION:**

Distance covered by A and C in successive seconds can be given as

| | | | | | | |
|---|---|---|---|---|---|---|
| A → | 10 + | 11 + | 12 + | 13 + | 14 + | 15 |
| C → | 15 + | 14 + | 13 + | 12 + | 11 + | 10 |
| A – C → | –5 | –3 | –1 | 1 | 3 | 5 |

A will overtakes C when Σ (A – C) = 0 which happens at the end of 6 seconds.

**(b) The correct option is (iii). EXPLANATION:**

| | | | | | | | | |
|---|---|---|---|---|---|---|---|---|
| B → | 5 + | 7 + | 9 + | 11 + | 13 + | 15 + | 17 + | 19 |
| C → | 15 + | 14 + | 13 + | 12 + | 11 + | 10 + | 9 + | 8 |
| B – C → | 10 | –7 | –4 | –1 | 2 | 5 | 8 | 11 |

B overtakes C when Σ (B – C) = 0 which happens between 7 and 8 seconds.

**(c) The correct option is (iii). EXPLANATION:**

| | | | | | | | | | |
|---|---|---|---|---|---|---|---|---|---|
| B → | 5 | 7 | 9 | 11 | 13 | 15 | 17 | 19 | 21 |
| D → | 20 | 18 | 16 | 14 | 12 | 10 | 8 | 6 | 4 |
| | –15 | –11 | –7 | –3 | 1 | 5 | 9 | 13 | 17 |

B overtakes D when Σ (B – D) = 0 which happens between 8 and 9 seconds.

**192.** If we denote five persons by P, Q, R, S, T, then we need to form a cyclic sequence P → Q → R → S → T → P where each persons take care of the persons just following him.

Now if A → B, then B → D, E and

If B → E, then D → C, B

$\therefore$ the various possibilities can be

A → B → D → E → C → A

A → B → D → C → E → A

A → B → E → D → C → A

**So the correct options for (a) and (b) are (ii).**

**193.** Note that 76 – 36 = 40 =

$\overline{k} + \overline{k+1}$ or $\overline{k} + \overline{k+1} + \overline{k+2}$ or $4k + 6$ or $5k + 10$

where k is the price of $y$th kg.

$\because$ $k$ is an integer $\therefore$ $40 = 5k + 10 \Rightarrow k = 6$ and

$\therefore$ $y - x = 5$.

And the price of packet of $x$th kg will be 6 + 5 = Rs 11.

Now 11 + 12 + 13 = 36

$\therefore$ $x = 3$ and $y = 8$.

**So the correct options for (a) and (b) are (iii) and (ii) respectively.**

**194.** Note that for transportation of 0 kg, 1 kg, 2 kg, 3 kg and 4 kg from A to B, the porter needs 12 minutes, 15 minutes 20 minutes, 30 minutes and 60 minutes. For transportation of unit kg (i.e. 1 kg) by four methods, he needs

| Weight | Minutes (A to B) | Minutes (A to B and then back without any weight) |
|---|---|---|
| 1 kg | 15 | (15 + 12)/1= 27 |
| 2 kg | 10 | (20 + 12)/2 = 16 |
| 3 kg | 10 | (30 + 12)/3 = 14 |
| 4 kg | 15 | (60 + 12)/4 = 18 |

**(a) The correct option is (i). EXPLANATION:**

For minimum time, the porter should carry 3 kg of weight three times and a kg of weight for fourth time.

$\therefore$ minimum time $= 14 \times 9 + 15$

$= 14 \times (10 - 1) + 15 = 141.$

**(b) The correct option is (i). EXPLANATION:**

For minimum time, the porter should carry

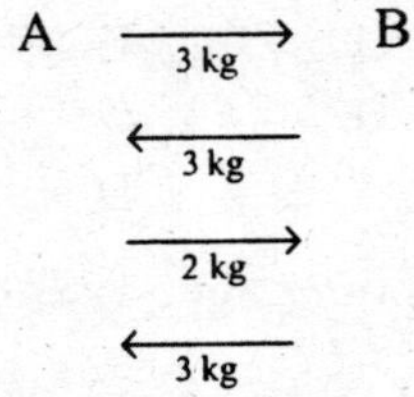


and minimum time will be

$30 \times 3 + 20 = 110$ minutes.

(c) **The correct option is (iii). EXPLANATION:**
The time for transportation of unit kg is least for 3 kg at a time.

**195.** Let $m$ be the number of red marbles bought, $n$ be the number of white marbles bought, $x$ be the cost of a red marble and $y$ be the cost of blue marble. Then

$mx + 2y + 5n + 2 \cdot 1 = 100$

$\Rightarrow mx + 2y + 5n = 98$

Case I: $n = 1$

Then $mx + 2y = 93 \Rightarrow x = \dfrac{93 - 2y}{m}$

Now $y$ must be greater than 7 than (otherwise one more blue marble could have been bought), let us put it equal to $8 + y'$.

Then $x = \dfrac{93 - 2 \cdot (8 + y')}{m} = \dfrac{77 - 2y'}{m}$

Now $m$ cannot be equal to 2 as $x$ is an integer.

And if $y' = 2$, $m$ can be equal to 3 but that makes $x = 25$ and in Rs 100, four red marbles can be bought.

$\therefore$ $m = 1$ is the only possibility.

Case II: $n = 2$

Then $mx + 2y = 88$

Now $y$ must be greater than 12 (otherwise one more blue marble could have been bought), let us put it equal to $8 + y'$.

Then $x = \dfrac{88 - 2(13 + y')}{m} = \dfrac{62 - 2y'}{m}$

If $m = 2$, then $x = 31 - y'$ and in this amount at least 3 red marbles could be bought. $\therefore$ $m = 1$ is the only possibility.

Case III: $n = 3$

Note that $y \geq 18$ and

$2y + 5n + 2 \geq 53$

and $mx \leq 47$.

But $(m + 1)\,x \geq 100$

$\Rightarrow \quad x \geq 53$

which cannot be possible

$\therefore \quad n = 3$ or $n \geq 3$ are not possible.

The maximum cost of a blue marble correspond to

$$x = \frac{93-y}{m} \qquad \text{...(Case I)}$$

and as $m = 1$,

$2x \geq 100$

$\therefore \quad 93 - 2y \geq 50$

$\Rightarrow \quad 2y \leq 43$

$\Rightarrow \quad y_{max} = 21.$

**So the correct options for (a), (b) and (c) are (i), (ii) and (iv) respectively.**

**196. (a) The correct option is (ii). EXPLANATION:**

2 1 6 7 4

Starting from 2, it will take ten trials to ascertain whether 2 is one of such number. [While checking 2 for 1, 6, 7, 4, the latter numbers are correspondingly changed to 2, otherwise they are not altered].

If 2 is not one of such number, it will take eight trials to check whether 1 is such a number (while checking, 2 and 1 are excluded). Similarly 7, 6 and 5 more trials are needed.

$\therefore$ total number of wrong calls after which

desired number is dialed $= 10 + 8 + 7 + 6 + 5 - 1$

$= 35$

**(b) The correct option is (iii). EXPLANATION:**

8 3 5 6 9 ⟶ Wrong calls
6 3 5 9 8 ⟶ Wrong calls
9 5 3 6 8 ⟶ Desired calls

From first and third numbers, the two numbers that could get exchanged are (8, 9) or (3, 5) while from second and third number, the numbers that could get exchanged are (6, 9) or (3, 5).

∴ (3, 5) is the required number as it is common to them.

**197.**

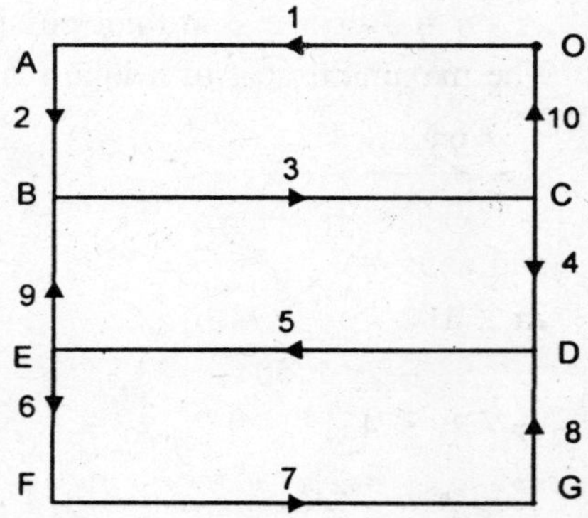


Let the two persons who run at the speeds of 1 m/s and 2 m/s be P and Q respectively.
Then the time taken by Q to reach G will be

$$\frac{2200}{2} = 1100 \text{ seconds.}$$

By this time P would have completed 1100 m and would be exactly between C and D. In next 100 seconds both P and Q will be at D. ∴ they meet after 1200 seconds. Now note that by the time P will be again at D (after next 1200 seconds), Q will also be at D. And in still next 1200 seconds, they will again meet at A and then the whole process gets repeated. ∴ they keep meeting at A and D.

**So the correct options for (a) and (b) are (i).**

**198. (a) The correct option is (iii). EXPLANTION:**

Had A, B, C, D had equal amount of money and the number of notes with them been $m$, $5m$, $10m$ and $25m$ respectively, then the total number of notes held by them would have been $41m$.

Now if $n = 250$, then the number of notes held by

D varies from $25m - 12$ to $25m + 12$ ($\because$ $12 \times 20 < 250$);

C varies from $10m - 5$ to $10m + 5$ ($\because$ $50 \times 5 \leq 250$);

B varies from $5m - 2$ to $5m + 2$ ($\because$ $100 \times 2 \leq 250$) and

A will be $m$.

$\therefore$ the total variation in total number of notes can be from $41m - 19$ to $41m + 19$, i.e. total variation of 38 notes.

$\because$ $38 < 41$ $\therefore$ $m$ can be uniquely determined.

For $n = 260$, total variation $= 40 < 41$, again $m$ can be uniquely determined.

For $n = 280$, total variation $= 42 > 41$. $\therefore$ A can have $m$ or $m + 1$ notes.

**(b) The correct option is (ii). EXPLANATION:**

For $x = 200$, the number of notes with D, C and B can vary from $(25m - 10)$ to $(25m + 10)$, $(10m - 4)$ to $(10m + 4)$ and $(5m - 2)$ to $(5m + 2)$ respectively.

$\therefore$ the total amount can vary from $(41m - 16)$ to $(41m + 16)$.

Now note that $180 = 41 \cdot 4 + 16$

$\therefore$ $m = 4$ and the number of notes held by C will be $10m + 4$, i.e. 44.

**(c) The correct option is (iii). EXPLANATION:**

Note that $230 = 41 \cdot 6 - 16$

From part (b), $m = 6$ and the number of notes held by B will be $5m - 2$, i.e. 28.

**199.** For person not possessing Rs 10 notes, he must possess $(5n_1)$ of Rs 20, $(2n_2)$ notes of Rs 50 and $n_3$ notes of Rs 100.

Now $18 \leq 5n_1 + 2n_2 + n_3 \leq 22$, $n_1, n_2, n_3 > 0$

Also $100n_1 + 100n_2 + 100n_3 = 500$

i.e. $n_1 + n_2 + n_3 = 5$

$\therefore$ $n_1 = 3$, $n_2 = 1$ and $n_3 = 1$

and total number of notes = 18 which is possessed by D.

For person not possessing Rs 20 notes, he must possess $(5n'_1)$ notes of Rs 10, $n'_2$ notes of Rs 50 and $n'_3$ notes of Rs 100 where $n'_1, n'_2, n'_3 > 0$. Now

$10 \geq 5n'_1 + n'_2 + n'_3 \leq 22$ and

$50n'_1 + 50n'_2 + 100n'_3 = 500$

i.e. $n'_1 + n'_2 + 2n'_3 = 10$

$\therefore n'_1 = 3, n'_2 = 1$ and $n'_3 = 3$

and total notes = 19 which is possessed by C.

Now let B got $x_1$ notes of Rs 10 and $x_2$ of Rs 20.

Then A got $(20 - x_1)$ notes of Rs 10 and $(20 - x_2)$ of Rs 20.

Also there are 2 notes of Rs 100 and 4 notes of Rs 50 which are equivalent to Rs 200 each and each can be with only one of A and B. $\therefore$ for B,

$10x_1 + 20x_2 = 500 - 200$ and for A,

$10(20 - x_1) + 20(20 - x_2) = 500 - 200$

which gives only one relation $x_1 + 2x_2 = 30$

Now $x_1 + x_2 + (2 \text{ or } 4) = 22$

$\Rightarrow x_2 = 30 - (20 \text{ or } 18) = 10 \text{ or } 12$

and consequently $x_1 = 10$ or 6

$\because$ there can be two values of $(x_1, x_2)$

$\therefore$ it cannot be determined which of A, B lacks in which of Rs 50, Rs 100.

**So the correct options for (a), (b), (c) and (d) are (iv), (iv), (ii) and (iii) respectively.**

**200. A.** Note that we cannot have

$A + B + C - D - E = C + D + E - A - B$

i.e. $A + B = D + E$ and for that matter, sum of no two of (A, B, C, D, E) can be equal to other two of them.

Also note that outside the three consecutive integers, no two integers should have differences of 1 or 2, otherwise the above condition would not be satisified

$\therefore$ the quintuplets can be

1, 2, 3, 5, (8 or 9) — Possible ; 1, 2, 3, 6, 9 — not possible ; 2, 3, 4 — not possible ;

1, 3, 4, 5, 9 — Possible ; 4, 5, 6 — not possible and other such

quintuplets which are obtained by subtracting all the above numbers by 10, i.e. the possible ones are 9, 8, 7, 5 (1 or 2) ; 9, 8, 7, 4, 1 and 9, 7, 6, 5, 1.

**So the correct options for (a), (b), (c) and (d) are (iii), (i), (iii) and (i) respectively.**

**B.** Note that there can be ${}^5C_3 = 10$ such sequences.

$\because$ A > B > C > D > E and four of such sequences are negative $\therefore$

$$C + D + E - A - B < 0 \quad \text{...(i)}$$
$$B + D + E - A - C < 0 \quad \text{...(ii)}$$
$$B + C + E - A - D < 0 \quad \text{...(iii)}$$
$$B + C + D - A - E < 0 \quad \text{...(iv)}$$

[Note that if $A + D + E - B - C < 0$ is taken, then together with (iii), it will give $2E < 0$ which cannot be possible]

Also note that the least value of B, C, D and E can be 4, 3, 2 and 1 and $\because$ $A + E > B + C + D$

$\therefore$ $A + 1 > 2 + 3 + 4$ $\Rightarrow A > 8$, i.e. A = 9, the only possible solution.

$\therefore$ (A, B, C, D, E) ≡ (9, 4, 3, 2, 1)

**So the correct options for (a), (b) and (c) are (iii), (iv) and (iii) respectively.**

**201.** Let $i$ was thrown up by the dice $x_i$ times where $i$ = 1, 2, 3, 4, 5 or 6. Then

$$x_1 + x_3 + x_5 = 5 \quad \text{...(i)}$$
$$x_2 + x_5 + x_6 = 9 \quad \text{...(ii)}$$
$$x_1 + x_2 + x_4 = 6 \quad \text{...(iii)}$$
$$x_3 + x_4 + x_6 = 8 \quad \text{...(iv)}$$

Now

$[(i) + (ii) - (iii) - (iv)]$ yields $2(x_4 - x_5) = 0$, i.e. $x_4 = x_5$

$[(i) + (iii) - (ii) - (iv)]$ yields $2(x_6 - x_1) = 6$, i.e. $x_6 - x_1 = 3$

$[(i) + (iv) - (ii) - (iii)]$ yields $2(x_2 - x_3) = 2$, i.e. $x_2 - x_3 = 1$

Now again, $x_1 + x_3 + x_4 = 5$ and $\because x_6 = 3 + x_1 \leq 4$
(according to the condition given) $\therefore x_1 = 1$ and $x_6 = 4$

The values of $x_2$, $x_3$, $x_4$, $x_5$ can be

| Cases | $x_2$ | $x_3$ | $x_4$ | $x_5$ |
|---|---|---|---|---|
| I | 2 | 1 | 3 | 3 |
| II | 3 | 2 | 2 | 2 |
| III | 4 | 3 | 1 | 1 |

**So the correct options for (a), (b) and (c) are (i), (iii) and (iv) respectively.**

**202.** We have

| | A | B | C | D |
|---|---|---|---|---|
| Initially: | 1 | 0 | 0 | 0 |
| After 1 cycle: | 2 | 1 | 1 | 0 |
| After 2 cycles: | 3 | 1 | 2 | 0 |
| After 3 cycles: | 4 | 2 | 2 | 1 |
| After 4 cycles: | 4 | 3 | 2 | 1 |
| After 5 cycles: | 4 | 4 | 3 | 2 |
| After 6 cycles: | 5 | 4 | 3 | 3 |
| After 7 cycles: | 5 | 4 | 4 | 4 |

If we take out 4 coins from each of them after 7 cycles, then the whole process will get repeated from initial stage as it did upto 7 cycles. $\therefore$ after $(7m + n)$ cycles $(0 < n < 7)$, the amount they will have will be $4m$ plus the amount they will have after n cycles.

**So the correct options for (a), (b), (c) and (d) will be (ii), (ii), (i) and (iii) respectively.**

**203. The correct option is (i). EXPLANATION:**

We have

| | | | |
|---|---|---|---|
| 2 C, 3 M | ——— | ----- | [C → Cannibal |
| 1 C, 2 M | ——→ | 1 C, 1 M | M → Man] |
| 1 C, 3 M | ←—— | 1 C | |
| 1 C, 1 M | ——→ | 1 C, 2 M | |
| 1 C, 2 M | ←—— | 1 C, 1 M | |
| 1 C | ——→ | 1 C, 3 M | |
| 2 C | ←—— | 3 M | |
| ----- | ——→ | 3 M, 2 C | |

From above, the minimum number of trips needed is 7.

**204.** Note that B cannot take 3rd period of class I.

∴ he will have to take 1st period of class I. Also D has to take 3rd period of class III. ∵ D teaches chemistry in 3rd period (to class III) ∴ to class III, C will teach Physics, B will teach Maths, A will teach English and E will teach Biology. So we can have the table as:

| Period/Class | I | II | III |
|---|---|---|---|
| 1 | B | (C/D) Chem | E (Bio) |
| 2 | C | — | A (Eng) |
| 3 | A/E | B (Phy/Maths) | D (Chem) |
| 4 | D | E/A (Eng) | B (Maths) |
| 5 | E/A (Eng) | — | C (Phy) |

We can have two cases for B teaching Physics or Maths to class II in period 3:

Case I:

| Period/Class | I | II | III |
|---|---|---|---|
| 1 | B (Phy) | C (Chem) | E (Bio) |
| 2 | C (Chem) | D (Bio) | A (Eng) |
| 3 | A (Maths) | B (Phy) | D (Chem) |
| 4 | D (Bio) | E (Eng) | B (Maths) |
| 5 | E (Eng) | A (Maths) | C (Phy) |

Case II:

| Period/Class | I | II | III |
|---|---|---|---|
| 1 | B (Maths) | D (Chem) | E (Bio) |
| 2 | C (Phy) | C (Phy) | A (Eng) |
| 3 | E (Bio) | B (Maths) | D (Chem) |
| 4 | D (Chem) | A (Eng) | B (Maths) |
| 5 | A (Eng) | E (Bio) | C (Phy) |

This case is not possible as each teacher takes at least one class of each subject he knows.

**So the correct options for (a), (b), (c), (d) and (e) are (i), (i), (ii), (i) and (iv) respectively.**

**205.** Note that E got Rs

$3 \times (70 + 80 + 90 + 100 + 110) - (220 + 250 + 280 + 310)$
$=$ Rs 290

Also each teacher takes one class of one subject and two of other subjects they know.

Now D got Rs 220 which only possible break up is Rs (70 + 70 + 80)

∴ D takes two classes of English and one class of Biology.

∵ one of them must take two classes of Biology, i.e. gets Rs 160 for Biology classes and third class he takes should give him Rs [(310, 250, 280, 290) – 160], i.e. Rs 150, 110, 120, 130 of which only Rs 110 is possible.

∴ B took two classes of biology and one class of chemistry. Now one of them must take two classes of chemistry, i.e. get Rs 180 from it. Only C or E can take two classes of chemistry (as 280, 290 – 180 = 100, 110)

Now only two classes of Maths can be taken by A or E only with third class they take giving them Rs 90 and Rs 70 respectively. But one class of chemistry (giving Rs 90) has already been taken by B. ∴ E takes two classes of Maths and consequently one class of English.

∴ we finally have, taking all teachers in consideration,

| | | | | |
|---|---|---|---|---|
| D | → | Eng (2) | + | Bio (1) |
| B | → | Bio (2) | + | Chem (1) |
| E | → | Maths (2) | + | Eng (1) |
| A | → | Physics (2) | + | Maths (1) |
| C | → | Chem (2) | + | Physics (1) |

**So the correct options for (a), (b), (c) and (d) are (iv), (ii), (i) and (ii) respectively.**

**206.** Note that switching of subjects by A affects all subjects as difference of money given for A, B and D, i.e. +30, +30 and –20 do not cancel each other. ∴ no two persons teach same pair of subjects. Now

A → Bigger subj (1) + Smaller subj (2)

B → Bigger subj (1) + Smaller subj (2) and

C → Bigger subj (2) + Smaller subj (1) = 280 = 100 + 100 + 80 (as 90 + 90 + 100 is not valid)

∴ $x$ = 20 (as Rs 100 and Rs 80 are switched)

Also the difference of money when put together must be zero.

∴ E would have got Rs 20 less.

Now, we can have

| Teacher | Difference of two subjects taught | Amount received | Subjects taught |
|---|---|---|---|
| A | Rs 30 | Rs 210 (60 × 2 + 90) | Eng (2) + Rs 90(1) |
| B | Rs 30 | Rs 240 (70 × 2 + 100) | Maths (1) + Rs 70(2) |
| C | Rs 20 | Rs 280 (100 × 2 + 80) | Maths (2) + Rs 80(1) |
| D | Rs 20 | | Rs 80 (2) + Rs 60 (1) |
| E | Rs 20 | | and Rs 90 (2) + Rs 70 (1) or vice versa |

∵ D teaches chemistry ∴ one gets Rs 80 per class for teaching chemistry and for teaching Bio/Phy, one gets Rs 70/Rs 90 or vice versa per class.

**So the correct options for (a), (b), (c) and (d) are (iii), (iii), (i) and (ii) respectively.**

**207.** Note that there are 5 males and 3 females.

∴ A, C have to be males.

∵ there are two couples in (A, C, E, D, B)

∴ D, E, G have to be females.

∵ there are all siblings in (A, D, F, G, H)

∴ E is the grandmother.

Out of (A, F, H) two are brothers and one of (D, G) is a sister. If (F, H) are brothers, then one of them has to be in the group of given two couples, viz. (C, E, A, D, B) which is not the case.

∴ A has to be one of the brother and that too married. Now he can be married to only D. ∴ (A, D) will be a couple. Consequently, G will be a sister; E will be married to one of (B, C) and one of (F, H) will be the unmarried brother.

**So the correct options for (a), (b) and (c) are (ii), (iii) and (iv) respectively.**

**208.** Note that Tony (M) — E (F)

Monica (F) — F (M)

Jane (F) — D (M)

Harrison (M) — A (F)

where ' — ' denotes 'married to'.

Now C is female ∴ B will be male and Tony.

Also Sheila can be A or E. But she cannot be married to Harison as he is not the father of C. ∴ Shiela is E. We can draw the relationship chart as

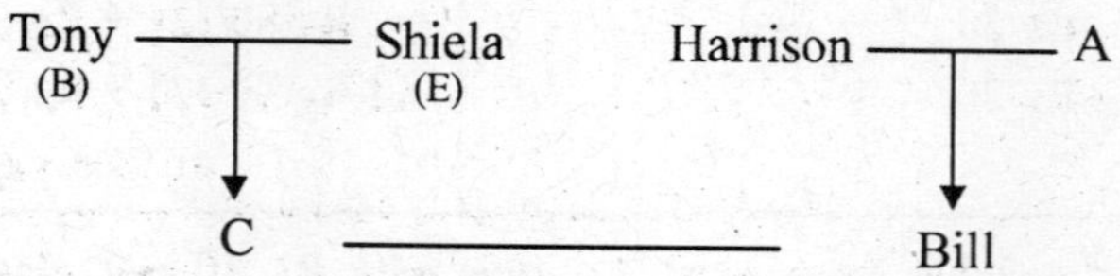


**So the correct options for (a), (b) and (c) are (i), (i) and (iii) respectively.**

**209.** We can draw a table as:

| | Non Leap | Leap |
|---|---|---|
| Jan | D | D |
| Feb | D + 3 | D + 3 |
| Mar | D + 3 | D + 4 |
| Apr | D + 6 | D |
| May | D + 1 | D + 2 |
| Jun | D + 4 | D + 5 |
| Jul | D + 6 | D |
| Aug | D + 2 | D + 3 |
| Sep | D + 5 | D + 6 |
| Oct | D | D + 1 |
| Nov | D + 3 | D + 4 |
| Dec | D + 5 | D + 6 |

where D denotes a particular day of the week.

Note that in 'Non Leap Year' only (D + 3) occurs thrice while in 'Leap Year' only D occurs thrice. ∴ these will correspond to Sunday.

**So the correct options for (a), (b), (c) and (d) are (ii), (i), (ii) and (iii) respectively.**

**210.** We can draw a chart as:

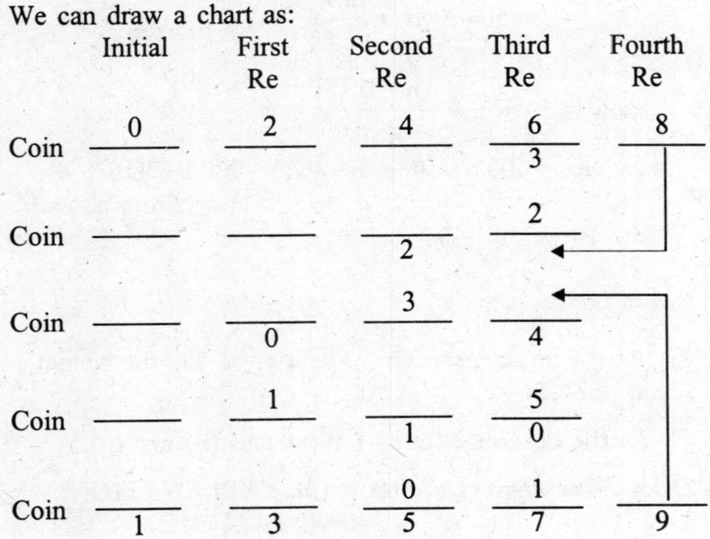

where 'Re' denotes 'Rearrangement'

**So the correct options for (a), (b) and (c) are (iii), (iii) and (iv) respectively.**

**211. The correct option is (ii). EXPLANATION:**

From arrangement

A C B D E F, it is deduced that A < C < B < E;

F D B C A E, it is deduced that F < D < B < E;

$\therefore$ we have

$(A, F) < (C, D) < B < E \quad \rightarrow \quad$ 4 possibilities

$$\left.\begin{matrix} A < C < F < D < B < E \\ F < D < A < C < B < E \end{matrix}\right\} \rightarrow \text{2 possibilities}$$

**212.** Let the average weight of girls be $w$ and their number be $n$. Then $n\,w + (10 - n)(w + 3) = 51 + \ldots\ 60 = 500 + 55 = 555$

$\Rightarrow 10w + 3(10 - n) = 555$

Let the weight of girls be

$$50 + \overline{x},\ 50 + \overline{x+1},\ \ldots\ 50 + \overline{x+(n-1)}$$

$$\text{Then } nw = 50n + \overline{x} + \overline{x+1} + \ldots\ \overline{x+(n-1)}$$

$$= 50n + nx + \frac{n(n-1)}{2}$$

$$\Rightarrow w = 50 + x + \frac{(n-1)}{2}$$

$$\therefore\ 10w = 500 + 10x + 5(n - 1) = 555 - 3(10 - n)$$

(from above)

$$\Rightarrow\ 10x = 30 - 2n$$

$$\Rightarrow\ x = \frac{1}{5}(15 - n)$$

As $x$ is an integer $\therefore$ $n = 5$ and $x = 2$ and the weight of girls are 52—56.

**So the correct options for (a) and (b) are (ii).**

**213. A. The correct option is (ii). EXPLANATION:**

Note that 2 is not against 3, 4, 1 or 6. ∴ it can be against 5 only.

**B.** One of the pair of each of the following triplets will denote the numbers on the opposite faces:

{(1, 2), (1, 4), (2, 4)} {(2, 3), (2, 5), (3, 5)}
and {(3, 4) (3, 6) (4, 6)}

The possibilities of numbers on opposite faces are

(1, 2); (3, 5); (4, 6) or (1, 4); (2, 5); (3, 6)

**So the correct options for (a) and (b) are (ii) and (iv) respectively.**

**214.** Let the starting position be A. Then

| | | | | | |
|---|---|---|---|---|---|
| 1 | 2 | 4 | 5 | 6 | |
| A | C | D | B | E | → Possible |
| | 3 | 4 | | | |
| | D | D | | | → Not possible |
| | 3 | 5 | | | |
| | D | C | | | → Not possible |

Let the starting position be B. Then

| | | | |
|---|---|---|---|
| 2 | 1 | 5 | |
| B | C | D | → Not possible |
| | 6 | 3 | |
| | D | A | → Not possible |
| | 6 | 1 | |
| | D | C | → Not possible |

Now from part (a), the options can be only (A, D). ∴ we need not check for C as the starting position. Let the starting position be D. Then

| | | | | | |
|---|---|---|---|---|---|
| 4 | 5 | 2 | | | |
| D | C | A | | | → Not possible |
| | 5 | 1 | | | |
| | C | B | | | → Not possible |
| 4 | 6 | 1 | 2 | 5 | |
| D | B | A | C | D | → Possible |
| | | 3 | | | |
| | | C | | | → Not possible |

$\therefore$ only two possible arrangements are

| | | | | | |
|---|---|---|---|---|---|
| 1 | 2 | 5 | 4 | 6 | |
| A | C | D | B | D | and |
| 4 | 6 | 1 | 2 | 5 | |
| D | B | A | C | D | |

**So the correct optoins for (a), (b), (c) and (d) are (ii), (iv), (i) and (iii) respectively.**

**215.** Let $m$, $n$, $p$ be the total numbers of 2 kg, 3 kg and 4 kg packets. Then

$$2m + 3n + 4p = 100 \text{ and } m + n + p = 30$$

$\Rightarrow$ $p = m + 10$ and $n = 2(10 - m)$

Let $m_1$, $n_1$, $p_1$ be the number of 2 kg, 3 kg and 4 kg packets respectively carried by porter A. Then $m_1 + n_1 + p_1 = 7$ and $2m_1 + 3n_1 + 4p_1 = 20$

$\Rightarrow p_1 - m_1 = -1$ and $n_1 = 2(4 - m_1)$

$\Rightarrow (m_1, n_1, p_1) \equiv (1, 6, 0); (2, 4, 1); (3, 2, 2); (4, 0, 3)$

$\because$ 0 is inadmissible

$\therefore (m_1, n_1\ p_1) \equiv (2, 4, 1)$ or $(3, 2, 2)$

Let $m_2$, $n_2$, $p_2$ be the number of 2 kg, 3 kg and 4kg packets respectively carried by porter B. Then

$$m_2 + n_2 + p_2 = 9 \text{ and } 2m_2 + 3n_2 + 4p_2 = 30$$

$\Rightarrow$ $p_2 = 3 + m_2$ and $n_2 = 2(3 - m_2)$

$\therefore$ $(m_2, n_2, p_2) \equiv (1, 4, 4)$ or $(2, 2, 5)$

Let $m_3$, $n_3$, $p_3$ be the number of 2 kg, 3 kg and 4 kg packets respectively carried by porter C.

Then $m_3 + n_3 + p_3 = 14$ and $2m_3 + 3n_3 + 4p_3 = 50$

$\Rightarrow p_3 = 8 + m_3$ and $n_3 = 2(3 - m_3)$

$\therefore (m_3, n_3, p_3) \equiv (1, 4, 9)$ or $(2, 2, 10)$

**So the correct options for (a), (b), (c) and (d) are (ii), (i), (ii) and (iii) respectively.**

**216. A.** We have three cases for each of the groups. We can form a chart as:

$$\underset{①}{\begin{bmatrix} B, A & E, F \\ B, F & A, E \\ B, E & A, F \end{bmatrix}} \quad \underset{②}{\begin{bmatrix} B, D & E, G \\ B, G & E, D \\ B, E & D, G \end{bmatrix}} \quad \underset{③}{\begin{bmatrix} B, C & F, H \\ B, F & C, H \\ B, H & C, F \end{bmatrix}}$$

If B, E are in the same group, then A, F, D, G has to be in one group but from ③, this is not possible.

If B, F are in the same group, then A, E, C, H has to be in one group but from ②, this is not possible.

∴ from ① A, B are in one group and E, F are in another group. The possible arrangements are

| | | | |
|---|---|---|---|
| I | A, B, D, C or H | and | E, F, G, H or C |
| II | A, B, G, C or H | and | E, F, D, H or C |

**So the correct options for (a) and (b) are (iv) and (iii) respectively.**

**B. (a) The correct option is (iv). EXPLANATION:**

| | {A, B, C, D} | {E, F, G, H} |
|---|---|---|
| X can have | (A, B), (A, C) or (A, D) | (E, F), (E, G), (E, H), (F, G), (F, H) or (G, H) |

$$\therefore X \equiv \left\{\begin{array}{r} A, B, E, G \\ F, G \\ G, H \end{array}\right\}, \left\{\begin{array}{r} A, C, E, F \\ E, H \\ F, H \end{array}\right\}, \left\{\begin{array}{r} A, D, E, F \\ E, H \\ F, H \end{array}\right\}$$

**(b) The correct option is (iii). EXPLANATION:**

As done in part (a), we can have similarly,

$$X \equiv \left\{\begin{array}{r} A, B \text{ or } D, E, F \\ E, H \\ F, G \\ F, H \\ G, H \end{array}\right\}, \quad \{A, C, F, H\}$$

**217.** There can be two cases:

G speaks French only.
H speaks English only.
I speaks Russian only.

$$\begin{array}{ll} \text{French} & G, D, F, \\ \text{English} & H, B, F, \\ \text{Russian} & I, B, D, \end{array} \begin{pmatrix} E \\ A \\ C \end{pmatrix} \text{ or } \begin{pmatrix} C \\ E \\ A \end{pmatrix}$$

H speaks French only.
G speaks Russian only.
I speaks English only.

$$\begin{array}{l} H, D, F, \\ I, B, F, \\ G, B, D, \end{array} \begin{pmatrix} E \\ A \\ C \end{pmatrix} \text{ or } \begin{pmatrix} C \\ E \\ A \end{pmatrix}$$

**So the correct options for (a) and (b) are (iv) and (i) respectively.**

**218.** Note that one of (C, H) is male and another female (∵ other possible pairs (A, D); (B, F) and (E, G) has one male and one female each). ∵ H is female ∴ C is male.

∵ there are only two Japanese delegates ∴ C will be one of them as can be seen from the given triplets.

Now we can have two cases for the six of given delegates ('+' is for male and '–' for female):

Case I:

| A | B | C | C | D | E | F | G | H |
|---|---|---|---|---|---|---|---|---|
| + | – | + | + | – | | + | | – |

G has to be '–' as it got to belong to Japan and consequently E '+'. Countrywise, they can be as

| A | B | C | C | D | E | F | G | H |
|---|---|---|---|---|---|---|---|---|
| + | – | + | + | – | + | + | – | – |
| En | Fr | J | J | Fr | En | Fr | J | En |

Case II:

| A | B | C | C | D | E | F | G | H |
|---|---|---|---|---|---|---|---|---|
| + | | + | + | + | – | | + | – |

F has to be '–' as it got to belong to Japan and consequently B '+'. Countrywise, they can be as

| A | B | C | C | D | E | F | G | H |
|---|---|---|---|---|---|---|---|---|
| – | + | + | + | + | – | – | + | – |
| | En | J | J | En | | J | | En |

This case is not possible as (E, G) cannot belong to France as they are given to belong to different countries. Note that this case may not be considered at all as there is no 'cannot be determined' in options but is given for clarification for those who start solving this problem with this case.

**So the correct options for (a), (b) and (c) are (i), (iv) and (iv) respectively.**

**219.** **(a) The correct option is (ii). EXPLANATION:**

The required number of ways will be simply the derrangement of 5 different things given as

$$\lfloor 5\left(\frac{1}{\lfloor 2}-\frac{1}{\lfloor 3}+\frac{1}{\lfloor 4}-\frac{1}{\lfloor 5}\right) = 5\cdot4\cdot3 - 5\cdot4 + 5 - 1 = 44$$

**(b) The correct option is (i). EXPLANATION:**

Note that the correct envelopes for the letters will be

$$\begin{matrix} A & B & C & D & E \\ \begin{pmatrix} G \\ I \\ J \end{pmatrix} & \begin{pmatrix} F \\ J \\ H \end{pmatrix} & \begin{pmatrix} I \\ G \\ F \end{pmatrix} & \begin{pmatrix} J \\ H \\ G \end{pmatrix} & \begin{pmatrix} H \\ F \\ I \end{pmatrix} \end{matrix}$$

and if A goes into G, then

| A | B | C | D | E |
|---|---|---|---|---|
| G | H, F | I | J | F, H |
| G | J | I | H | F |
| G | H | F | J | I |
| G | J | F | H | I |

So the envelopes can be tried in five ways.

**(c) The correct option is (ii). EXPLANATION:**

We have

| A | B | C | D | E |
|---|---|---|---|---|
| I | J | F | G | H |
| I | J, H | G | H, J | F |
| I | F | G | J | H |

So the envelopes can be tried in four ways.

**(d) The correct option is (iv). EXPLANATION:**

We have

| A | B | C | D | E |
|---|---|---|---|---|
| J | F | G | H | I |
| J | F | I | G | H |
| J | H | F, I | G | I, F |

∴ if E goes into F, it implies that B, C, D go into H, I and G respectively.

**220.** Note that the three triplets can be only

[1, 2, 3] [4, 5, 6] [7, 8, 9] or
[0, 1, 2] [4, 5, 6] [7, 8, 9] or
[0, 1, 2] [3, 4, 5] [7, 8, 9] or
[0, 1, 2] [3, 4, 5] [6, 7, 8]

∴ B > D > G > I will be respectively 9, 6, 3 and 0.

Now the sequence I A F E H B D G C J is

O A F E H 9 6 3 C J which can be only
0 1 2 7 8 9 6 3 4 5

**So the correct options for (a) and (b) are (i) and (iv) respectively.**

**221.** Let four of them won $m$ matches each while fifth won $n$ matches. Then

$4m + n = 29$. $\because$ $m, n \leq 10$ $\therefore$ $(m, n) \equiv (5, 9)$ or $(6, 5)$ or $(7, 2)$

Now the persons who can win the match will be $A_k$ where $k$ (assumed to be > 10) will be few of $(m, m, m, m, n) + 1$

$\therefore$ for $(m, n) \equiv (5, 9)$, $k = 11, 15, 16, 20, 21, 25, 26$
for $(m, n) \equiv (6, 5)$, $k = 12, 13, 18, 19, 24, 25$
for $(m, n) \equiv (7, 2)$, $k = 15, 17, 22, 24, 29$

Now $X_{18}$ can be winner only for $(m, n) \equiv (6, 5)$ and
$\because$ $(6 + 6 + 5) + 1 = 18$ $\therefore$ next winner will be $X_{24}$

**So the correct options for (a), (b) and (c) are (iv), (iii) and (ii) respectively.**

**222. A. The correct option is (iv). EXPLANATION:**
Note that $(P_1, P_2)$ cannot be of blood group AB. Also $P_1$ cannot be of blood group O as $P_2$ and $P_3$ will also be of the same blood group which cannot be possible. Now if $P_1$ is of blood group A, then $P_2$ will be of blood group O or A while $P_3$ will be of blood group B or AB. Now $P_2$ will not be able to take blood from $P_3$ $\therefore$ the given conditions are not possible together.

**B.** From statement (V), we have

$P_5 \equiv$ O ($P_2 \not\equiv$ O) or B ($P_2 \not\equiv$ O or B)

and from statement (IV), we have

$P_5 \equiv$ O ($P_5 \not\equiv$ O) or A ($P_5 \not\equiv$ O or A)

From the above two conditions, we conclude that $P_5 \equiv$ B
From statement (III), we have

$P_3 \equiv$ O or A or B (only if $P_2$ is of blood group AB)

From statement (I), we have

$P_1 \equiv$ AB or B [as it can take blood from $P_5$ ($\equiv$ B)]

$\because$ $P_3$ and $P_1$ are of different blood groups

$\therefore$ $P_3 \equiv$ O or A only

From statement (II), we have

$P_2 \equiv$ AB or B (only if $P_4 \equiv$ O)

Now $P_2 \not\equiv$ O or B from statement (V)

$\therefore$ $P_1 \equiv$ AB

**So the correct options for (a), (b), and (c) are (iv), (iii) and (iii) respectively.**

**223. A.** We are given:

| A | B | C | D | E | F | G | H |
|---|---|---|---|---|---|---|---|
| F | M | F | F | M | M | F | M |

If D, E is a couple, then another couple must be from A, B; B, C; F, G or G, H. Let us assume A, B to be a couple. Then C must be married to F or H and G will be married to H or F accordingly. As there will be three couples together $\therefore$ this case is not possible and A, B cannot be a couple. Similarly B, C; F, G or G, H cannot be a couple. $\therefore$ D, E cannot be a couple.

Now if D is married to B, then there cannot be two couples who can be together. $\therefore$ D, B also cannot be a couple.

**So the correct options for (a) and (b) are (ii).**

**B.** We are given:

| A | B | C | D | E | F | G | H |
|---|---|---|---|---|---|---|---|
| | M | | F | M | | F | |

There can be two cases:

Case I: D, E is a couple. Another couple can be A, B; B, C; F, G or G, H, i.e. the couple being together cannot be known.

Case II: If D, E is not a couple, then the couples who are together can be determined only if C, D and E, F are couples and A, H are male and female respectively represented as:

| A | B | C | D | E | F | G | H |
|---|---|---|---|---|---|---|---|
| M | M | M | F | M | F | F | F |

**So the correct option will be (ii).**

**C.** We have,

| | | | | | | | |
|---|---|---|---|---|---|---|---|
| A | B | C | D | E | F | G | H |
| | M | F | | | | F | M |

There can be only two possibilities:

| | | | | | | | | |
|---|---|---|---|---|---|---|---|---|
| A | B | C | D | E | F | G | H | |
| M | M | F | F | M | F | F | M | or |
| F | M | F | M | F | M | F | M | |

**So the correct option is (iv).**

**224. (a) The correct option is (ii). EXPLANATION:**

This given condition is only possible only if the four terms are $x$, 100, $x$, $x$ where $0 < x \leq 100$

**(b) The correct option is (ii). EXPLANATION:**

Consider the series

$x, y, x + y, x + 2y, 2x + 3y, 3x + 5y, 5x + 8y, 8x + 13y...$

where a term (third term onward) is equal to the sum of its two preceding terms.

$\therefore$ if $A_0 = x$, $A_1 = y$, then

$A_3 = x + 2y - 100n$ and

$A_6 = 5x + 8y - 100m$

where $n$, $m$ are suitable positive integers.

$\Rightarrow$ $x + 2y = 40 + 100m$ and

$5x + 8y = 100\ (n + 1)$

$\Rightarrow$ $x = 100\ (n + 1) - 160 - 400m$

$= 100\ (n + 1 - 4m) - 160$

Now $0 < x \leq 100$

$\therefore$ $n + 1 - 4\ m = 2$

and $x = 40$

**(c) The correct option is (i). EXPLANATION:**

As done in part (b),

$2x + 3y = 30 + 100m \qquad \times 13$

and $8x + 13y = 70 + 100n \qquad \times 3$

On subtraction, we get

$2x = (390 - 210) + 100(13m - 3n)$

$\Rightarrow$ $x = 90 + 50\ (13m - 3n)$

Now $13m - 3n$ can be 0 or $-1$.

But for $13m - 3n = 0$

$n$ should be equal to 13 which is not possible.

$\therefore x = 90 - 50 = 40$

**225.** Note that $x_{n+2} = 4x_n - 1$ if $x_n$ is odd.
$= 4x_{n-2}$ if $x_n$ is even.

$\Rightarrow (x_{n+2} - 1/3) = 4(x_n - 1/3)$ if $x_n$ is odd
and $(x_{n+2} - 2/3) = 4(x_n - 2/3)$ if $x_n$ is even.

**(a) The correct option is (iv). EXPLANATION:**
Note that $(x_{n+2} - 2/3) = 4(x_n - 2/3)$

$$\Rightarrow \quad x_n - 2/3 = 4(x_{n-2} - 2/3) \qquad \times 4^1$$
$$\vdots \qquad \vdots \qquad \vdots$$
$$x_2 - 2/3 = 4(x_0 - 2/3) \qquad \times 4^{n/2}$$

Adding, we get

$$(x_{n+2} - 2/3) = (4^1 + 4^2 + \ldots 4^{n/2+1})(x_0 - 2/3)$$

$$\Rightarrow x_{n+2} - \frac{2}{3} = \frac{4(4^{n/2+1} - 1)}{3}\left(x_0 - \frac{2}{3}\right)$$

$$\Rightarrow x_{100} = \frac{2}{3} + \frac{4(2^{100} - 1)}{3}\left(x_0 - \frac{2}{3}\right)$$

$\therefore \; x_0 = 2 + 2/3 = 7/3$

**(b) The correct option is (ii). EXPLANATION:**

We have similarly, $x_{101} = \dfrac{1}{3} + 4\left(\dfrac{2^{100} - 1}{3}\right)\left(x_0 - \dfrac{1}{3}\right)$

$\therefore \; x_0 = 1 + 1/3 = 4/3$

**226.** Note that
A must follow B or C only;
B must follow C or D only;
C must follow D or A only;
D must follow A.

**(a) The correct option is (iv). EXPLANATION:**
The sequence can be B A D B A D ... or C A C A ...

**(b) The correct option is (i). EXPLANATION:**
We can form branches of sequence as:

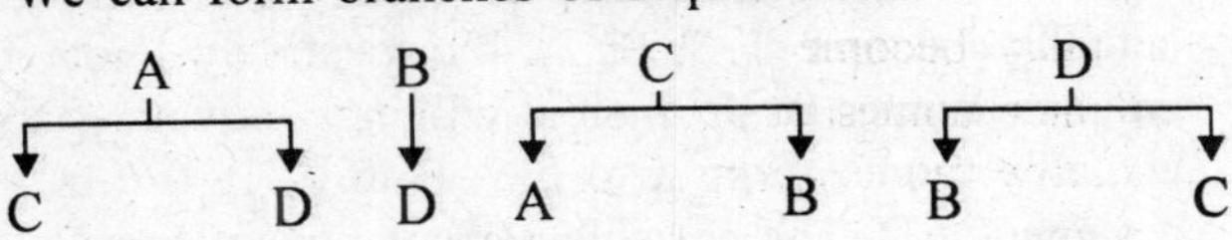

and the whole sequence as:

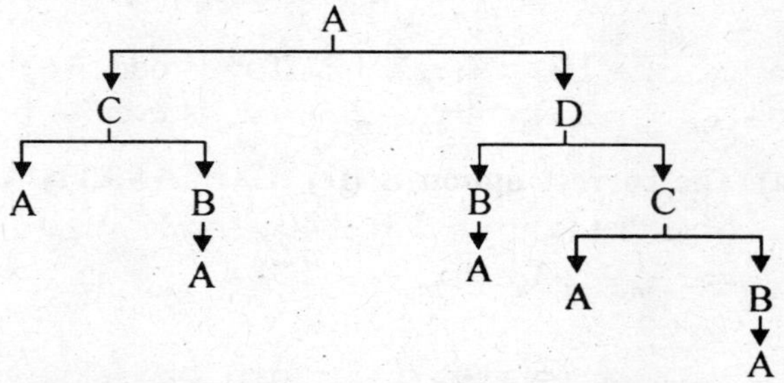


**(c) The correct option is (iv). EXPLANATION:**

As done in part (b), we have,

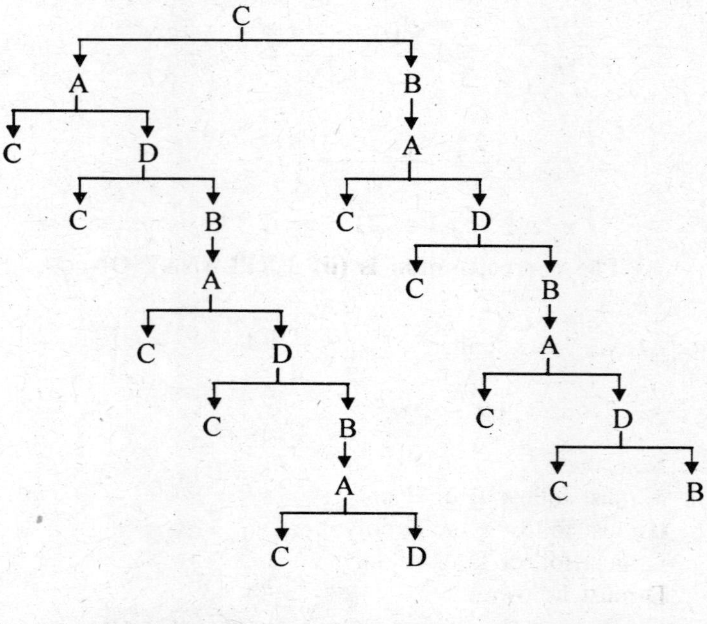


**227.** Note that the movement of counter is cyclic which gets repeated after it moves around the pentagon once. ∴ it does not matter if we we subtract multiple of 5 from the number assigned to A, B, C, D and E. And 11, 13, 15, 17, 19 will actually become 1, 3, 0, 2, 4 respectively. Note that if the counter comes at 0, then it will not move. ∵ the counter actually moved from A to E to B to C. ∴ 0 (i.e. 15) will be assigned to D. The possible permutations when 11 is assigned to A can be:

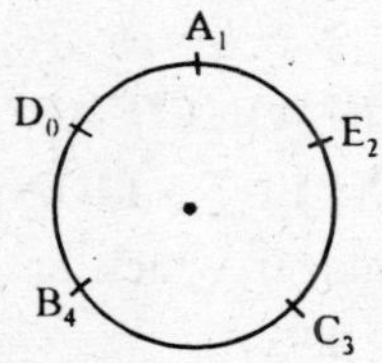


or

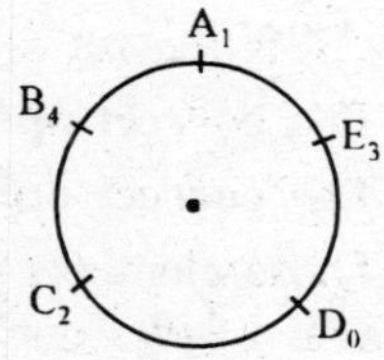


**So the correct options for (a) and (b) are (i).**

**228.** Let $t_n = E$

Then $t_{n+1} = A$

$t_{n-1} = E - A,$

$t_{n+2} = 2A$ if $2A \le E,$

$= 2A - E$ if $2A > E,$

$t_{n-2} = E - 2A$ or ...(i)

$2E - 2A$ ...(ii)

$t_{n+3} = 3A$ if $3A \le E$ ...(iii)

$$\left.\begin{array}{l} = 3A - E \text{ if } 2A \le E < 3A \\ = 3A - E \text{ if } 2A > E \text{ and } 3A - E \le E \end{array}\right\} = 3A - E \text{ if } 1.5A \le E \le 3A \quad \text{... (iv)}$$

$= 3A - 2E$ if $2A > E$ and $3A - E > E$ ...(v)

Now, $t_{n-2} = t_{n+3}$

$\therefore$ $E = 5A$, $E \ge 3A$ [(i) and (iii)] $\Rightarrow$ valid

$E = 2.5A$, $1.5A \le E < 3A$ [(i) and (iv)] $\Rightarrow$ valid

$E = 5/3A$, $E < 1.5A$ [(i) and (v)] $\Rightarrow$ not valid

$E = 2.5A$, $E \ge 3A$ [(ii) and (iii)] $\Rightarrow$ not valid

$E = 5/3A$, $1.5A \le E \le 3A$ [(ii) and (iv)] $\Rightarrow$ valid

$E = 5/4A$, $E < 1.5A$ [(ii) and (iv)] $\Rightarrow$ valid

$\Rightarrow$ $E = 5A$ and the terms are $3A$, $4A$, $5A$, $A$, $2A$ or

$= 2.5A$ and the terms are $.5A$, $1.5A$, $2.5A$, $A$, $2A$ or

$= 5/3A$ and the terms are $4/3A$, $2/3A$, $5/3A$, $A$, $A/3$ or

$= 5/4A$ and the terms are $1/2A$, $1/4A$, $5/4A$, $A$, $3/4\,A$

**So the correct options for (a), (b), (c) and (d) are (ii), (ii), (iv) and (iii) respectively.**

**229.** $S \equiv \{1, 3, 5, 7\}$

Let $S''$ be the set of averages of two numbers from the set S.

Then $S'' \equiv \{2, 3, 4, 4, 5, 5, 6, 6, 7, 8\}$

Now S′ is the set of averages of two numbers from set S″.

**(a) The correct option is (i). EXPLAINED ABOVE.**

**(b) The correct option is (iii). EXPLANATION:**

Those elements of set S′ are integer which are the averages of two numbers from the groups

(2, 4, 4, 6, 6, 8) or (3, 5, 5, 7)

and the number of these elements is 15 + 6 = 21

**(c) The correct option is (ii). EXPLANATION:**

The distinct elements of set S″ are

(2, 3, 4, 5, 6, 7, 8). Now

$8 + 5 = 7 + 6,$

$7 + 5 = 6 + 6 = 8 + 4,$

$8 + 3 = 7 + 4 = 6 + 5,$

$5 + 5 = 6 + 4 = 7 + 3 = 8 + 2,$

$5 + 4 = 6 + 3 = 7 + 2,$

$5 + 3 = 6 + 2$

$3 + 4 = 5 + 2$

∴ total number of elements =

3 (4, 5, 6 may be selected twice) +

21 (two distinct numbers are selected) –

12 (those sums which are repeated above) = 12

**230.**

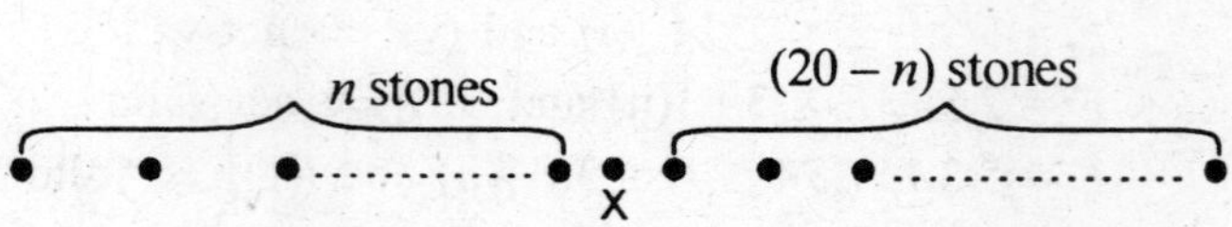


Let the man has to bring all the stones to X. Then,

$d_X = 2(1 + 2 + 3 + \ldots + n) + 2\,\{1 + 2 + 3 + \ldots (20 - n)\}$

$= 2\dfrac{n(n+1)}{2} + 2\dfrac{(20-n)(21-n)}{2}$

$= n^2 + n + n^2 - 41n + 420$

$= 2n^2 - 40n + 420$

$= 2(n^2 - 20n + 100 + 110)$

$= 2(\{n - 10)^2 + 110\}$

**(a) The correct option is (ii). EXPLANATION:**

If $d_C = 2\{(m - 10)^2 + 110\}$, then

$d_D + d_B - 2d_C = 2\{(m - 9)^2 + (m + 11)^2 - 2(m - 10)^2\}$

$= 2(81 + 121 - 200) = 4$

**(b) The correct option is (iii). EXPLANATION:**

If B is $m$th stone, then

$d_B = 2\{(m - 1 - 10)^2 + 110\} = 22000$ ... given

$\Rightarrow (m - 11)^2 + 110 = 110$

$\Rightarrow m = 11$

**(c) The correct option is (iii). EXPLANATION:**

He will carry two consecutive stones at a time

$\therefore$ he will have to travel

$2(2 + 4 + 6 + ... 20)$

$= 4(1 + 2 + ... 10)$

$$= 4 \cdot \frac{10 \cdot 11}{2} = 220m$$

**231.** Note that those who do not want to be together can be (G, A); (G, B); (G, C); (G, E); (H, E); (F, B) and (D, A)

$\because$ we need three exclusive pairs

$\therefore$ it comes out to be (H, E), (D, A) and (B, G)

(as C, F are forbidden from these pairs)

**(a) The correct option is (iii). EXPLANATION:**

Let (H, E) be both males

(D, A) be both females and

B be male and G, female

Then the committees can be

C, F, (H or E or B), (D or A or G) $\rightarrow$ 8 ways excluding the committee (C, F, B, G)

C, one of (H, E), one of (D, A), G $\rightarrow$ 4 ways

F, one of (D, A), one of (H, E), B $\rightarrow$ 4 ways

$\therefore$ total of 16 such committees are possible.

**(b) The correct option is (ii). EXPLAINED ABOVE.**

**(c) The correct option is (iv). EXPLANATION:**

From part (a), note that two males or two females who do not want to be together can be found in at most 7 different committees each while the male and the female who do not want to be together in a committee can be in at most 6 different committees each.

∴ from given conditions (A, D) will be of same sex, (H, E) will be of opposite sex and corollarily (B, G) will be of same sex. Also sex of (A, D) will be opposite of that of (B, G).

**232. (a) The correct option is (i). EXPLANATION:**

Note that the two males can be selected from four couples in $^4C_2$, i.e. 6 ways while the females of other two couples can be selected in just 1 way. ∴ total number of different ways in which the committee can be formed will be 6.

**(b) The correct option is (iv). EXPLANATION:**

We have,

| Male | | Female | |
|---|---|---|---|
| A | ⟷ | — | ['⟷' denotes being couple] |
| C | ⟷ | — | |
| – | ⟷ | B | |
| – | ⟷ | F | |

which on further development becomes

| | | |
|---|---|---|
| A | ⟷ | D |
| C | ⟷ | E |
| G | ⟷ | B |
| H | ⟷ | F |

**233.** Note that those who want to be together can be (A, E); (B, F); (C, D) and (G, H) while those who do not want to be together can be (A, B); (A, F); (B, E); (C, G); (C, H); (D, G); (D, H) and (E, F)

We can have following cases:

| Those who want to be together | Those who do not want to be together |
|---|---|
| A, E | (C, G); (C,H); (D, G) or (D, H) |
| B, F | (C, G); (C,H); (D, G) or (D, H) |
| C, D | (A, B); (A, F); (B, E) or (E, F) |
| G, H | (A, B); (A, F); (B, E) or (E, F) |

**So the correct options for (a), (b) and (c) are (ii), (i) and (iii) respectively.**

**234.** Note that a cyclic sequence of eight given letters can be formed such that no person represented by a letter want to be in a committee with persons represented by the adjacent letters. Let us start the sequence as

B D — — — — — E B which can be developed further as following cases:

| Cases | B | D | — | — | — | — | — | E | B |
|---|---|---|---|---|---|---|---|---|---|
| I | | | C | | F | | | | |
| II | | | C | | | | F | | |
| III | | | F | | C | | | | |
| IV | | | F | | | | C | | |
| V | | | | C | | | F | | |
| VI | | | | F | | | C | | |

Now note that (A, G), (A, H), (C, H), (F, H), (E, A) and (E, H) cannot be neighbours. ∴ only possibility comes out to be (from case VI):

B D H G F A C E B

If committees of four persons are formed, then it can be either (B, H, F, C) or (D, G, A, E)

**So the correct options for (a), (b), (c), (d) and (e) are (i), (iv), (iv), (i) and (iv) respectively.**

**235. (a) The correct option is (i). EXPLANATION:**

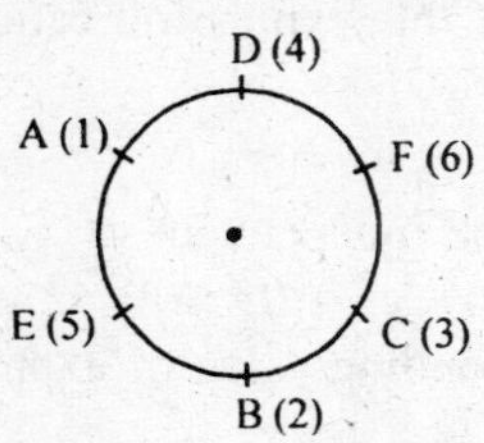


(Note that movement of E does not make any difference as it will retain its initial position)

We can get the sequence A B C D E F A if the letters B, C and F moved in that order.

**(b) The correct option is (ii). EXPLANATION:**

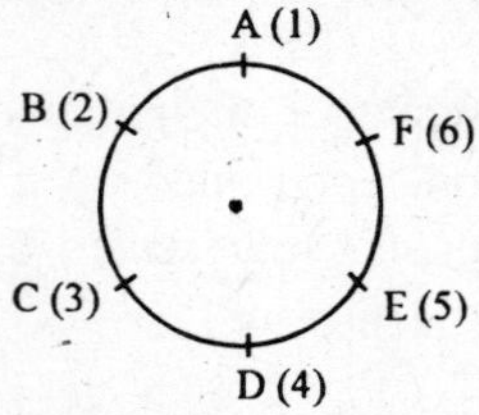


We can get the sequence A B C D E F A if the letters A, B, C and D moved in that order.

**(c) The correct option is (ii). EXPLANATION:**

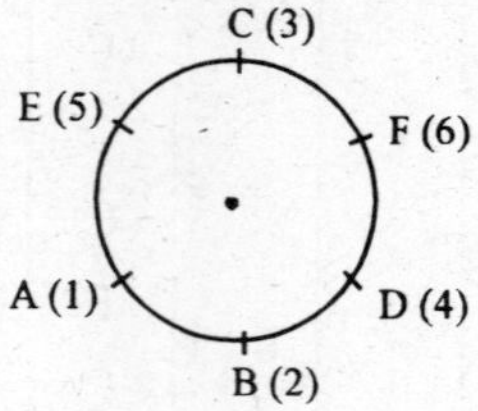


Note that only option (ii) is amenable as the desired sequence can be get by moving letters A, B, D and F in that order.

**236.** $$\frac{x_1x_2 + x_4x_5 + x_3 + x_2}{x_1 + x_2 + x_1x_2 + x_1x_4 + x_2x_5}$$

For the above expression to be independent of $x_1$, either $x_2 = 0$, $x_4 = -1$ or $x_4x_5 + x_3 + x_2 = 0$, $x_2 + x_2x_5 = 0$ and the corresponding value of expression will be $\frac{x_3 - x_5}{0}$ (indeterminate, $\therefore$ not possible)

and $\frac{x_2}{1 + x_2 + x_4}$ (The value of this expression cannot be non zero constant $\therefore$ rejected)

For the above expression to be independent of $x_2$, either $x_1 = -1$, $x_5 = 0$ or $x_4x_5 + x_3 = 0$, $x_1(1 + x_4) = 0$ and the corresponding value of expression will be $\frac{x_3}{-(1 + x_4)}$ (rejected, as it is not a constant) and $\frac{1 + x_1}{1 + x_1 + x_5}$, which will be equal to a non zero constant if $x_5 = 0$.

From option (a), we need not check for any other $x_i$.

**So the correct options for (a), (b) and (c) are (ii), (iv) and (iii) respectively.**

**237. (a) The correct option is (ii). EXPLANATION:**

Note that the branches after every one process of division (branching) increases by 2 and number of lateral branches are sequentially $2^1, 2^2, 2^3, \ldots$

Now $2 + 4 + 8 + 16 + 32 + 64 > 100$.

$\therefore$ lateral branches just above $A_{100}$ will be upto $A_m$ where

$$m = 2 + 4 + 8 + 16 + 32 = 62$$

and if $A_{100}$ is the direct branch of $A_{30 + n}$ where

$$62 + 2x = 100 \quad \Rightarrow \quad x = 19$$

$\therefore$ $A_{100}$ will be the direct branch of $A_{49}$.

**(b) The correct option is (iii). EXPLANATION:**

In a way similar to as done in part (a),

$A_{200}$ will be the direct branch of

$A_{62 + x}$ where $126 + 2x = 200$

$\Rightarrow x = 37$, i.e. $A_{99}$.

**(c) The correct option is (iv). EXPLANATION:**

Let $A_m$ will be the direct branch of lateral branches which ranges from $2^k - 1$ to $2^{k+1} - 2$.

$\therefore$ $A_m$ will be the direct branch of $A_{2^k - 2} + x$ where

$2^{k+1} - 2 + 2x = m$ or $m + 1$ according as $m$ is even or odd.

$$\Rightarrow 2^k + x = \frac{m}{2} + 1 \text{ or } \frac{m+1}{2} + 1$$

Now $n = 2^k - 2 + n$,

$$\Rightarrow n = \frac{m}{2} - 1 \text{ or } \frac{m+1}{2} - 1$$

Similarly $p$ can be expressed in terms of $n$ and

$$\therefore p = \frac{m-2}{4} \text{ or } \frac{m}{2} \text{ or } \frac{m+1}{4} \text{ or } \frac{m-1}{2}$$

**238.** Note that $G_5$ is the only one to be not given in pairs of statement II. $\therefore$ $G_5$ is the parent group with 8 elements. Also exactly one of each pairs of statement will be the group with one element.

From groups ($G_5$, $G_7$) and ($G_5$, $G_{14}$),
$G_7$ and $G_{14}$ will be the one having one element and consequently $G_{12}$ and $G_3$ will be the groups having more than one element. Now from the six remaining pairs, six different groups has to come. $\therefore$ $G_6$ and $G_{10}$ will be the groups having more than one element and consequently $G_1$, $G_8$, $G_{13}$, $G_9$ will have one element each. Now we are remained with only two groups ($G_2$, $G_{15}$) and ($G_4$, $G_{11}$).

**So the correct options for (a), (b) and (c) are (iv), (ii) and (i) respectively.**

**239. (a) The correct option is (iii). EXPLANATION:**

Note that the last number of $n$th group will be $A_k$ where

$$k = 1 + 2 + 3 \ldots + n = \frac{n(n+1)}{2}$$

For $n = 13$ and 14, $k = 78$ and 105 respectively.

$\therefore$ $A_{100}$ will be found in 14th group.

**(b) The correct option is (ii). EXPLANATION:**

Note that the last number of $n$th group will be $A_k$ where
$k = 1 + 3 + 5 + \ldots + (2n - 1) = n^2$

$\therefore$ $A_{1000}$ will lie in 32nd group.

**240. (a) The correct option is (ii). EXPLANATION:**

Note that $n$ elements are found in $n$th group and upto $n$ groups, the number of elements are

$$1 + 2 + 3 + \ldots + n = \frac{n(n+1)}{2}$$

For $n = 24$, this sum is 300.

$\because$ the elements of even numbered groups are placed in reverse order $\therefore$ the position of $A_{300}$ will be

$$\frac{23 \cdot 24}{2} + 1 = 277\text{th}$$

**(b) The correct option is (iii). EXPLANATION:**

Note that $n$th groups ends in

$A_{1+2+3+\ldots(n+1)+1}$, i.e. $A_{\frac{(n-1)n}{2}+1}$

and $(n+1)$th group starts in

$A_{1+2+3+\ldots(n+1)}$, i.e. $A_{\frac{(n+1)(n+2)}{2}}$

From given conditions of the problem,

$$\frac{(n-1)n}{2}+1 = m \text{ and}$$

$$\frac{(n+1)(n+2)}{2} = m + 200$$

$\Rightarrow 2n = 200 \quad \Rightarrow n = 100$

and $m = 99 \cdot 50 + 1 = (100 - 1) \cdot 50 + 1 = 4951$

**(c) The correct option is (ii). EXPLANATION:**

Note that there are $(2n - 1)$ elements in $n$th group and upto $n$th group, there are

$1 + 3 + \ldots + (2n - 1) = n^2$ elements

$\therefore$ 200 lies in 15th group and

( ___ $\underline{198}$ ___ $\underline{200}$ .................... $\underline{199}$ ___ $\underline{197}$ )

$\therefore$ the position of 200 will be (196 + 4)th, i.e. 200th.

**241.** ABCDA = 3

Note that if A is 0, then BCD cannot be equal to 3.

If A = 1, then there can be three cases satisfying ABCDA = 3, viz.

| | | | | |
|---|---|---|---|---|
| Case I: D = '–' | B = 3 | C = 0 | and | E = 2 |
| Case II: C = '–' | B = 3 | D = 2 | and | E = 1 |
| Case III: B = '–' | C = 2 | D = 3 | and | E = 0 |

Out of which only case III satisfies the another given condition, i.e. ACBEA = 4.

$\because$ there are no 'cannot be determined' in the options $\therefore$ there will be only one solution corresponding to case III. (Note that the cases pertaining to A = 2 or 3 may be ruled out if these are taken prior to the case where A = 1)

**So the correct options for (a), (b) and (c) are (iv), (iv) and (i) respectively.**

**242.** Note that if in toss number 4, D got H, then D would have either got no points or two points. ∴ it has to be T and the table will become as:

| Toss Number | A | B | C | D |
|---|---|---|---|---|
| 1 | T | T | H | H |
| 2 | | | | T |
| 3 | | | | H |
| 4 | H | T | T | T |
| 5 | T | T | H | T |
| 6 | T | H | T | T |

Note that in the above table, B would have got point in fifth toss only. Note that A, C can get a point in third or fourth toss.

**So the correct options for (a), (b) and (c) will be (iv), (iii) and (iv) respectively.**

**243.** The table can be drawn as below:

| Toss Number | A | B | C | D |
|---|---|---|---|---|
| 1 | H | | | |
| 2 | | T | | T |
| 3 | | | T | |
| 4 | | | H | H |
| 5 | T | T | | |
| | | 2H | 2H | 3H |

∵ total heads tossed up was 10. ∴ A tossed up 3 H.

Now first, second, third and fourth column will have only one T, T, H and T respectively.

In fourth toss, A and B could not have simultaneously tossed up T as there would be no 4T.

Regarding part (c), we have

| Toss Number | A | B | C | D |
|---|---|---|---|---|
| 1 | H | H | T | H |
| 2 | H | T | H | T |

| | | | | |
|---|---|---|---|---|
| 3 | T | T | T | H/T |
| 4 | H | H | H | H |
| 5 | T | T | T | T/H |

and regarding part (d), we have

| Toss Number | A | B | C | D |
|---|---|---|---|---|
| 1 | H | H/T | T | H |
| 2 | T | T | H | T |
| 3 | H | T/H | T | H |
| 4 | H | H | H | H |
| 5 | T | T | T | T |

**So the correct options for (a), (b), (c) and (d) are (iii), (iv), (ii) and (iv) respectively.**

**244.**

| | A | B | C | D | E | F | |
|---|---|---|---|---|---|---|---|
| Round 1: | 1 | 1 | –1 | –1 | 1 | –1 | → 2H, 4T |
| Round 2: | –1 | 1 | 1 | 1 | –1 | 1 | → 3H, 3T |
| Round 3: | 1 | –1 | 1 | –1 | 1 | –1 | → 4H, 2T |

From Round 1: Only one of A, B, E can be male
∴ (A, B, E) → 1M and (C, D, F) → 2M

From Round 2: Two to B, C, D, F will be male
∴ (B, C, D, F) → 2M and (A, E) → 1M

From Round 3: Only one of A, C, E can be female
∴ (A, C, E) → 2M and (B, D, F) → 1M

∵ (C, D, F) → 2M and (B, C, D, F) → 2M ∴ B is female

∵ (A, E) → 1M and (A, C, E) → 2M ∴ C is male

and consequentely (D, F) → 1M

Note that in rounds one, two and three, males tossed heads once, twice and twice respectively. ∴ the total number of times the males turned up heads was 5.

**So the correct options for (a), (b), (c) and (d) are (ii), (ii), (iv) and (ii) respectively.**

**245.** First we should start with F (as its distances from three other persons are given).

If we take D and B to be on the same side of F, then it can be shown that there is no feasible solution. Taking D and B on the opposite sides of F, we will get the distance between them as

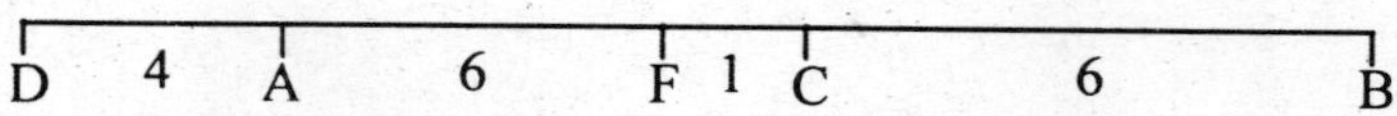


, the position of E can be either right to B or left to D. Now the extreme persons will move at least two steps or at most 4 steps towards each other. If $5n$ be the number of total steps between them initially, then it should be, after movement, $5n - (2, 3, 4)$.

Now if E is left to D, then the distance between extreme persons will be 19 and when added to (2, 3, 4) it must be divisible by 5 which is not the case. ∴ E is right to B and the distance between extreme persons is 22 which, when added to 3, gives 25, i.e. $n = 5$.

Now for the distance between C, F to be 5, they must have moved 2 steps each ∴ both are males and F is married to one of (B, E) while C is married to one of (A, D). Also B must have moved 1 step towards C while E must have moved one steps towards C. ∴ E and B are females. Similarly A must have moved 1 step toward F and D must have moved 2 steps towards F. ∴ A is female and D is male. ∴

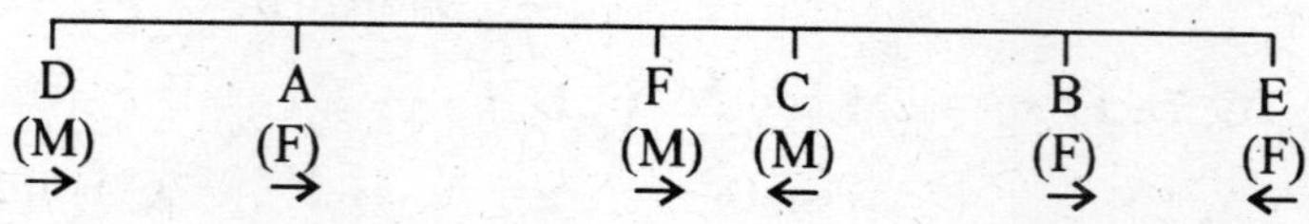


and the couples are (C, A) and (B, D), (F, E) or (B, F), (D, E).

**So, the correct options for (a), (b), (c), (d) and (e) are (ii), (ii), (iii), (i) and (i) respectively.**

**246.** Note that one each of (A, E), (C, D) and (B, F) is male and another female. Now the numbers thrown up by (A, E) can be 5, 3 or 2, 6;

(C, D) can be 4, 3 or 5, 2;

(B, F) can be 1, 5 or 4, 2

which together implies that

B, F → (1, 5) as 1 is not in any of the other groups;

A, E → 2, 6 and C, D → 3, 4

Now E, F are 3 steps away ∴ the number thrown up by them can be respectively 2, 1 or 2, 5 according as they are of opposite sex or same sex. Also the maximum distance between extreme ones can be 11 steps. ∴ the steps moved by A, F are (2, 5) or (6, 1). The number thrown by A cannot be 2 (as it has already been thrown by E) ∴ the numbers thrown by A, F, E, B will be 6, 1, 2 and 5 respectively and their respective positions will be

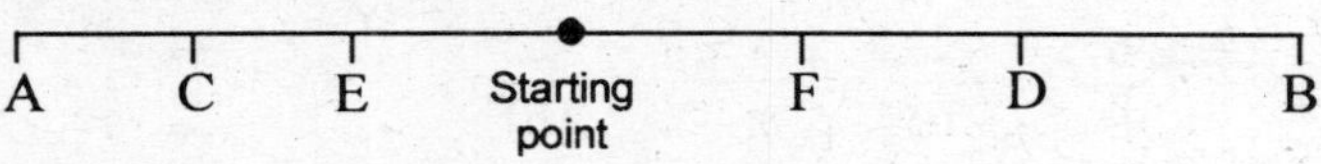


∵ E is west to D and E = 2, D = 3 or 4 ∴ D is in the east.

∵ F is east of E and E = 2, F = 1 ∴ F is in the east.

**So the correct options for (a), (b), (c), (d) and (e) will be (iv), (iv), (iv), (ii) and (iii) respectively.**

**247.** There can be two possible ways of arrangements of males and females:

(I)

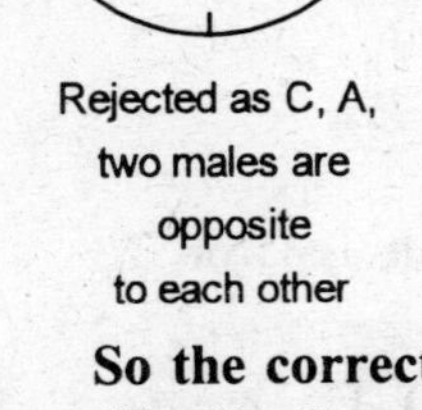


Rejected as C, A, two males are opposite to each other

(II)

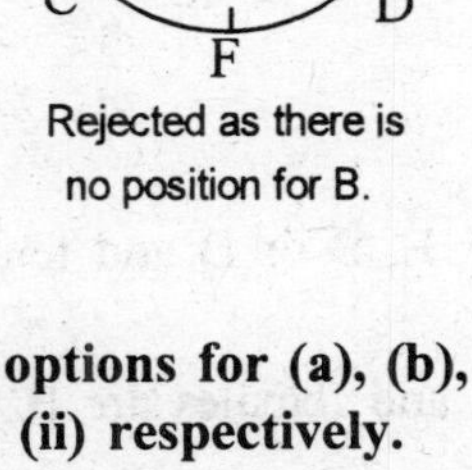


Rejected as there is no position for B.

(III)

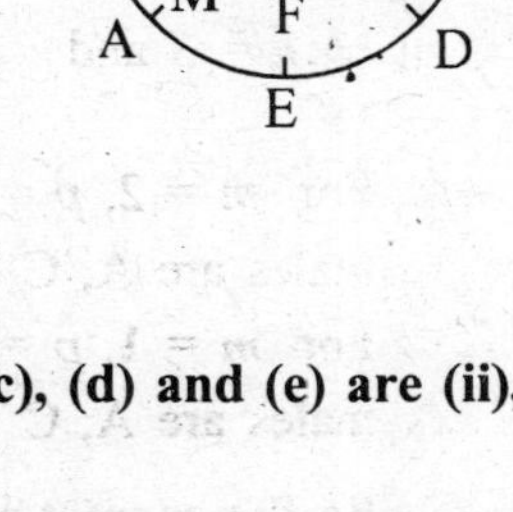


**So the correct options for (a), (b), (c), (d) and (e) are (ii), (ii), (i), (i) and (ii) respectively.**

**248.** Let a male and a female can do the work in M and F days respectively. Let there be *m*, *n* and *p* males in groups (A, B, D), (A, C, F) and (B, C, D, E) respectively. Then

$$\frac{m}{M}+\frac{3-m}{F}=\frac{1}{42};\ \frac{n}{M}+\frac{3-n}{F}=\frac{1}{35}\text{ and }\frac{p}{M}+\frac{4-p}{F}=\frac{1}{30}$$

$$\Rightarrow\ (m-n)\left(\frac{1}{M}-\frac{1}{F}\right)=\frac{1}{42}-\frac{1}{35}=-\frac{1}{210}$$

$$\Rightarrow\ \frac{1}{M}-\frac{1}{F}=-\frac{1}{210(m-n)}\qquad ...(i)$$

$$\text{Also }(m+n)\left(\frac{1}{M}-\frac{1}{F}\right)+\frac{6}{F}=\frac{1}{42}+\frac{1}{35}=\frac{11}{210}$$

$$\Rightarrow\ \frac{6}{F}=\frac{11}{210}+\left(\frac{m+n}{m-n}\right)\cdot\frac{1}{210}$$

$$\therefore\ p\left(\frac{1}{M}-\frac{1}{F}\right)+\frac{4}{F}=\frac{1}{30}$$

$$\Rightarrow\ -\frac{p}{210(m-n)}+\frac{4}{6}\left(\frac{11}{210}+\frac{m+n}{m-n}\cdot\frac{1}{210}\right)=\frac{1}{30}$$

$$\Rightarrow\ p+\frac{2}{3}\,[11(n-m)-(m+n)]=7(n-m)$$

$$\Rightarrow\ 3p+2(10n-12m)=21(n-m)$$

$$\Rightarrow\ 3p=n+3m$$

$\because$ $1/M > 1/F$ $\therefore$ $m > n$ [using (i)]

$$\Rightarrow\ 3(p-m)=n$$

$\Rightarrow n = 3$ and $m = 2, p = 3$ or

$m = 1, p = 2$

For $m = 2, p = 3$,

males are A, C, F, E, B or D and female is D or B.

For $m = 1, p = 2$,

males are A, C, F and females are B, D, E.

**So the correct options for (a), (b), (c) and (d) are (iii), (iv), (i) and (ii) respectively.**

**249.** Let there be $m$ males and $(7 - m)$ females.

Two heads: if only males gets it, then

$2 + (7 - m) = 3 \Rightarrow m = 6$

: if only females get it, then

$7 - m - 2 = 3 \Rightarrow m = 1$

: if one male , one female gets it, then

$1 + 7 - m - 1 = 3 \Rightarrow m = 4.$

First two cases are rejected and only third case is valid. Now

(A, C, E) $\rightarrow$ Two heads $\rightarrow$ 1M, ( 3 – 1) F $\equiv$ 1M, 2F

(C, D, F, G) $\rightarrow$ Three heads $\rightarrow$ $x$M, $(3 - y)$ F $\rightarrow x + y = 3$,

$x + 3 - y = 4$

$\therefore x = 2$ and $y = 2$

(A, B, G) $\rightarrow$ Four heads $\rightarrow$ $x$M, $(3 - y)$ F $\rightarrow x + y = 4$,

$x + 3 - y = 3$

$\therefore x = 2$ and $y = 2$

(B, D, E, F) $\rightarrow$ Five heads $\rightarrow$ $x$M, $(3 - y)$ F $\rightarrow x + y = 5$,

$x + 3 - y = 4$

$\therefore x = 3$ and $y = 2$

For (A, C, E) $\rightarrow$ M, 2F there will be three cases:

Case I: A $\rightarrow$ male, (C, E) $\rightarrow$ females. On examination of fourth group, B, D, F $\rightarrow$ males. On examination of third group, 4 persons are female. Also second group is verified.

Case II: C $\rightarrow$ male (A, E) $\rightarrow$ females. From fourth group, B, D, F $\rightarrow$ males. From third group, G $\rightarrow$ male. This case is rejected as second group has two females.

Case III: E $\rightarrow$ male, (A, C) $\rightarrow$ females. On examination of third group, B,G $\rightarrow$ males and on examination of other two groups, one of D, F $\rightarrow$ male and another female.

$\therefore$ we will have finally two valid cases:

| | Males | Females |
|---|---|---|
| Case I: | (A, B, D, F) | (C, E, G) |
| Case III: | (B, G, E, F/D) | (A, C, D/F) |

**So the correct options for (a), (b), (c), (d), (e) and (f) are (iii), (ii), (i), (ii), (ii) and (iii) respectively.**

**250.** In first toss, there are (4H, 2T) or (4T, 2H).

Also C → (2H, 2T) , D → (2H, 2T), E → (3H, T)
F → (3T, H) , A → (3H, T) or (3T, H) and
B → (3H, T) or (3T, H)

After second toss, $G_2$ have only one person, i.e. either 4 of the persons in $G_2$ changed their sides or all 5 changed their groups and one in $G_1$ also changed their sides but it requires 6T which is not possible. ∴ only 4 of the persons changed their groups and subsequently in IInd toss A → T, D → T and in first toss, we have, A → T, D → H.

∴ we have

| Toss | A | B | C | D | E | F |
|---|---|---|---|---|---|---|
| First | T | | | H | | |
| Second | T | T | H | T | H | T |
| Third | H | | T | T | | T |
| Fourth | H | H | | H | H | |

Note that there will be two cases either C is in $G_2$ or E is in $G_2$ after second toss.

Case I: C is in $G_2$ ∴ E was in $G_1$ and others were in $G_2$ before second toss. We have

after first toss: $G_1$ → E and $G_2$ → A, B, C, D, F;
after second toss: $G_1$ → A, B, D, E, F and $G_2$ → C
after third toss: $G_1$ → A, C and $G_2$ → D, F, B, E;
after fourth toss: $G_2$ must have A, D, E, B but after fourth toss, each group will have three persons only (∵ C, D exchanged their original groups while other remained in their original groups) ∴ this case is rejected.

Case II: E is in $G_2$ ∴ C was in $G_1$ and other were in $G_2$ before second toss. We have

after first toss: $G_1$→ C and $G_2$ → A, B, E, D, F;
after second toss: $G_1$ → A, B, D, C, F and $G_2$ → E;
after third toss: $G_1$→ A, (B or E) and $G_2$ → C, D, F, (E or B);
after fourth toss: $G_1$→ C, (B or E), F and $G_2$ → A, D, (E or B).

**So the correct options for (a), (b), (c), (d), (e) and (f) are (i), (iv), (ii), (iii), (ii) and (i) respectively.**

**251.** Given that

| Toss | | | | $G_1$ | | | |
|---|---|---|---|---|---|---|---|
| 3 | → | K | B | L | D | H | E |
| 4 | → | G | A | I | C | B | D |
| 6 | → | G | A | B | D | H | E |

Note that in $G_1$ corresponding to 4 and 6, two letters are uncommon. ∴ between the tosses which threw up 4 and 6, there is one more toss. Similarly between 3 and 6, there is one more toss. Between 4 and 6, (I, C) and (H, E) are exchanged. ∴ 5 is between them (as I is exchanged when 5 is tossed up). Between 3 and 6, (K, L) and (G, A) are exchanged ∴ 1 is between them (as K is exchanged when 1 is tossed up) Now we have five consecutive toss as

31654 or 45613

Also ∵ I → 5 ∴ C → 4 or 6 according as which followed and ∵ K → 1 ∴ L → 3 or 6 according as which followed.

**So the correct options for (a), (b), (c) and (d) are (iv), (iii), (i) and (iv) respectively.**

**252.** Note that (G, H, I), i.e. (architect, professor, engineer) will have one person in each of the groups. Consequently (doctor, accountant, actor) will have one person in each of the groups.

∵ doctor, actor are in $G_1$, $G_2$ respectively

∴ accountant will be in $G_3$. ∵ lawyer is in $G_1$

∴ B, i.e. chemist can be in $G_2$ only. And we can have

| (A | B | C) | (D | E | F) |
|---|---|---|---|---|---|
| ↓ | ↓ | ↓ | ↓ | ↓ | ↓ |
| $G_3$ | $G_2$ | $G_1$ | $G_3$ | $G_1$ | $G_2$ |
| (Art) | (Chem) | (Law / Doc) | (Acc) | (Doc / Law) | (Act) |

| (G | H | I) |
|---|---|---|
| ↓ | ↓ | ↓ |
| $G_2$ | $G_1$ | $G_3$ |

**So the correct options for (a), (b) and (c) are (iii), (iv) and (iii) respectively.**

**253.** The different cases can be
(A, G) or A
(B, F), (B, H) or B [The pairs denote couples]
(C, I) or C
(D, F), (D, G) or D
(E, I), (E, F) or E
Note that ∵ only one of them is a bachelor ∴ (B, H) has to be a couple. The only exclusive combination will be (A, G), (B, H), (D, F), (C, I) + E

**So the correct options for (a), (b) and (c) are (iii), (ii) and (i) respectively.**

**254.** There can be four different cases:

| | | | |
|---|---|---|---|
| Case I: | B → Female | ; | E, I, D → Males |
| | A → Female | | C, H → Males |
| | F, G → Females | | |
| Case II: | E → Female | ; | B, I, D → Males |
| | A C → Females | ; | G, F → Males |
| | H → Female | | |
| Case III: | I → Female | ; | B, E, D → Males |
| | A, C → Females | ; | H → Male |
| | F, G → Females | | |
| Case IV: | D → Female | ; | B, E, I → Males |

one of A, C → Male
one of F, G, H → Male } which imply
one of C, H → Male

Males → C,(F or G)
Females → H, A, (G or F) } or Males → H, A
Females → C, F, G

**So the correct options for (a), (b), (c) and (d) are (i), (ii), (i) and (ii) respectively.**

**255.** ∵ A, B, C, F have no couples ∴ let the couples be (A, ) ; (B, ) ; (C, ) and (F, ). We have
D, F, G, H → no couple (∵ A, B, C, F have no couple)
H, E, G, C → one couple (Given)
B, D, G, E → one couple (Given)

Compounded with fourth possibility, i.e. A, H, D, F (and corollarily B, E, C, G) have no couple, we have

H, E, G, C → C, H is a couple

B, D, G, E → B, D is a couple

and the other couples can be (A, E), (F, G) or (A, G), (F, E).

Regarding part (c), if A is a male, then one of (E, G) will be female and another male as (C, H, E, G) has two males and two females and further (C, H) is a couple.

**So the correct options for (a), (b), (c) and (d) are (ii), (i), (ii) and (iii) respectively.**

**256.** We have,

(B, C, G, H)→ one couple

(A, D, E, H)→ one couple

(C, E, F, G) → one couple

(B, D, E, G)→ one couple

(A, F, G, H) → no couple

For first group, we can have three cases:

Case I: Let B, C be of same sex, say male, Then G, H will be female. From last group, A, F will be male and from third group, E will be female and from second group, D will be male.

∵ from last group, A, F are not married to G, H

∴ we can have following sub cases:

I. (A, E) ; (C, G) are couples → Not possible

II. (F, E) ; (D, H) and (B, G) are couples.

III. (D, E) ; (C, G) are couples.

IV. (D, H) ; (C, E) and (B, G) are couples.

V. (D, H) ; (C, G) and (B, E) are couples.

Case II: Let B, G be of the same sex, say male. Then (C, H) will be female. From fourth group, (D, E) will be female. But D, E, H cannot be female in second group. ∴ this case is rejected.

Case III: Let B, H be of same sex, say male. Then C, G will be female. From third group, E, F will be male and from second group A, D will be female. ∴ the numbers of males and females are equal ∴ this case will also be rejected.

**So the correct options for (a), (b), (c) and (d) are (i), (i), (i) and (ii) respectively.**

**257.** Note that (A, F), (C, G), (B, D) and (I, L) cannot be couples. There can be four cases:

Case I: (A, G) and (B, H) are couples. Then (C, F) and (D, J) cannot be couples. But two of (C, F, D, J) must be couples (because in the group of any four persons who do not want to be together, there has to be one couple). Looking at other committees which are not possible, only (C, J) is one of the possible couple and others are (F, K) and (E, L), (D, I) or

(E, I), (D, L). ∴ the couples are

(A, G); (B, H); (C, J); (F, K) ; $\begin{cases}\text{(D, I) and (E, L)}\\ \text{(D, L) and (E, I)}\end{cases}$

Case II: (A, G) and (B, J) are couples. As done for case I, the couples will be

(A, G); (B, J); (F, H); (C, E); $\begin{cases}\text{(D, I) and (K, L)}\\ \text{(D, L) and (K, I)}\end{cases}$

Case III: (A, C) ; (B, H); (G, J); (F, K); $\begin{cases}\text{(D, I) and (E, L)}\\ \text{(D, L) and (E, I)}\end{cases}$

Case IV: (A, C); (B, J); (F, H); (G, E); $\begin{cases}\text{(D, I) and (K, L)}\\ \text{(D, L) and (K, I)}\end{cases}$

**So the correct options for (a), (b), (c), (d) and (e) are (iv), (i), (iv), (i) and (iv) respectively.**

**258.** Let H, T denote the head and tail of a coin. Then sum of (4T, H) = –5 ⇒ sum of (4H, T) = 5
Also sum of (4H, T) = 7

$$\therefore \text{ sum of three of } (a, b, c, d, e) = \frac{7+5}{2} = 6 = 1 + 2 + 3$$

[Had the sum been $a + b + c + d - e$ and $a + b + c - d + e$, then sum of both of them would have been $2(a + b + c)$]

$$\therefore a = 1, b = 2, c = 3 \text{ and } e - d = \frac{7-5}{2} = 1$$

Now sum of (3H, 2T) = $-3$

This is not possible if the coins of values $d$ and $e$ turn up opposite faces.

$\therefore\ 1 + 2 + 3 - (d + d + 1) = -3$

$\Rightarrow 9 = 2d + 1 \Rightarrow d = 4$ and subsequently $e = 5$.

Now (2H, 3T) = $-1$ which can be possible in two different ways: $-1 - 2 + 3 + 4 - 5 = -1$ or

$-1 + 2 - 3 - 4 + 5 = -1$.

**So the correct options for (a), (b), (c) and (d) are (ii), (iv), (i) and (i) respectively.**

**259.** A → (3, 4)
B → (2, 6)
C → (3, 6)
D → (1, 5)
E → (2, 4)

Note that in A, D and E, 6 can be against 1, 4 and 5.

$\therefore$ 6 has to be against 4 in D and subsequently

D → (1, 5), (4, 6), (2, 3)

Case I: Let 6 be against 1 in A. Then we will have
A → (3, 4), (1, 6), (2, 5)
B → (2, 6), (3, 5), (1, 4)
C → (3, 6), (2, 1), (4, 5)
D → (1, 5), (4, 6), (2, 3)
E → (2, 4), (5, 6), (1, 3)

Case II: Let 6 be against 1 in E. Then we will have
A → (3, 4), (5, 6), (1, 2)
B → (2, 6), (4, 5), (1, 3)
C → (3, 6), (2, 5), (1, 4)
D → (1, 5), (4, 6), (2, 3)
E → (2, 4), (1, 6), (3, 5)

**So the correct options for (a), (b) and (c) are (iv), (i) and (i) respectively.**

**260. A.** For 4 and 6 (sum of numbers shown up and that of hidden numbers), the cases for two dices are

$$\begin{Bmatrix} (1,2) & ; & (1,4) & \text{or} & (2,3) \\ (3,4) & & (3,2) & & (2,3) \end{Bmatrix}$$

where (...) denotes the numbers on two opposite faces of a dice. Also any dice may have upper or lower values. For 9 and 9, the cases are

$$\begin{Bmatrix} (5,4) & ; & (6,3) & ; & (5,3) & \text{or} & (5,6) \\ (4,5) & & (3,6) & & (4,6) & & (4,3) \end{Bmatrix}$$

For 8 and 5, the cases are

$$\begin{Bmatrix} (4,2) & ; & (4,3) & ; & (5,4) & ; & (5,1) & ; & (5,3) & ; & (6,1) & ; & (6,4) & \text{or} & (6,2) \\ (4,3) & & (4,2) & & (3,1) & & (3,4) & & (3,2) & & (2,4) & & (2,1) & & (2,3) \end{Bmatrix}$$

So the possible cases may be

I: (1, 2) ; (4, 3)
(3, 4) ; (5, 6) → Not possible

II: (1, 4) ; (5, 3) ; (6, 2)
(3, 2) ; (4, 6) ; (5, 1) → Possible

[Note that (6, 2) and (2, 3) correspond to the third toss]

III: (2, 3) ; (5, 4)
(2, 3) ; (4, 5) → Not possible

**So the correct options for (a), (b), (c) and (d) are (iii), (ii), (iii) and (iv) respectively.**

**B.** There can be three cases relating to the sum of hidden numbers when the sum of numbers shown up is 4.

Case I: The implied numbers are 4, 8. Then the (number shown up, hidden number) for two dices can be
(2, 4) and (2, 4) → Not possible [as other sums
or (1, 6) and (3, 2) → Not possible cannot be
or (1, 2) and (3, 6) → Not possible accounted for]

Case II: The implied numbers are (4, 9). Then the (number shown up, hidden number) for two dices can be
(1, 5) and (3, 4) → Possible
or (1, 4) and (3, 5) → Not possible

Case III: The implied numbers are (4, 10). Then the (number shown up, hidden number) for two dices can be
(2, 5) and (2, 5) → Possible, other pairs of number on opposite faces can be (1, 6) and (3, 4)

or (1, 6) and (3, 4) → Possible
or (1, 4) and (3, 6) → Not Possible

**So the correct options for (a), (b), (c) and (d) are (i), (iv), (i) and (iv) respectively.**

**261. (a) The correct option is (ii). EXPLANATION:**

Numbers showed up : 1, 2, 3, 4, 4, 5, 6, 6
Number recorded : 1, 2, 2, 3, 4, 5, 5, 6

Note that there are two extra numbers showed up (4, 6) and recorded (2, 5) which do not match. But since tails turned up four times ∴ let the corresponding numbers
showed up be : A, B, 4, 6 and
recorded be : A, B, 2, 5.

Now if 4 (or 6) is against A, then A is also against 4 (or 6) which is only possible if B is also 4 (or 6) and which, in turn, can be possible only if A is equal to one of 2, 5. ∴ 1 will be against 3 as they are exclusive to above pair of four numbers.

If (4, 6) is against (2, 5) , then only possibility is that 1 will be against 3.

∴ in any case, 1 will be against 3.

**(b) The correct option is (iii). EXPLANATION:**

Number showed up : 1, 1, 2, 2, 3, 4, 5, 6
Number recorded : 1, 2, 4, 4, 5, 5, 6, 6

∵ tails showed up seven times, they can be rearranged as:

$$\begin{matrix} \text{Numbers showed up}: \\ \text{Numbers recorded}\ : \end{matrix} \begin{pmatrix} 1, 2, 4, 6 \\ 1, 2, 4, 6 \end{pmatrix} \begin{pmatrix} 1, 2, 3 \\ 5, 4, 6 \end{pmatrix}$$

[Note that 5 turned up when head turned up]

The second bracket has 3, 5 which are not found in first bracket. ∴ 3 and 5 will be against each other.

**262.** Note that when the dice showed up 4 once, it will keep showing it up successively and when the dice showed up 2, it will show up the number opposite to 2 next time.

So there will be six cases cases:

| | Initially | H | T | H | T |
|---|---|---|---|---|---|
| I | 1 | 2 | 3 | 5 | 4 |
| II | 1 | 2 | 5 | 3 | 4 |
| III | 1 | 3 | 2 | 5 | 4 |
| IV | 1 | 3 | 5 | 2 | 4 |
| V | 1 | 5 | 2 | 3 | 4 |
| VI | 1 | 5 | 3 | 2 | 4 |

For cases I and II:

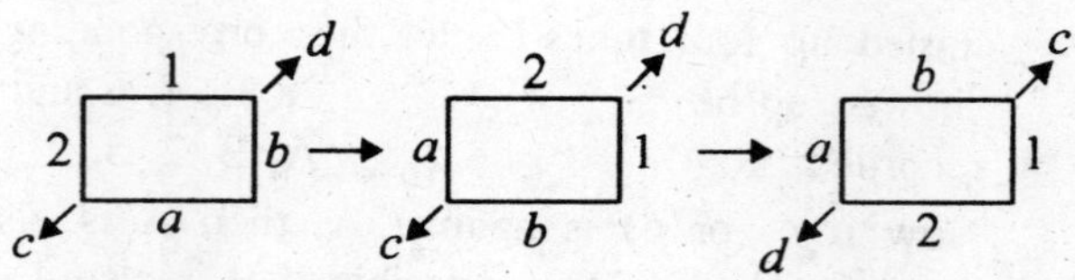

Now b cannot be equal to 3 as as it will bring 1 up in next toss. ∴ $b = 5$ and in next toss it will show up $a$, i.e. 3 and then it will show up $c$, i.e. 4. ∵ there are no 'cannot be determined' in the options ∴ other cases will be rejected. However for those who start solving problem with these cases, explanations are given below:

For cases III and IV:

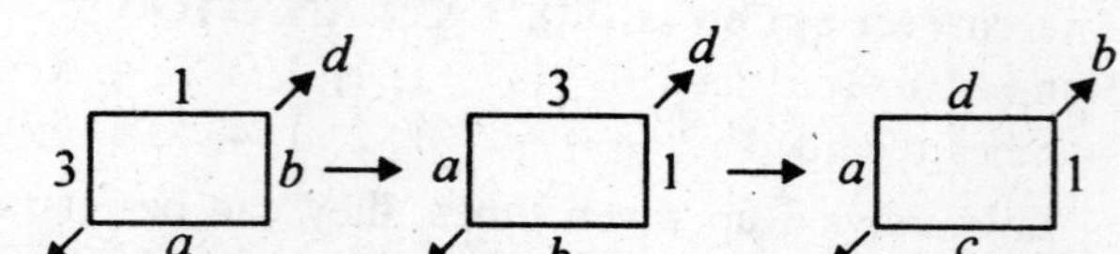

For case III, $d = 2$ and dice after third toss will be

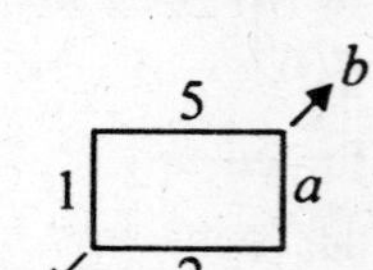

∵ the next toss will bring up 3
∴ this case is rejected.

For case IV, $d = 5$ and dice after third toss will be

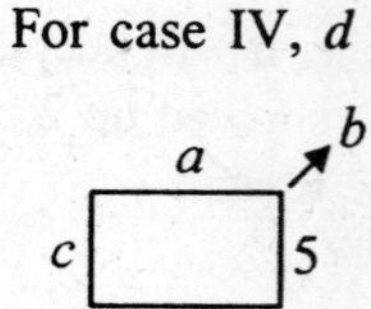

where $a = 2$. ∵ the next toss will bring up 1
∴ this case is also rejected.

For cases V and VI:

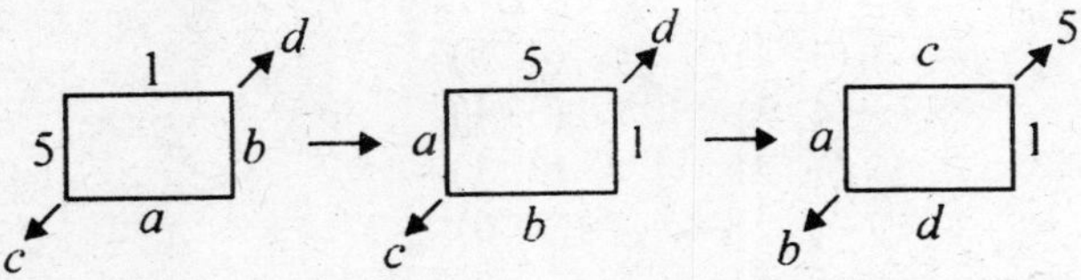


For case V, $c = 2$ and dice after third toss will be

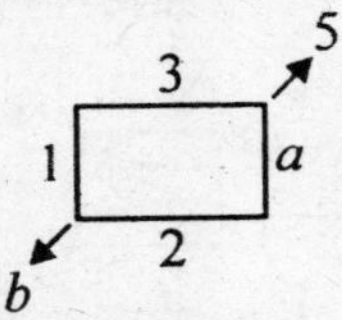


∵ the next toss will bring up 5.
∴ this case is rejected.

For case VI, $c = 3$ and dice after third toss will be

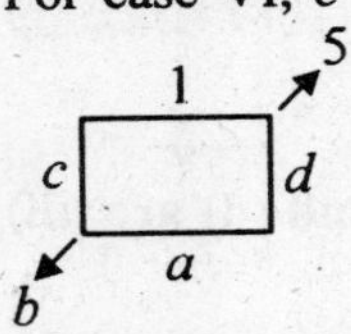


∵ 1 cannot be on top
∴ this case is also rejected.

**So the correct options for (a), (b) and (c) are (ii), (iii) and (i) respectively.**

**263.** Let the opposite set of numbers for A, B, be given as

| A | hidden number | B |
|---|---|---|
| 3 | $w$ | 5 |
| 1 | $x$ | 6 |
| 2 | $y$ | 3 |
| 4 | $z$ | 1 |

Now $w$ = 1, 2, 4 or 6

Case I: $w = 1$

| A | B |
|---|---|
| (3,1) | (1, 5) |
| (1, 3) | (3, 6) |
| (2, 6) | (3, 6) |
| (4, 5) | (2, 4) → {(1, 5) and (3, 6) are already there} |

Now $w$ = 1, 2, 4 or 6

Case II: $w = 2$ But $y$ cannot be equal to 3.
∴ this case is rejected.

Case III: $w = 4$

| A | B |
|---|---|
| (3, 4) | (4, 5) |
| (4, 3) | (3, 1) |
| (1, 2) | (3, 1) |
| (1, 2) | (2, 6) |
| (5, 6) | |

[as (1, 2), (3, 4) are already there]

Case IV: $w = 6$

| A | B |
|---|---|
| (3, 6) | (6, 5) |
| (1, 5) | (5, 6) |
| (2, 4) | (4, 3) and (1, 2) |

[as (1, 5), (3, 6) are already there]

**So the correct options for (a), (b), (c) and (d) are (iii), (iv), (i) and (iii) respectively**

**264.** The positions after second and fourth tosses are (4, 3) and (10, 8). Note that $10 - 4 = 6$ and $8 - 3 = 5$, i.e. in third and fourth toses, 5 and 6 are thrown up. Now let the initial position and position after sixth toss be $(4 - a, 3 - b)$ and $(10 + x, 8 + y)$ where $a$, $b$ denote the numbers thrown up in first and second tosses while $x$, $y$ denote the numbers thrown up in fifth and sixth tosses.

$\because$ $(4 - a, 3 - b)$, $(4, 3)$ are $(10 + x, 8 + y)$ are in a line

$$\therefore \quad \frac{4-(4-a)}{3-(3-b)} = \frac{4-(10+x)}{3-(8+y)} \Rightarrow \frac{a}{b} = \frac{x+6}{y+5}$$

$\Rightarrow \quad a\,(5 + y) = b\,(6 + x)$

Now $a, b, x, y$ are 1, 2, 3, 4

$\therefore$ on inspection,

$a = 4, y = 1, b = 3$ and $x = 2$.

So the initial position is (0, 0) while the position after sixth toss is (12, 9).

The object moved in $x$ direction for numbeis 4, 6 and 2.

The distance between the initial and final position is

$$\sqrt{(12-0)^2+(9-0)^2} = 3\sqrt{4^2+3^2} = 15 \text{ unit}$$

**So the correct options for (a), (b) and (c) are (ii), (ii) and (iv) respectively.**

**265. A.** Let (A, B), (C, D), (E, F) be three pairs of opposite faces which sums are respectively 36, 40 and 41.

Now $33 + 43 = 76 = 36 + 40 = A + B + C + D$ and
$39 + 38 = 77 = 36 + 41 = A + B + E + F$

Let $A + C = 33$. Then
$B + D = 43$ and
$B = 36 - A, C = 33 - A, D = 7 + A,$

$$\begin{cases} E = 39 - A, & F = 2 + A \text{ or} \\ E = 3 + A, & F = 38 - A \end{cases}$$

**(a) The correct option is (i). EXPLANATION:**

Note that if the difference of two numbers is odd, then their sum also must be odd.

$\therefore \quad |E - F| = 5$ and $E + F = 41$

$\Rightarrow \quad E, F = 18, 23$ and

A can be equal to $\underbrace{16, 21}_{F = 2 + A}$, $\underbrace{15, 20}_{E = 3 + A}$ and

correspondingly B = 20, 15 , 21, 16 .

$\because$ the difference of one of pairs on the opposite faces is 14, and as it cannot be $|A - B|$ $\therefore$ it has to be $|C - D|$

$\therefore |C - D| = 2\ |13 - A| = 14$ which is only possible when $A = 20$ and correspondingly C = 13, D = 17.

$\therefore$ the least number inscribed on the dice will be 13.

**(b) The correct option is (iv). EXPLANTION:**

The obvious possible differences are
$D - A = 7$ and $B - C = 3$.
Now if we take $E = 39 - A$ and $F = 2 + A$, then
$E - B = 3, E - C = 6, F - A = 2$ and $D - F = 5$
If we take $E = 3 + A$ and $F = 38 - A$, then

E – A = 3, D – E = 4, F – B = 2 and F – C = 5

The common differences of the two cases are 2 and 5.

∴ the differences can be 2, 3 5 or 7.

(c) **The correct option is (i). EXPLANATION:**

As explained in part (b).

(d) **The correct option is (iv). EXPLANATION:**

Let E = 39 – A and F = 2 + *A*.

Then C + F = 37 and E + D = 46.

For the other case, the sum 37 is not possible.

∴ when one of the sum is 37, then one of the other sum must be 46.

**B.** Let $(a, 11 - a)$, $(b, 12 - b)$ and $(c, 13 - c)$ be the numbers on their opposite faces. Also let $a$, $b$, $c$ be the number that turned up. Now

$a + 11 - a + b + 12 - b = 23 = 10 + 13$

$\therefore \quad a + b = 10$

$a + 11 - a + c + 13 - c = 24 = 15 + 9$

$\therefore \quad a + c = 15$

Similarly $b + c = 11$

$$\therefore \quad a + b + c = \frac{10+15+11}{2} = 18$$

and $a = 7$, $b = 3$, $c = 8$

$11 - a = 4$, $12 - b = 9$, $13 - c = 5$

**So the correct options for (a) and (b) are (iii) and (i) respectively.**

**266.** (a) **The correct option is (iv). EXPLANATION:**

There can be two possible cases:

$X_6$ did not play ⇒ $Y_6$ played

⇒ $Y_5$ played and lost or $X_5$ played and won

| ⇓ | ⇓ |
|---|---|
| $Y_4$ played and lost or one of $(Y_1, Y_2, Y_3)$ played with $X_4$ and lost. | $X_4$ played and lost or one of $(X_1, X_2, X_3)$ played with $Y_4$ and lost |

**(b) The correct option is (ii). EXPLANATION:**

Note that both $X_1$, $Y_1$ played at least one game and exactly one of $(X_i, Y_i)$, i = 2, 3, ...8, played game.

$\because$ five of first group played game

$\therefore$ 1 + (7 – 4), i.e. 4 of second group played game.

**(c) The correct option is (iii). EXPLANATION:**

We have

| | | ✓ | | ✗ | | ✓ | |
|---|---|---|---|---|---|---|---|
| $X_1$ | $X_2$ | $X_3$ | $X_4$ | $X_5$ | $X_6$ | $X_7$ | $X_8$ |
| $Y_1$ | $Y_2$ | $Y_3$ | $Y_4$ | $Y_5$ | $Y_6$ | $Y_7$ | $Y_8$ |

Either $X_3$ won $\Rightarrow$ $X_3$, $Y_4$ played $\Rightarrow$ $X_3$ won

$\Rightarrow$ $X_3$, $Y_5$ played

$\Rightarrow$ → $X_3$ won $\Rightarrow$ $X_3$, $Y_6$ played $\Rightarrow$ $Y_6$ won

→ $X_3$ lost $\Rightarrow$ $Y_5$, $X_6$ played $\Rightarrow$ $Y_5$ won

or $X_3$ lost $\Rightarrow$ $X_4$ won $\Rightarrow$ $X_4$, $Y_5$ played

$\Rightarrow$ → $X_4$ won $\Rightarrow$ $X_4$, $Y_6$ played $\Rightarrow$ $Y_6$ won

→ $Y_5$ won $\Rightarrow$ $Y_5$, $X_6$ played $\Rightarrow$ $Y_5$ won

**267.** Note that we need to arrange A, B, C, D, E, F and G in circular sequence, denoting them by $P_1$, $P_2$, ...$P_7$ for the sake of clarity, as:

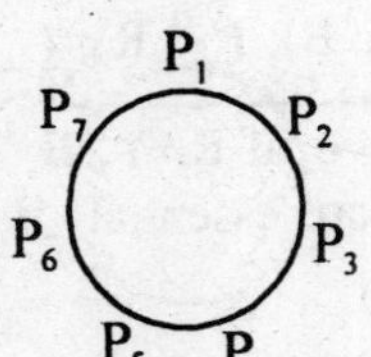


or

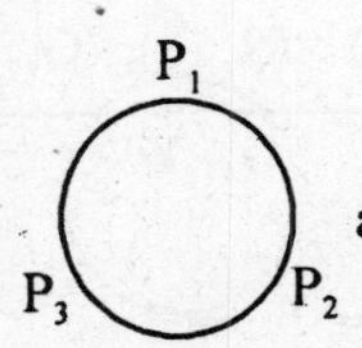


and

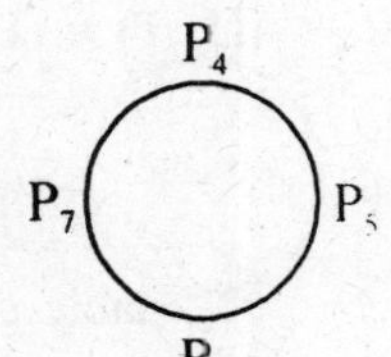


where each person can go out with the persons adjacent to him. Now we can have, from given conditions, following arrangements:

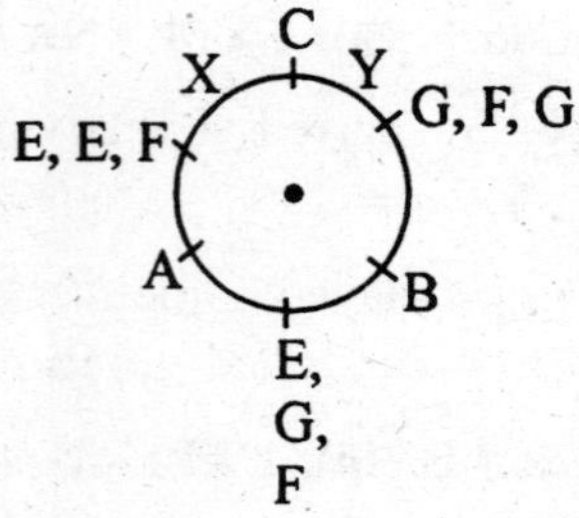


[D can be at X or Y]

or

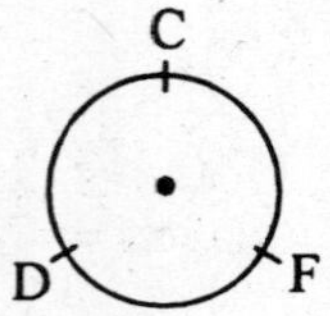


and

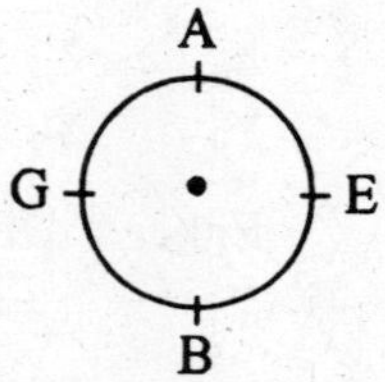


∴ we will have total of 7 cases.

Also A and B cannot go out with D.

**So the correct options for (a), (b) and (c) are (ii), (i) and (i) respectively.**

**268.** Note that one colour is painted on three coins. Using first toss, we can write Head (H), Tail (T) as:

(H, T) ≡ (B, _ ) ; (R, _ ); (G, _ ); ( _, B); ( _, R); ( _, Y)

Using second toss, we have

(H, T) ≡ (B, _ ) ; (R, _ ); (G, _ ); ( _, B); ( _, R); ( _, Y)

G, Y — Two of R, Y, B are essential

∴ a table can be formed as:

| | | | | | |
|---|---|---|---|---|---|
| B, G | R, Y | G, R | Y, B | B, R | G, Y |
| B, Y | R, G | G, B | R, B | Y, R | G, Y |
| B, G | R, G | G, Y | (R, Y), B | (Y, B), R | (B, R) Y |
| B, G | R, G | G, Y | (R, Y), B | (Y, B), R | (B, R) Y |

**So the correct option for (a), (b), (c) and (d) are (iii), (ii), (iii) and (ii) respectively.**

**B.** There can be four different cases:

| | | | | | | | | |
|---|---|---|---|---|---|---|---|---|
| | H | $\longrightarrow$ | B | B | R | R | G | Y |
| I | T | $\longrightarrow$ | G | Y | B | G | Y | R |
| II | T | $\longrightarrow$ | G | Y | B | Y | R | G |
| III | T | $\longrightarrow$ | G | R | Y | G | Y | B |
| IV | T | $\longrightarrow$ | Y | R | Y | G | B | G |

**So the correct options for (a) and (b) are (i) and (iv) respectively.**

**269.** Note that each colour is used in colouring three different coins. Now the sum of values of coins coloured with blue =

$2 \times (1 + 2 + 3 + 4 + 5 + 6) - (11 + 12 + 13)$
$= 42 - 36 = 6.$

$\because$ $6 = 1 + 2 + 3$ is the only possibility

$\therefore$ the coins of values 1, 2, and 3 are coloured with blue.

Now, Red $\equiv$ 13 = one of (1, 2, 3) + two of (4, 5, 6)

Possibilities : (3, 4, 6) or (2, 5, 6)

Green $\equiv$ 12 = one of (1, 2, 3) + two of (4, 5, 6)

Possibilities : (1, 5, 6) or (2, 4, 6) or (3, 4, 5)

Yellow $\equiv$ 11 = one of (1, 2, 3) + two of (4, 5, 6)

Possibilities : (1, 4, 6) or (2, 4, 5)

So we can have two cases :

Red; Green; Yellow $\equiv$ (3, 4, 6) ; (1, 5, 6) ; (2, 4, 5) or
(2, 5, 6) ; (3, 4, 5) ; (1, 4, 6)

**So the correct options for (a), (b) and (c) are (i), (ii) and (iv) respectively.**

**270.** Note that

$8 = 1 + 2 + 5$ or $1 + 3 + 4$

$9 = 1 + 2 + 6$ or $1 + 3 + 5$ or $2 + 3 + 4$

$10 = 1 + 3 + 6$ or $1 + 4 + 5$ or $2 + 3 + 5$

Now the numbers can be grouped into three groups, each group having numbers of opposite faces and above sums are sum of three numbers, one from each group. The various groups that can be formed so as to get the sum of 8, 9, 10 as shown above can be done in following ways :

For 8 = 1 + 2 + 5, the groups can be

(1, –) ; (2, –) and (5, – )

Checking for 9 and then subsequently for 10, the groups can be

| | | | | | |
|---|---|---|---|---|---|
| (1, 3) | ; | (2, 4) | ; | (5, 6) | or |
| (1, 4) | ; | (2, 3) | ; | (5, 6) | or |
| (1, 4) | ; | (2, 6) | ; | (5, 3) | or |
| (1, 3) | ; | (2, 6) | ; | (5, 4) | |

Similarly for 8 = 1 + 3 + 4, the various groups can be

| | | | | | |
|---|---|---|---|---|---|
| (1, 5) | ; | (3, 2) | ; | (4, 6) | or |
| (1, 5) | ; | (3, 6) | ; | (4, 2) | or |
| (1, 2) | ; | (3, 6) | ; | (4, 5) | or |
| (1, 2) | ; | (3, 5) | ; | (4, 6) | |

Note that such sums as 8, 9, 10 can be 21 – (8, 9, 10), i.e. 13, 12, 11. Also such sums can be 6 [when the groups are (1, 4) (2, 6) (5, 3)] or 7 [when the groups are (1, 3), (2, 6), (5, 4)]

**So the correct options for (a), (b), (c) and (d) are (iv), (iii), (ii) and (iv) respectively.**

**271.** Let R, B, G, Y, $B_K$ and W denote red, blue, green, yellow, black and white respectively. Then (2, Y), (3, W) and (5, R) will be opposite faces. We can have four cases :

Case I: (2, Y) ; (3, W) and (5, R) are distinct. Then the opposite faces can be

(2, 4) ; (3, 1) and (5, 6) or

(2, 6) ; (3, 4) and (5, 1)

and the corresponding colours will be

| | | | | |
|---|---|---|---|---|
| (2, 4) | ; | (3, 1) | ; | (5, 6) |
| B, Y | ; | $B_K$, W | ; | G, R |
| $B_K$, Y | ; | G, W | ; | B, R |

| | | | | | |
|---|---|---|---|---|---|
| and (2, 6) | ; | (3, 4) | ; | (5, 1) | |
| G, Y | ; | B, W | ; | $B_K$, R | |
| B, Y | ; | $B_K$, W | ; | G, R | |

Case II: (2, Y) and (3, W) are same.

Then one of the group will be (2, 3) while other two groups will be (4, –) and (5, –). Now blue cannot be found in the pair with 1, green cannot be found in the pair with 4 and black cannot be found in the pair with 6 which cannot be possible together. $\therefore$ this as well as similar subsequent cases are not possible.

**So the correct options for (a), (b) and (c) are (iv), (iii) and (i) respectively.**

**272. (a) The correct option is (ii). EXPLANATION:**

Note that 3 – 11 in S can be obtained as

$3 \rightarrow 1 + 2$

$4 \rightarrow 1 + 3$

$5 \rightarrow 1 + 4, \quad 2 + 3$

$6 \rightarrow 1 + 5, \quad 2 + 4$

$7 \rightarrow 1 + 6, \quad 2 + 5, \quad 3 + 4$

$8 \rightarrow 2 + 6, \quad 3 + 5$

$9 \rightarrow 3 + 6, \quad 4 + 5$

$10 \rightarrow 4 + 6$

$11 \rightarrow 5 + 6$

For 3 – 11 to be in set S, the pairs of numbers on opposite faces must be selected from 5, 6, 7, 8 and 9 in the above table. Such pairs can be

(3, 2) ; (6, 1) ; (4, 5) or
(4, 1) ; (2, 5) ; (6, 3) or
(4, 2) ; (6, 1) ; (5, 3) or
(5, 1) ; (4, 3) ; (6, 2)

**(b) The correct option is (i). EXPLANATION:**

Note that if S lacks in 5, then two of the pair of numbers on the opposite faces will be (3, 2) and (4, 1). Corollarily (6, 5) will be the third such pair which implies that S will lack in 11 also.

**(c) The correct option is (ii). EXPLANATION:**

If S lacks in 9, then two of the pair of numbers on the opposite faces will be (6, 3) and (5, 4). Corollarily (1, 2) will be the third such pair which implies that S will lack in 3 also.

If S lacks in 10, then one of the pair of numbers on the opposite faces will be (6, 4) and the sum of numbers in other two such pairs will be

1 + 2 + 3 + 4 + 5 + 6 − 10 = 11

which means that other pairs can be (3, 2) and (5, 1). So S can lack in just 10.

**273.** Let us disregard the correct spacing of the points around the circle. We can draw the relevant figures as:

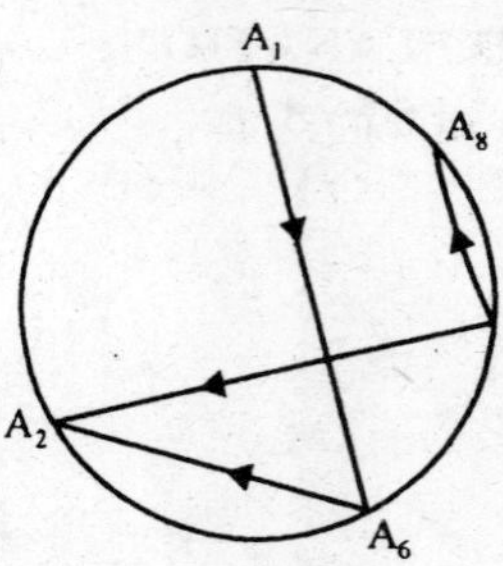


Case I: [Not possible as there is no place for $A_3$]

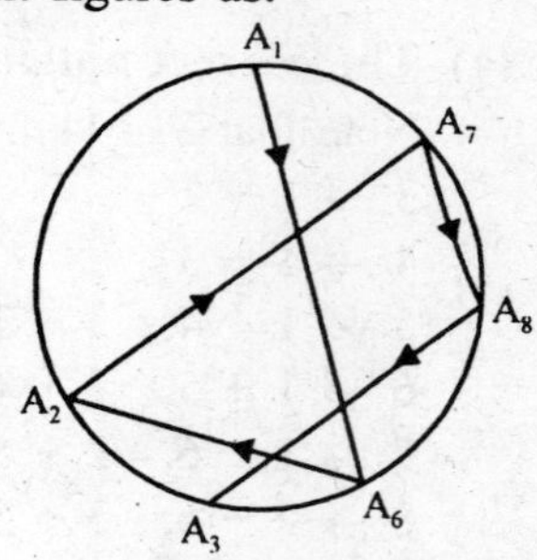


Case II: [$A_4$ can be between ($A_2$, $A_3$) or ($A_3$, $A_6$). But if $A_4$ is between ($A_2$, $A_3$), then there will be no position for $A_5$. So $A_4$ has to be between ($A_3$, $A_6$) and $A_5$ between ($A_7$, $A_8$).

The final figure can be drawn as:

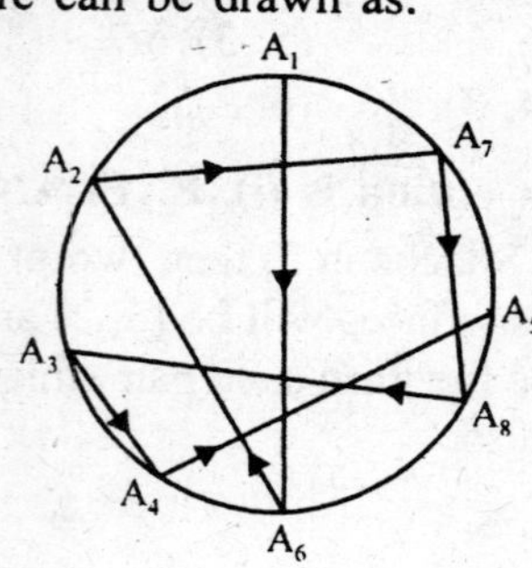

**So the correct options for (a), (b), (c) and (d) are (ii), (iv), (i) and (iii) respectively.**

**274.** Let A, B, C, D, E also represent the weight (in kg) of persons they represent. Then

$C = 2 + E, \quad B = 8 + A \quad \text{and} \quad D = 78$

Also the total weight of couples $= 2 \times (79 + 82) = 322$ kg

and that of all persons $= 5 \times 80 = 400$ kg

$\therefore$ the weight of unmarried person $= 400 - 322$

$= 78$ kg

which is that of D.

Now $8 + A + C = B + 2 + E$

$\Rightarrow 6 + A + C = B + E$

$\Rightarrow (B + E) - (A + C) = 6$

Also the difference between the weights of couple is

$2 \times (82 - 79) = 6.$

As weight of no two persons are same

$\therefore$ (B, E) and (A, C) will be couples.

**So the correct options for (a) and (b) are (ii) and (iii) respectively.**

**275.** Note that F, A, D are single siblings. The two exclusive siblings cannot be (A, C), (A, F), (A, G) or two of (F, A, D). Note that the relations are as

| | | | | | | |
|---|---|---|---|---|---|---|
| Male | couple | Female | and | Male | couple | Female |
| | | ↓ | | ↓ | | ↓ |
| | | Female (sister) | | Male (brother) | | Male (brother) |

$\therefore$ there cannot be siblings from (B, C, E, G)

So the possibilities are

| Bros. and Sis. | Brothers | Sisters |
|---|---|---|
| A, E | B, F | D, G |
| A, E | C, F | D, G |

**So the correct options for (a), (b) and (c) are (iv), (iv) and (ii) respectively.**

**276.** From statements

II and III : G is mother as II have both mothers.

I and II : D is daughter.

I and III : E is son (as it cannot be parent and III contains only sons)

II and IV : J is mother and D is her daughter. Also C, G are married couple.

I and IV : J is mother of D and A, and E, H are brother-sister.

I : B is brother of E.

∴ the two families are

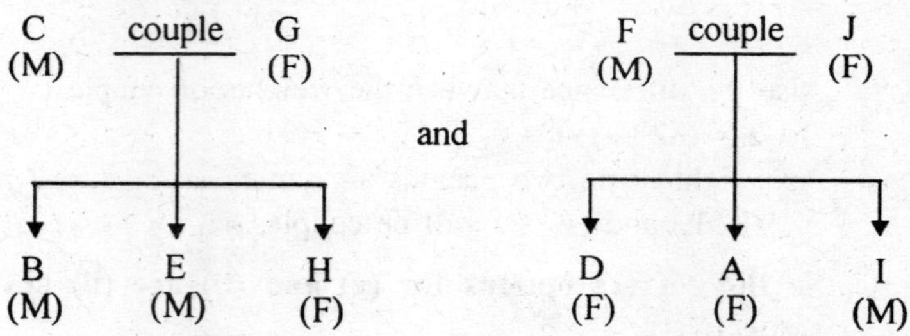


**277.** As there are two couples in (A, B, C, D) ∴ another two will be in (E, F, G, H). Now the format of husband-wife (H, W) should be H > W > H > W > H > W > H > W

∴ (A, B), (C, D), (G, F), (E, H) can't be couple. There will be four cases:

Case I: (A, C), (B, D), (G, E), (F, H) are couples. Then (G, E) > (A, C) > (F, H) > (B, D)

Case II: (A, C), (B, D), (G, H), (F, E) are couples. But (G, H) > (E, F) or (G, H) < (E, F) are not possible.

Case III: (A, D), (B, C), (G, E), (F, H) are couples. But (A, D) > (B, C) or (A, D) < (B, C) are not possible.

Case IV: (A, D), (B, C), (G, H), (F, E) are couples. But (G, H) > (E, F) or (G, H) < (E, F) are not possible.

∴ only case I is valid.

**So the correct options for (a), (b) and (c) are (ii), (iii) and (ii) respectively.**

**278.** According to the statements by persons, the couples are (A, F), (B, G), (C, H), (D, F), (E, A), (F, C), (G, D) and (H, B).

∴ A, C, D, B will be of one sex and
F, G, E, H of another sex.

Now at least one each of (E, A), (H, B), (F, C), (G, D) speaks lie. ∵ only four persons speak lie ∴ one each of the given pairs speaks lie. So the couples can be one of

(A, F) or (E, A)
(B, G) or (H, B)
(C, H) or (F, C)
(D, F) or (G, D)

So exclusive pairs can be

(E, A), (B, G), (C, H), (D, F) or
(E, A), (H, B), (F, C), (G, D)

where first of each pair speaks truth and second speaks lie.

**So the correct options for (a), (b) and (c) are (ii), (i) and (iii) respectively.**

**279.** Note that A, B, F are males and C, D, E, G are females.

∵ there cannot be two male brothers ∴ (VI) has to be wrong.

Now one of (I) and (III) ; (II) and (IV) ; (I) and (VII) has to be wrong.

∴ (I) has to be wrong and one of (II), (IV) will be wrong.

We can have two cases:

Case I: (II), (I) and (VI) are wrong. Then
C is mother of G, D is married to A, E is daughter of F.
∴ we have relationships as

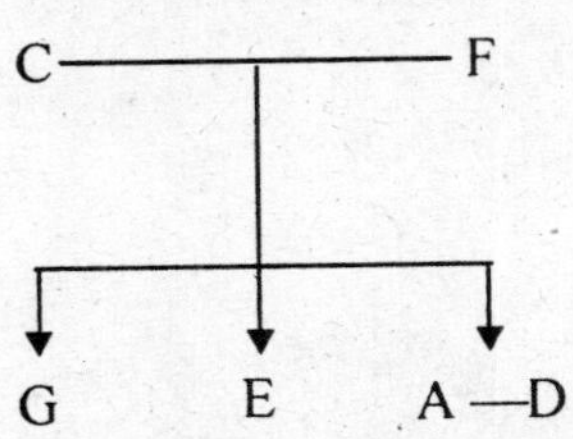


where (C, F) are parents, (A, D) are couple,
(G, E) are daughters, one of whom is married to B.

Case II: (IV) (I) and (VI) are wrong. Then we can have relationships as

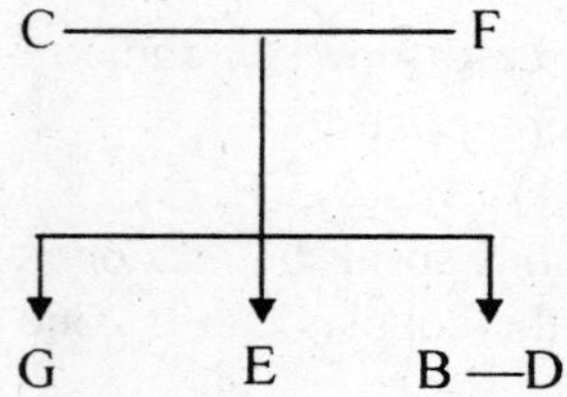


where (C, F) are parents, (B, D) are couple,
(G, E) are daughters, one of whom is married to A.

**So the correct options for (a), (b), (c) and (d) are (iii), (iv), (iii) and (i) respectively.**

**280. (a) The correct option is (ii). EXPLANATION:**

R E A D I N G
I G N R D A E

Note that (N, A), (E, G) are exchangeable which will take two processes. Also (I, R, D) are to be mutually exchanged which will take another two processes.

**(b) The correct option is (i). EXPLANATION:**

M A N A G E M E N T
A E G E M N A N T M

Note that for setting n distinct letters which are at each other's place (none at the place it should be), usually (n – 1) process is needed. Now

| | | |
|---|---|---|
| A is at M's place; | 1 | |
| E is at A's place; | | 6 |
| G is at N's place; | 3 | |
| E is at A's place; | 5 | |
| M is at G's place; | 2 | |
| N is at E's place; | 4 | |
| A is at M's place; | | 7 |
| N is at E's place; | | 10 |
| T is at N's place; | | 9 |
| M is at T's place; | | 8 |

We can form a group: A, M, G, N, E (1, 2, 3, 4, 5) which are at each other's place and another similar group: E, A, M, T, N (6, 7, 8, 9, 10)

$\therefore$ minimum of 4 + 4 = 8 processes will be needed.

**281.** We have

$$\begin{array}{cccc} \vec{A}_1 & A_2 & A_3 & A_4\downarrow \\ A_5 & \vec{A}_6 & A_7\downarrow & A_8 \\ A_9 & A_{10}\downarrow & \vec{A}_{11} & A_{12} \\ A_{13}\downarrow & A_{14} & A_{15} & \vec{A}_{16} \end{array}$$

where arrow associated with a person denotes that its spouse is in the same row/column.

Note that each row will have exactly one couple and each column will have exactly one couple accounting for all eight couples. Now we can have four cases:

Cases I: ($A_1$, $A_2$) and ($A_6$, $A_5$) are couples. Then the other couples will be
($A_{13}$, $A_9$), ($A_{10}$, $A_{14}$), ($A_{11}$, $A_{12}$), ($A_{16}$, $A_{15}$), ($A_7$, $A_3$) and ($A_4$, $A_8$)

Cases II: ($A_1$, $A_2$) and ($A_6$, $A_8$) are couples. Then the other couples will be
($A_{10}$, $A_{14}$), ($A_4$, $A_{12}$), ($A_{11}$, $A_9$), ($A_{16}$, $A_{15}$), ($A_7$, $A_3$) and ($A_{13}$, $A_5$)

Cases III: ($A_1$, $A_3$) and ($A_6$, $A_5$) are couples. Then the other couples will be
($A_{13}$, $A_9$), ($A_7$, $A_{15}$), ($A_{11}$, $A_{12}$), ($A_{10}$, $A_2$), ($A_{16}$, $A_{14}$) and ($A_4$, $A_8$)

Cases IV: ($A_1$, $A_3$) and ($A_6$, $A_8$) are couples. Then the other couples will be
($A_2$, $A_{10}$), ($A_7$, $A_{15}$), ($A_4$, $A_{12}$), ($A_{16}$, $A_{14}$), ($A_{11}$, $A_9$) and ($A_{13}$, $A_5$).

**So the correct options for (a), (b), (c) and (d) are (iv), (iv), (i) and (ii) respectively.**

**282.** Note that blue balls can be B, D, F, H, I only while Red balls can be A, C, E, G, I only.

∴ we can form a table as:

| Possibilities | A | B | C | D | E | F | G | H | I |
|---|---|---|---|---|---|---|---|---|---|
| Green | G | G | G | G | G | G | G | G | G |
| Red | R | R | | R | | | R | R | |
| Blue | | B | B | | B | B | | | B |

Note that out of (B, C) and (E, F), only one of each pair will be blue ball. As there are three blue balls

∴ I has to be a blue ball.

Similarly out of (A, B) and (G, H), only one of each pair will be red ball. As there are three red balls

∴ D has to be a red ball.

Now there will be one blue and one red ball in each of the groups (A, B, C) and (E, F, G, H)

∴ A B C can be R G B, R B G or G R B

and E F G H can be G B G R, B G R G or G B R G.

The total number of possibilities for balls will be $3 \times 3 = 9$.

**So the correct options for (a), (b) and (c) are (iii), (ii) and (iii) respectively.**

**283.** Let A, E, I $\xrightarrow{\text{be denoted by}}$ O

C, D, H $\longrightarrow$ X

B, F, G $\longrightarrow$ —

Then we can have two possibilities:

| | | | | | | | | |
|---|---|---|---|---|---|---|---|---|
| Department: | I | II | III | | I | II | III |
| Boss: | O | X | – | | O | – | X |
| Sect: | – | O | X | or | X | O | – |
| Clerk: | X | – | O | | – | X | O |

**(a) The correct option is (iii). EXPLANATION:**

There are three positions for each of the groups and each group can occupy these positions in 6 ways.

∴ total number of possibilities $= 2 \times 6 \times 6 \times 6 = 432$

**(b) The correct option is (iv). EXPLANATION:**

Note that the given condition correspond to second configuration. ∴ '—' cannot be secretary to 'X' (clerk)

**(c) The correct option is (iv). EXPLANATION:**

Note that the given condition correspond to first configuration and all the given conditions are possible.

**284. (a) The correct option is (ii). EXPLANATION:**

Note that if $n$ different things occupy $n$ distinct places, then the number of ways in which they can be arranged so that none of them occupy their previous position is given by derrangement formula as:

$$\lfloor\!\underline{n}\left\{1-\frac{1}{\lfloor\!\underline{1}}+\frac{1}{\lfloor\!\underline{2}}-\frac{1}{\lfloor\!\underline{3}}+\ldots\ldots\frac{(-1)^n}{\lfloor\!\underline{n}}\right\}$$

where, for any positive integer r,

$\lfloor\!\underline{r} = 1\cdot 2\cdot 3\cdot \ldots r$

∴ the answer here will be

$$\lfloor\!\underline{4}\left(1-\frac{1}{\lfloor\!\underline{1}}+\frac{1}{\lfloor\!\underline{2}}-\frac{1}{\lfloor\!\underline{3}}+\frac{1}{\lfloor\!\underline{4}}\right)$$

$$= 4\cdot 3\cdot 2\left(\frac{1}{1\cdot 2}-\frac{1}{1\cdot 2\cdot 3}+\frac{1}{1\cdot 2\cdot 3\cdot 4}\right)$$

$$= 4\cdot 3 - 4 + 1 = 9$$

**(b) The correct option is (ii). EXPLANATION:**

| | | | |
|---|---|---|---|
| A | B | C | D |
| E | G | F | H |
| H | F | G | E |

Note that right envelope for
A can be F or G only;
B can be E or H only;
C can be E or H only;
D can be F or G only;

So the possibilities for right envelopes can be

| A | B | C | D |
|---|---|---|---|
| F | E | H | G |
| F | H | E | G |
| G | E | H | F |
| G | H | E | F |

Also if (A, D) and (B, C) are chosen, then the envelops they are presently in can be mutually exchanged without altering the given condition.

**285.** Note that

those who want to sit together ≡ BE, AF, CA or GH;
those who do not want to sit at the ends ≡ A, C, D, F;
those who want to be in different groups: (A, D) or one of (F, B, E) and one of (C, G, H).

There can be three cases pertaining to the questions asked, viz. (B, E), (A, F) and (C, A) wanting to sit together.

Case I: B, E want to sit together.

Those who do not want to sit at the ends cannot be (F, A) or (F, D) as there cannot be any valid pair for the category of those who want to be in different groups. Let it be (F, C). Then those who want to be in different groups will be (A, D) and consequently those who do not want to sit together will be (G, H) which cannot be possible.

∴ those who do not want to sit at the ends can be (A, C), (A, D) or (C, D).

So we can have following subcases:

| | (A, C) | (A, D) | (C, D) |
|---|---|---|---|
| Those who do not want to be together in a group: | (F, G) or (F, H) | (F, C) or (F, G) or (C, H) | (F, G) or (F, H) |
| Those who do not want to sit together: | (D, H) → P; (D, G) → N. P | (G, H) → N. P; (C, H) → N. P; (C, G) → P | (A, H) → P; (A, G) → P |

where P stands for 'possible' and
N.P for 'Not possible'.

Case II: A, F want to sit together.
It implies that C, D are the ones who do not want to sit at the ends. ∴ those who do not want to be in the same group can be (B, G), (B, H) (C, E) or (E, H) and the persons who do not want to sit together will be correspondingly by (E, H), (E, G), (B, H) and (B, G), all being possible case.

Case III: C, A want to be together.
Then it implies that those who do not want to sit at the ends will be (D, F). For other categories, it will be same as in case II.

**So the correct options for (a), (b), (c) and (d) are (iv), (iii), (iv) and (iv) respectively.**

**286.** Note that from two arrangements, the couples who want to sit together can be

(A, G); (G, B); (B, E); (E, F); (F, H); (H, D); (D, C) **and**

(G, B); (B, E); (E, D); (D, H); (H, F); (F, C); (C, A)

The common to them are (G, B; (B, E); (F, H) and (H, D)
and uncommon to them are (A, G); (E, F); (D, C); (D, E); (F, C) and (C, A)

So we can have the possible cases:

| Cases | Couples who want sit together | Couples who do not want to sit together |
|---|---|---|
| I. | (B, G) and (F, H) | (A, D) and (C, E) |
| II. | (B, G) and (H, D) | (A, F) and (C, E) |
| III. | (B, E) and (F, H) | (A, D) and (C, G) |
| IV. | (B, E) and (H, D) | (A, F) and (C, G) |

**So the correct options for (a), (b) and (c) are (ii), (i) and (iv) respectively.**

**287.** We are given:

$P_3$ × A ✓ $P_1$ ['×' denotes 'not in'
$P_5$ × B ✓ $P_2$ '✓' denotes 'occupied by']
$P_4$ × C
$P_1$ × D
$P_2$ × E

Also ($P_1$, $P_3$) and ($P_2$, $P_5$) are together in a flat. So we can have

| | | Case I | Case II | Case III |
|---|---|---|---|---|
| A | → | $P_1$ | $P_1$ | $P_1$ |
| B | → | $P_2$ | $P_2$ | $P_2$ |
| C | → | ($P_1$, $P_3$) | – | ($P_2$, $P_5$) |
| D | → | ($P_2$, $P_5$) | ($P_2$, $P_5$) | – |
| E | → | – | ($P_1$, $P_3$) | ($P_1$, $P_3$) |

**(a) The correct option is (ii). EXPLANATION:**
If ($P_3$, $P_4$) share a flat, then only case I will be valid and ($P_3$, $P_4$) will share E, ($P_5$, $P_1$) will share A and ($P_2$, $P_4$) will share B.

**(b) The correct option is (i). EXPLANATION:**
If ($P_4$, $P_5$) share a flat, then for

Case I: ($P_4$, $P_5$) share E and ($P_1$, $P_4$) share A.

Case III: ($P_4$, $P_5$) share D and ($P_1$, $P_4$) share A.
(Note that case II is not possible)

**288.** There can be two cases for the scheduled day of exams:

Case I: Mon Tue Thur Sat Mon Wed Fri
Not possible as exams culminates on Saturday.

Case II:

| | Mon | Wed | Fri | Sat | Tue | Thur | Sat |
|---|---|---|---|---|---|---|---|
| | Phy | Chem. | Comp | Bio | Maths | Econ. | Eng. |
| or | Chem. | Comp. | Phy/Maths | Bio | Eng | Econ. | Maths/Phy |
| or | Eng | Econ | Maths | Bio | Chem | Comp | Phy |
| or | Phy/Math | Econ | Eng | Bio | Maths/Phy | Chem | Comp. |

The filling is done in sequence
Bio → (Chem, comp) → _ _ _

**So the correct options for (a), (b), (c), (d) and (e) are (iv), (i), (iv), (ii) and (iv) respectively.**

**289.** We have

| Question | Responses (9 of them will be wrong) | | | |
|---|---|---|---|---|
| 1 | A | C | D | → Two wrong. |
| 2 | B | A | B | → At least one wrong. |
| 3 | C | A | A | → At least one wrong. |
| 4 | D | B | C | → Two wrong. |
| 5 | C | B | B | → At least one wrong. |
| 6 | A | C | C | → At least one wrong. |

We can have

| Cases for correct response | | | | | Responses of students | | |
|---|---|---|---|---|---|---|---|
| 1 | | | | | A | C | D |
| 2 | B | B | B | A | B | A | B |
| 3 | A | A | C | A | C | A | A |
| 4 | | | | | D | B | C |
| 5 | B | C | B | B | C | B | B |
| 6 | A | C | C | C | A | C | C |

- Fourth case → Not possible as it makes second student make 4 correct answers
- Third case → The responses for first and fourth questions can be (A, B) or (C, D)
- Second case → The responses for first and fourth questions can be (A, B) or (C, D)
- First case → The responses for first and fourth questions can be (A, B) or (C, D)

**So the correct options for (a), (b), (c), (d) and (e) are (i), (i), (iv), (ii) and (ii) respectively.**

**290.**

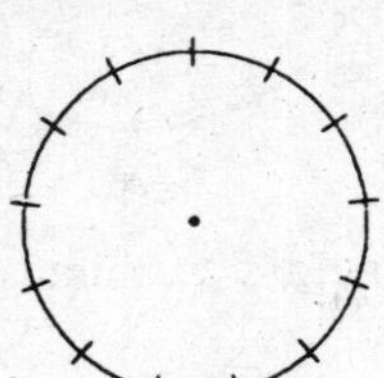

In the given subquestions, we need to name these vertices.

**(a) The correct option is (i). EXPLANATION:**

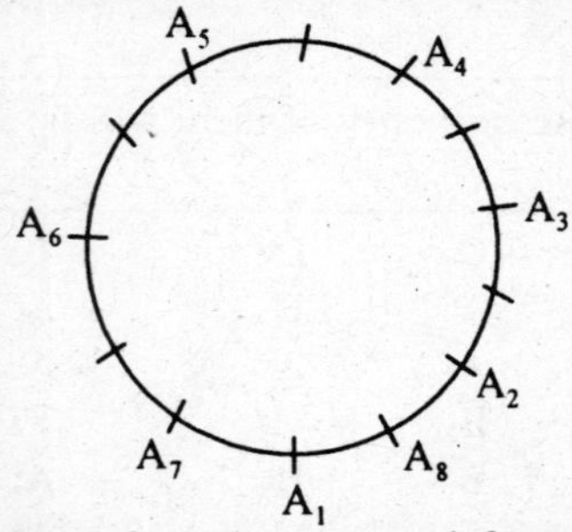


(The naming of vertices started from $A_1$)

**(b) The correct option is (ii). EXPLANATION:**

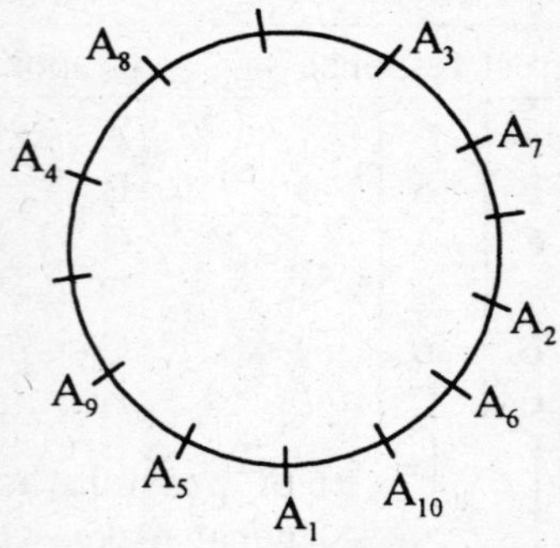


(The naming of vertices started from $A_1$)

**(c) The correct options is (iv). EXPLANATION:**

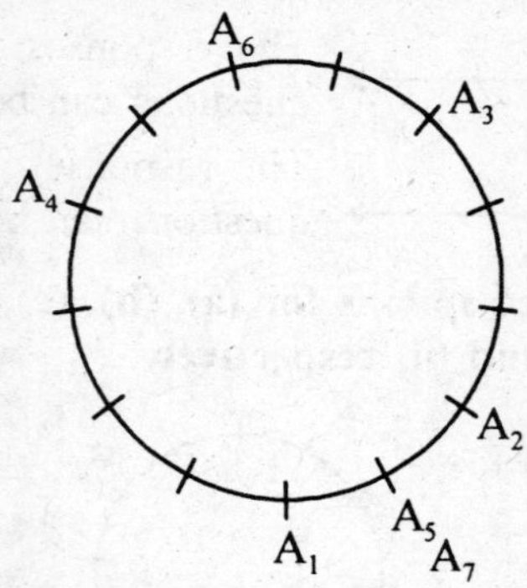


$\because$ $A_5$, $A_7$ coincides $\therefore$ this case is not possible.

**291.** Note that a coin can be completely surrounded by six identical coins. The only possible arrangement will be

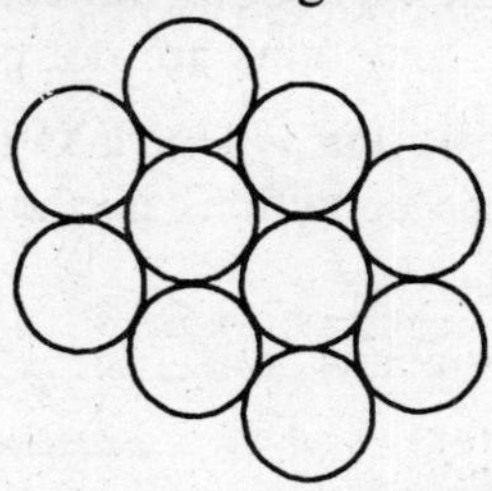

Note that *n* corresponds to two middle coins which will be equal to 6 and C, F has to be in the middle. So the numbering of coins will be

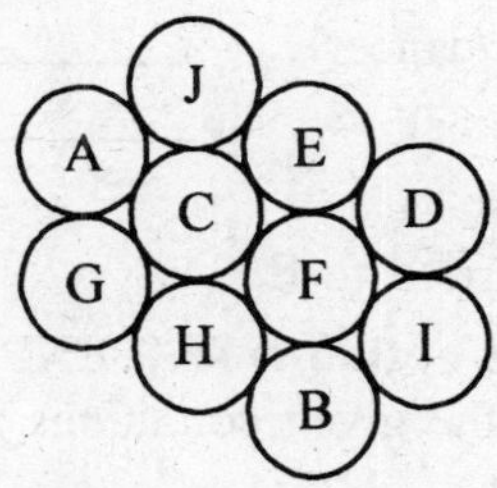


**So the correct options for (a), (b) and (c) are (iv), (ii) and (iv) respectively.**

**292.** Note that there can be three cases:

Case I:

| Male | | Female |
|---|---|---|
| Accountant | married to | Teacher |
| C | ______ | Doctor |
| D | ______ | B |

Case II:

| Male | | Female |
|---|---|---|
| Accountant | ______ | Doctor |
| C | ______ | B |
| D | ______ | Teacher |

Case III:

| | | | Male | | Female | | |
|---|---|---|---|---|---|---|---|
| C | D | – | Accountant | ______ | ○ | – | – |
| D | – | D | ○ | ______ | Teacher | B | – |
| – | C | C | ○ | ______ | Doctor | – | B |

A total of six subcases (3 × 2) in this case.

**(a) The correct option is (iv). EXPLANTATION:**

On putting the conditions, no case is found to be valid.

∴ the given conditions are not possible.

**(b) The correct option is (ii). EXPLANATION:**

On putting the conditions in above cases, we get

Case I:

| Male | | Female |
|---|---|---|
| A/E (accountant) | ________ | E/A (teacher) |
| C (actor) | ________ | F (doctor) |
| D (lawyer/dancer) | ________ | B (dancer/lawyer) |

Case II:

| Male | | Female |
|---|---|---|
| A/E (accountant) | ________ | E/A (doctor) |
| C (lawyer/dancer) | ________ | B (dancer/lawyer) |
| D (actor) | ________ | F (teacher) |

Case III: Not Feasible

∴ A is married to E.

**(c) The correct option is (iii). EXPLANATION:**

On putting the given conditions in above cases, we get

Case I: Not Feasible

Case II: Not Feasible

Case III:

| Male | | | | Female |
|---|---|---|---|---|
| A | (accountant) | ________ | | (lawyer) |
| D | | ________ | B | (teacher) |
| C | (dancer) | ________ | F | (doctor) |

or

| Male | | | | Female |
|---|---|---|---|---|
| F | (accountant) | ________ | | (dancer) |
| D | | ________ | B | (teacher) |
| C | (lawyer) | ________ | A | (doctor) |

or

| Male | | | | Female |
|---|---|---|---|---|
| F | (accountant) | ________ | | (dancer) |
| D | (lawyer) | ________ | A | (teacher) |
| C | | ________ | B | (doctor) |

or

| Male | | | | Female |
|---|---|---|---|---|
| A | (accountant) | ________ | | (lawyer) |
| D | (dancer) | ________ | F | (teacher) |
| C | | ________ | B | (doctor) |

∴ E is married to accountant and

actor is married to B

**(d) The correct option is (i). EXPLAINED ABOVE.**

**293.** Note that A, C, E lives in the middle and further A lives in the centre as E, C has T, Q to their adjacent positions. ∴ we can have

| | B/D | C | A | E | D/B |
|---|---|---|---|---|---|
| | T | S | Q | P | R |
| | yellow | red / blue | white | blue / red | green |
| or | R | S | T | P | Q |
| | white | red / blue | green | blue / red | yellow |

**So the correct options for (a), (b) and (c) are (i), (i) and (iii) respectively.**

**294.** We have

$$\left.\begin{array}{lcl} \text{Prof.} & \equiv & 100 + D \\ \text{Acc.} & \equiv & C - 100 \\ \text{Art.} & \equiv & 2A \\ \text{Doc.} & \equiv & B - 200 \end{array}\right\}$$

⇒ Prof. + Acc. ≡ C + D

∴ either Prof., Acc. ≡ C, D respectively

or A, B if A + B ≡ C + D

Now in any case,

Art. + Doc. ≡ A + B (as each of A, B correspond to one of the given profession)

∴ 2 A + B − 200 ≡ A + B

⇒ A ≡ 200

Now we can have three cases:

Case I: Doct. ≡ A, B ≡ 400 ≡ Art., Prof. ≡ C, Acc. ≡ D (their money cannot be determined)

Case II: C ≡ Art. ≡ 400, Acc. ≡ 300 ≡ B, Prof. ≡ A

D ≡ 100 ≡ Doct.

Case III: D ≡ 400 ≡ Art., Prof. ≡ B ≡ 500, Doct. ≡ C ≡ 300

Acc. ≡ A

**So the correct options for (a), (b), (c) and (d) are (ii), (iv), (i) and (iii) respectively.**

**295.** Note that

Painter cannot be D

Doctor cannot be A, B

Wrestler cannot be C, D

Also amount with (Law. + Paint.) = that of (Doc. + Wrest.)

Now we can have

| Cases: | I | II | III | IV | V | VI |
|---|---|---|---|---|---|---|
| Doctor | C | C | D | D | D | D |
| Wrestler | A | B | A | A | B | B |
| Painter | B | A | B | C | A | C |
| Lawyer | D | D | C | B | C | A |

For

Case I: $2C = A + B$ , $2A = C + D$ , $D = 2B$

$$\Rightarrow 3C = 4B, \quad \Rightarrow C = \frac{4}{3} B \quad \text{and } A = \left(\frac{2}{3} + 1\right) B = \frac{5}{3} B$$

Case II: $2C = A + B$ , $2B = C + D$ , $D = 2A$

$$\Rightarrow 3C = 4A \quad \Rightarrow C = \frac{4}{3} A \quad \text{and consequently } B = \frac{5}{3} A$$

Case III: $2D = A + B$, $2A = C + D$, $D = 2B$

$\Rightarrow A = 3B$ and $C = 4B$

Case IV: $2D = A + B$, $2A = C + D$, $D = 2C$

$$\Rightarrow A = \frac{3C}{2} \quad \text{and } B = \frac{5C}{2}$$

Case V: $2D = A + B$, $2B = C + D$, $D = 2A$

$\Rightarrow B = 3A$ and $C = 4A$

Case VI: $2D = A + B$, $2B = C + D$, $D = 2C$

$$\Rightarrow B = \frac{3C}{2} \quad \text{and } A = \frac{5C}{2}$$

**So the correct options for (a), (b), (c), (d) and (e) are (i), (ii), (i), (iii) and (iv) respectively.**

**296.** By scaling down the given amounts by a factor of 10,000, we have

A ≡ Prof. + 1 ≡ Law. – 1,
B ≡ Doc. – 1 ≡ Art. – 3 and
D ≡ E + 1 ≡ Chem. – 1

We can have three cases pertaining to A being doctor, chemist or artist.

Case I: A ≡ Doc.

Then B ≡ A – 1 ⇒ A ≡ B + 1 ≡ Prof. + 1

∴ B ≡ Prof. and ∵ D, E cannot be chemist

∴ C ≡ Chem.

Now B ≡ A – 1

⇒ Art. – 3 ≡ Law. – 2

⇒ Art. ≡ Law + 1

∴ D ≡ Art. and E ≡ Law.

Case II: A ≡ Chemist

Then D ≡ A – 1 ≡ Proff.

Now ∵ B cannot be doctor or artist ∴ B ≡ Law. and

B ≡ A + 1 = D + 2 ≡ E + 3 ≡ Doc. – 1
≡ Art. – 3

Now E cannot be doctor or artist

∴ this case is rejected.

Case III: A ≡ Artist

Now B cannot be doctor or artist, neither professor nor lawyer. ∴ it has to be a chemist.

Now B ≡ Doc. – 1 ≡ A – 3,
D ≡ E + 1 ≡ B – A and
A ≡ Prof. + 1 ≡ Law. – 1

⇒ E + 1 = Doc. – 2 ≡ A – 4
≡ Prof. – 3 ≡ Law. –5

∵ E cannot be doctor, professors or lawyer

∴ this case is also rejected.

**So the correct options for (a), (b), (c) and (d) are (i), (ii), (ii) and (ii) respectively.**

**297. A.** Scaling down the given amounts by factor of 100, we have

| | | | | |
|---|---|---|---|---|
| Artist | ≡ C, D + 1 | –(i) | Artist, Chemist = A – 1 | –(v) |
| Chemist | ≡ A, D – 1 | – (ii) | Doctor, Artist = B + 1 | –(vi) |
| Lawyer | ≡ B, C – 1 | – (iii) | Lawyer, Doctor = C + 1 | –(vii) |
| Doctor | ≡ B, A + 1 | – (iv) | Chemist, Lawyer = D – 1 | –(viii) |

From (i) and (vi),

Artist cannot be B + 1 (as A, B, C, D are different)

∴ Doctor ≡ B + 1 – (ix)

From (vii) and (ix),

Lawyer ≡ C + 1 –(x)

From (iii) and (x),

Lawyer ≡ B – 1 –(xi)

From (viii) and (x),

Chemist ≡ D – 1 (xi)

From (v) and (xi),

Artist ≡ A – 1 – (xii)

∴ we can have two cases:

$$\left.\begin{array}{llll} \text{Artist} & \equiv C & \equiv & D+1 \\ \text{Lawyer} & \equiv A & \equiv & D+2 \\ \text{Chemist} & \equiv B & \equiv & D+3 \\ \text{Doctor} & \equiv D & & \end{array}\right\} \text{ or } \left.\begin{array}{llll} \text{Artist} & \equiv B & \equiv & D+1 \\ \text{Lawyer} & \equiv D & & \\ \text{Chemist} & \equiv C & \equiv & D-3 \\ \text{Doctor} & \equiv A & \equiv & D+2 \end{array}\right\}$$

**So the correct options for (a), (b), (c) and (d) are (ii), (iv), (iv) and (ii) respectively.**

**B.** We have

Lawyer ≡ (B, D) + 100 ≡ (A, C) – 100, –(i)

Doctor ≡ (A, C) + 100 ≡ (B, D) – 100 and –(ii)

Chemist ≡ Lawyer, Artist – 100 –(iii)

Let the amount with lawyer be $x$. Then there will be two persons with amounts $x$ – 100 and $x$ + 100.

∵ there are only four persons. ∴ the amount with doctor will be $x$ – 100 or $x$ + 100. Now we can have two cases:

Case I: Lawyer → $x$, Doctor → $x$ – 100

Artist → $x$ + 100 and Chemist → $x$ – 200

This case is rejected as equation (iii) is not satisfied.

Case II: Lawyer $\rightarrow x$, Doctor $\rightarrow x + 100$

Chemist $\rightarrow x - 100$ and Artist $\rightarrow x + 200$.

Then (Lawyer, Doctor) = A, C or C, A and

(Chemist, Artist) = B, D or D, B

**So the correct options for (a), (b) and (c) are (ii), (i) and (iii) respectively.**

**298.** $\because$ A likes blue, teacher likes yellow, one who lives on ground floor likes green and doctor lives just above A $\therefore$ the doctor likes red and $\because$ artist lives on second floor $\therefore$ lawyer likes green and lives on ground floor. Consequently, artist like blue. $\therefore$ we have

| A | B | C/D | D/C |
|---|---|---|---|
| Blue | Green | Red | Yellow |
| Artist | Lawyer | Doctor | Teacher |
| Second | Ground | Third | First |

**So the correct options for (a), (b) and (c) are (i).**

**299.** Carefully note that each of the elements of the quadruplets

(A, artist, yellow, second floor),

(B, lawyer, blue, top floor),

(C, doctor, green, first floor) and

(D, teacher, red, ground floor)

corresponds to different persons/professions/likes/the floor occupied.

Let us start with A being lawyer. Then, there can be three cases:

Case I:

| A | B | C | D |
|---|---|---|---|
| Lawyer | Artist | Teacher | Doctor |
| { Green | Red | Blue/Yellow | Yellow/Blue |
| Red | Green | Blue/Yellow | Yellow/Blue |

Case II:

| A | B | C | D |
|---|---|---|---|
| Lawyer | Teacher | Artist | Doctor |
| { Green | Yellow | Red | Blue |
| Red | Green | Blue | Yellow |

Case III:

| | A | B | C | D |
|---|---|---|---|---|
| | Lawyer | Doctor | Teacher | Artist |
| | Green | Red | Yellow | Blue |
| | Red | Yellow | Blue | Green |

Similarly there will be eight possibilities each for A being teacher and doctor. ∴ total number of possibilities will be 24. Note that in each of the column of any of the above cases, there are three elements from three different quadruplets. ∴ the fourth row corresponding to floors will be automatically from the corresponding fourth quadruplet.

Regarding part (d) and (e), if B is artist, then there will be similarly three cases of which first will be same as above and other two cases will be

Case I:

| | A | B | C | D |
|---|---|---|---|---|
| | Teacher | Artist | Lawyer | Doctor |
| { | Blue | Green | Red | Yellow |
| | Green | Red | Yellow | Blue |

Case II:

| | A | B | C | D |
|---|---|---|---|---|
| | Doctor | Artist | Teacher | Lawyer |
| { | Blue | Red | Yellow | Green |
| | Red | Green | Blue | Yellow |

**So the correct options for (a), (b), (c) (d) and (e) are (i), (ii), (ii), (iii) and (iii) respectively.**

**300.** We have

| | | | | | |
|---|---|---|---|---|---|
| Doctor | → | (R, G) | | (R, Y) | [R, B, G, Y denote |
| Actor | → | (B, R) | or | (B, G) | red, blue, green |
| Lawyer | → | (Y, B) | | (Y, R) | and yellow respectively |
| Proffessor | → | (G, Y) | | (G, B) | and '→' signifies 'likes'] |

**(a) The correct option is (iv). EXPLANATION:**

In a way similar to above, we have

| | | | | |
|---|---|---|---|---|
| A | → | (G, R) | | (G, Y) |
| B | → | (R, G) | or | (R, C) |
| C | → | (B, Y) | | (B, G) |
| D | → | (Y, B) | | (Y, R) |

$\because$ (A, B, C, D) and (Doctor, Actor, Lawyer, Professor) denote same set of four persons and none of the columns corresponding to them matches $\therefore$ this case is not possible.

**(b) The correct option is (i). EXPLANATION:**

We have

$$\left.\begin{array}{lll} A & \rightarrow & (R,B) \\ B & \rightarrow & (Y,G) \\ C & \rightarrow & (B,Y) \\ D & \rightarrow & (G,R) \end{array}\right\} \text{ or } \left.\begin{array}{l} (R,Y) \\ (Y,R) \\ (B,G) \\ (G,B) \end{array}\right\}$$

Now, we can have two valid cases:

A, B, C, D ≡ Actor, Professor, Lawyer, Doctor (in order)

[From first columns corresponding to them]

or A, B ≡ Doctor, Lawyer or vice versa

and C, D ≡ Actor, Professor or vice versa

[From second columns corresponding to them]

**(c) The correct option is (i). EXPLANATION:**

We have

$$\left.\begin{array}{lll} A & \rightarrow & (R,B) \\ B & \rightarrow & (B,Y) \\ C & \rightarrow & (Y,G) \\ D & \rightarrow & (G,R) \end{array}\right\} \text{ or } \left.\begin{array}{l} (R,G) \\ (B,R) \\ (Y,B) \\ (G,Y) \end{array}\right\}$$

$\because$ these two columns matches with the first column (Doctor, Actor, Lawyer, Professor) $\therefore$ we can have two cases, viz.

A, B, C, D ≡ Actor, Lawyer, Professor, Doctor (in order)

or

Doctor, Actor, Lawyer, Professor (in order)

**301.** Note that the last two digit will remain same. Now each of successive groups

(4, 7), (3, 6), (4, 9), (5, 6) and (1, 4) will have at least one digit as one of the last two digits of the original number [Note that 49 and 56 cannot be first two digits as from given options of part (a), 700 is not there]. Also one of (3, 6) or one of (5, 6); one of (4, 7) or one of (4, 9); and one of (4, 9) or one of (1, 4) will be one of the last two digits of the original number. ∴ 4 has to be one of the last two digits of the original number [deduced from (4, 7), (4, 9) and (1, 4)] while second of the last two digits will be one of 3, 5 or 6.

Case I: 3 is one of the last two digits.
Then we will have the first two numbers as

(7 __ __ __ and __ 6 __ __ )

or ( __ 7 __ __ and 6 __ __ __ )

This case is rejected due to digits (5, 6) of third successive sum.

Case II: 5 is one of the last two digits. Then we will have the first two numbers as __ 7 __ __ and 63 __ __ .
And the next three sums should be (addendum being 600) 69 __ __ , 75 __ __ and 81 __ __
Note that 75 __ __ is not possible.
∴ this case is rejected.

Case III: 6 is one of the last two digits. Then the numbers can be only

__ 7 __ __ , __ 3 __ __ , __ 9 __ __ , __ 5 __ __ and __ 1 __ __ ,

(the other possibilities being not found valid)

**So the correct options for (a), (b), (c) and (d) are (iv), (ii), (ii) and (ii) respectively.**

**302.** $abcd + dabc + cdab + bcda = 1111\ (a + b + c + d)$
If $a + b + c + d = x\,y$, a two—digit number, then
$1111 \times x\,y = a\,e\,e\,c\,d$

Note that if $x + y < 10$, then $c = e$.

∴ $x + y$ must be $\geq 10$. Also $x + y \leq 30$

∴ $x\,y$ can be equal to 19, 28 or 29 and the corresponding number will be 21109, 31108 and 32219 respectively. Now

∵ $b$ is a single digit integer ∴ only $x\,y = 19$ and $a\,e\,e\,c\,d$ = 21109 is retained. And $b = 19 - (2 + 0 + 9) = 8$.

**So the correct options for (a), (b) and (c) are (iv), (ii) and (ii) respectively.**

**303.**

$$\begin{array}{cccc} & a & b & c \\ + & d & e & f \\ + & g & h & i \\ \hline a & a & a & a \end{array}$$

Note that $a$ has to be 1. Now

$$\left.\begin{array}{ll} c+f+i & =21 \\ b+e+h & =9 \\ a+d+g & =10 \end{array}\right\} \quad \text{or} \quad \begin{array}{l} 11 \\ 10 \\ 10 \end{array}$$

$\because$ only seven of them are from (1 – 9)

$\therefore$ two of them are 0.

Also 1 + 2 + 3 + ... 9 = 45

Now $a + b + ... + i = 40$ or $31 = (45 - 5)$ or $(45 - 14)$

$\because$ the missing numbers can be from groups (4, 6, 7, 8, 9) and (1, 2, 3, 5) and sums of them are 5 or 14

$\therefore$ they can be (1, 4) or (9, 5). But a = 1

$\therefore$ only (9, 5) is valid.

**So the correct options for (a) and (b) are (iv).**

**304.** Note that the sum of all numbers is $222\ (A + B + C)$.

$\therefore$ $1150 + 1231 + 139\,x = 222\ (A + B + C)$

$\Rightarrow$ $222\ (A + B + C) = 3771 + x$

Now $222 \times 17 = 3774$

$\therefore$ $x = 3$ and $A + B + C = 17$

**(a) The correct option is (ii). EXPLAINED AS ABOVE.**

**(b) The correct option is (ii). EXPLANATION:**

$\because$ only one of the numbers (4, 5, 6, 7) is not a member of set $\{A, B, C\}$ $\therefore$ $A, B, C$ each are a number from the set (4, 5, 6, 7) $\because$ $A + B + C = 17$ and $4 + 6 + 7 = 17$

$\therefore$ 5 is the required answer.

**305.** Observing the last digits of the sum, note that $(C, F) \equiv$ (2, 4), (1, 5), or (9, 7)

$(A, D) \equiv (5, 4), (6, 3), (7, 2)$ or $(8, 1)$

$(B, E) \equiv (1, 4), (2, 3), (7, 8)$ or $(9, 6)$

From last sum, $C + F < 10$ $\therefore$ $C, F \equiv (9, 7)$ is rejected. Now $C + F = 6$. Also as $A + D = 9$ and the last sum is $n\ 0\ 5$ $\therefore$ $n = 7$ and $B + E = 15$. And consequently, $(B, E) \equiv (1, 4)$ or $(2, 3)$ are rejected. The possible solutions are

$(C, F), (B, E), (A, D) \equiv$

- $(2, 4)$
  - $(7, 8) - (6, 3)$
  - $(9, 6) - (8, 1)$
- $(1, 5)$
  - $(7, 8) - (6, 3)$
  - $(9, 6) - (7, 2)$

Considering the order of pairs in the bracket, the total number of possible solutions will be $2 \times 2 \times 2 \times 4 = 32$.

**So the correct options for (a), (b), (c) and (d) are (ii), (i), (iii) and (i) respectively.**

**306.** Note that

| | | | | | |
|---|---|---|---|---|---|
| $B+C+D$ | = | 10 | or | 20 | sums of last digits |
| $D+C+A$ | = | 8 | or | 18 | |
| $A+B+C$ | = | 16 | or | 15 | sums of first digits |
| $B+D+C$ | = | 21 | or | 20 | |

$\because$ first and fourth equations are same

$\therefore$ first set of values are rejected. Now

$B - A = 2$, $D - A = 5$, $2A + C = 13$ and

$A$ cannot be equal to 1 ($\because$ $C$ is a single digit integer) or 5 ($\because$ $D$ is a single digit integer).

$\because$ $B + C + D = 20$ $\therefore$ $A + B + C + D$ cannot be equal to 25.

**So the correct options for (a), (b) and (c) are (iv), (iii) and (iii) respectively.**

**307.** Note that the maximum value of product of any two distinct single digit positive integers is 72; and other few numbers in decreasing orders are 63, 56, 54, 48, 45, 42 40 and 36.

Now $CB \geq 136 - 72 = 64$

$\therefore$ $C$ can be equal to 6, 7, 8 or 9.

When $C = 9$, $CB = 136 - 56 = 80 \rightarrow$ not possible or
$= 136 - 48 = 88 \rightarrow$ not possible or
$= 136 - 42 = 94$ or
$= 136 - 40 = 96$

Checking for $C \times B + AD = 112$, we find that

$9 \times 4 + 76 = 112$ and $9 \times 6 + 58 = 112$

$\therefore \quad (A, B, C, D) \equiv (7, 4, 9, 6)$ or $(5, 6, 9, 8)$

When $C = 8$, $CB = 136 - 54, 48 = 82, 88$ (not possible as digits are distinct).

Now $C \times B + AD = 16 + 96 = 112$

$\therefore \quad (A, B, C, D) \equiv (9, 2, 8, 6)$

When $C = 7$, $CB = 136 - 63 = 73$

Now $C \times B + AD \neq 112 \quad \therefore$ this case is rejected.

When $C = 6$, $CB = 136 - 72 = 64$

Now $C \times B + AD = 24 + 89 = 113$

So this case is also rejected. But for part (d), it is relevant and $D = 9$ is the greatest of all integers.

**So the correct options for (a), (b), (c) and (d) are (iii), (iv), (ii) and (iv) respectively.**

**308. The correct option is (ii). EXPLANATION:**

$x = A\,B\,C + D\,E\,F + G\,H\,I$

$= 100\,(A + D + G) + 10\,(B + E + H) + (C + F + I)$

Note that there will be only $6 \times 6 \times 6$ values of $(A, B \ldots I)$ only if the sum of elements of one of $(A, D, G)$, $(B, E, H)$ or $(C, F, I)$ is $6\ (1 + 2 + 3)$ and that of elements of another is $24\ (7 + 8 + 9)$. For minimum value of $x$,

$A + D + G = 6$, $B + E + H = 15$ and $C + F + I = 24$

$\therefore \quad x = 774 = 9 \cdot 86 = 9 \cdot 2 \cdot 43$

**309.** Let the numbers be $a, b, c, d, e, f, g, h$ and $i$ such that the digits of three-digit numbers are $(a, b, c)$, $(d, e, f)$ and $(g, h, i)$.

**(a) The correct option is (i). EXPLANATION:**

$$\text{If } \left.\begin{aligned} c+f &= i \\ b+e &= h \\ a+d &= g \end{aligned}\right\}, \text{ then } \left.\begin{aligned} c+f+i &= 2i \\ b+e+h &= 2h \\ a+d+g &= 2g \end{aligned}\right\}$$

$\therefore$ in each triplets, there are either two odd numbers and one even number or three even numbers and they cannot give four even numbers and five odd numbers.

**(b) The correct option is (i). EXPLANATION:**

Let us assume

$c + f = i + x$, $b + e = h + y$ and $a + d + 1 = g$
(even, even, even) (odd, odd, even) (odd, odd, odd)

where one of $x$, $y$ is 10 and other 0 to account for one carry (+1). Now we can have $c + f = i + x$ as

I. $2 + 4 = 6$. Then $y = 10$ and one of $b$, $e$, say, $b = 8$
$\therefore$ $e - h = 2$ and $a + d = g - 1$. No value of $(e, h, a, d, g)$ from (1, 3, 5, 7, 9) is possible.

II. $2 + 6 = 8$. Then y = 10. Then either $b + e = 14$ or $b$ (or $e$) $= 6 + h$. But $(a, d, g) \rightarrow$ not possible

III. $8 + 6 = 14$. Then y = 0.
$\therefore$ $b$ (or $e$) $- h = 2 \rightarrow$ not possible from case I.

IV. $8 + 4. = 12$ Then y = 0.
$\therefore$ $b$ (or $e$) $+ 6 = h$ (Not possible from case II.) or $b + e = 6$ $(a, d, g) \rightarrow$ not possible

**(c) The correct option is (i). EXPLANATION:**

Let $c + f + i = 2(i + 5)$
$b + e + h = 2(h + 5) - 1$
$a + d + g = 2g - 1$

$\because$ $(c, f, i) \Rightarrow$ odd, odd, even or even, even, even
$(b, f, h) \Rightarrow$ odd, even, even, or odd, odd, odd
$(a, d, g) \Rightarrow$ odd, even, even, or odd, odd, odd

they cannot give four even numbers and five odd numbers.

**(d) The correct option is (i). EXPLANATION:**

Let $c + f + i = 2(i + 10)$
$b + e + h = 2(h - 1)$
$a + d + g = 2g$

$\because$ in each triplets, there are either two odd numbers and one even number or three even numbers and they cannot give four even numbers and five odd numbers.

**310.** Let $x$ be the number. Then

$$4x = 3072 \text{ or } 3076 \text{ or } 3700 \text{ or } 3704 \text{ or } 3708$$

$$\Rightarrow x = 768 \text{ or } 769 \text{ or } 925 \text{ or } 926 \text{ or } 927$$

$$\Rightarrow 3x = \underbrace{2304 \text{ or } 2307}_{\text{only this is valid}} \text{ or } 2775 \text{ or } 2778 \text{ or } 2781$$

$$\Rightarrow 5x = \underbrace{3840}_{\text{only this is valid}} \text{ or } 3845 \qquad \therefore x = 768$$

$$\therefore \quad x = 768 \text{ or } 769$$

**So the correct options for (a) and (b) are (iii) and (ii) respectively.**

**311.** There can be three cases for first digits of each number.

$$\begin{array}{l} 1\,\_\_\;\_\_ \\ 3\,\_\_\;\_\_ \end{array} \quad \text{or} \quad \begin{array}{l} 2\,\_\_\;\_\_ \\ 2\,\_\_\;\_\_ \end{array} \quad \text{or} \quad \begin{array}{l} 1\,\_\_\;\_\_ \\ 2\,\_\_\;\_\_ \end{array}$$

$$\left\{\begin{array}{ccc} 1 & 2 & 5 \\ 3 & 4 & 1 \end{array}\right. \updownarrow \qquad \left\{\begin{array}{ccc} 2 & 1 & 9 \\ 2 & 4 & 7 \end{array}\right. \updownarrow \updownarrow \qquad \left\{\begin{array}{ccc} 1 & 9 & 3 \\ 2 & 7 & 3 \end{array}\right. \updownarrow \text{ or } \begin{array}{c} 2 \\ 4 \end{array} \text{ or } \begin{array}{c} 5 \\ 1 \end{array}$$

$$\left\{\begin{array}{ccc} 1 & 5 & 2 \\ 3 & 1 & 4 \end{array}\right. \updownarrow \qquad \left\{\begin{array}{ccc} 1 & 9 & 8 \\ 2 & 6 & 8 \end{array}\right. \updownarrow \text{ or } \begin{array}{c} 7 \\ 9 \end{array} \updownarrow$$

$$\left\{\begin{array}{ccc} 1 & 3 & 9 \\ 3 & 2 & 7 \end{array}\right. \updownarrow \qquad \left\{\begin{array}{ccc} 1 & 7 & 7 \\ 2 & 8 & 9 \end{array}\right.$$

$$\left\{\begin{array}{ccc} 1 & 4 & 9 \\ 3 & 1 & 7 \end{array}\right. \updownarrow$$

where $\updownarrow$ denotes the interchangeability of digits.

**So the correct options for (a), (b) and (c) are (iv), (iii) and (iv) respectively.**

**312.** Let the number be $ABC$. Then $A + B + C = 10$. Also $A < 3$.

$2A + 2B + 2C = 20$. Now sum of digits of $2(ABC)$ is 11.

$\therefore$ only one of $B$, $C$ must be 5 or greater than 5.

($\because$ $2 \cdot 10 - 10 + 1 = 11$). Again $3A + 3B + 3C = 30$ and the sum of digits of $3(ABC)$ is 21 $(30 - 10 + 1)$.

$\therefore$ only one of them must be greater than 3 and it should be less than 7 (as it makes the sum 12 or 22).

$\therefore$ the digits can be

$$\underset{A}{(1, 3, 6)}, \qquad \underset{A}{(2, 2, 6)} \qquad \text{or} \qquad \underset{A}{(2, 3, 5)}$$

and the numbers can be 163, 226, 262 or 253.

**So the correct options for (a), (b) and (c) are (ii), (iii) and (ii) respectively.**

**313.** $xy \times yx = xxab$

Note that when $xxab$ is divided by $xy$, then the quotient must be less than 100 but close to it.

$\because$ from part (a), $x \geq 5$ $\therefore$ $y$ has to be 9.

And $x9 \times 9x = xxab$

$\Rightarrow (10x + 9)(90 + x) = xxab$

$\Rightarrow xxab = 10x^2 + 909x + 810$

$$\Rightarrow 11x \simeq \frac{x^2}{10} + 9x + 8 \quad \text{(neglecting few irrelevant terms)}$$

$$\Rightarrow 2x \simeq \frac{x^2}{10} + 8$$

$$\Rightarrow x \simeq 4 + \frac{x^2}{20}$$

Checking $x = 5, 6, ....$, we have

$95 \times 59 = 95 \times (60 - 1) = 5700 - 95 = 5605$ ... rejected

$96 \times 69 = 96 \times (70 - 1) = 6720 - 96 = 6624$ ... retained

**So the correct options for (a), (b) and (c) are (ii), (i) and (ii) respectively.**

**314.** Note that from $zx \times y =$ __ __ 1, $x$, $y$ can be odd and $(x, y) = (3, 7)$ or $(7, 3)$.

Now $xy \times z =$ __ 8 __

$$\therefore \begin{cases} 37 \times z = \text{—}8\text{—} \Rightarrow z = 5 \\ 73 \times z = \text{—}8\text{—} \Rightarrow z = 8 \end{cases}$$

Also $yz \times x = 2$ __ __

The cases $75 \times 3 = 225$ and $38 \times 7 = 266$ are verified.

$\therefore$ $(x, y, z) = (3, 7, 5)$ or $(7, 3, 8)$

**So the correct options for (a) and (b) are (iv) and (i) respectively.**

**315. A.** $3x \times y7 = 1a3b$

Note that y can be only 3, 4 or 5.

$\therefore$ digit at ten digit place of

$(30 + x)(10y + 7)$ is 3

$\Rightarrow$ $10\, x \cdot y + 10 + 7x$ is 3

$\Rightarrow$ $x \cdot (10y + 7)$ is 2

$\Rightarrow$ $x \times 37, 47$ or $57$ is 2

$x \times (40 - 3), (50 - 3)$ or $(60 - 3)$ is 2

$\therefore$ $x$ can be equal to 6, 9 or 4 respectively.

Now $3x \times y7 = 1a3b$

$3x \times y7 = 1a3b$

$36 \times 37 = 1332$

$39 \times 47 = 1833$ and

$34 \times 57 = 1938$

**So the correct options for (a), (b), (c) and (d) are (iii), (iv), (ii) and (iii) respectively.**

**B.** $w87 \times 15w = x92yz$.

Note that 687 × 150 is a six-digit number.

$\therefore$ Checking for $w = 1, 2, 3, 4, 5$, we get the product as 28237, 43624, 59211, ...

$\therefore$ $w = 3, x = 5, y = 1, z = 1$

(we need not check $w = 4, 5$ as from part (a), (b) there are unique values of $x$, $y$)

**So the correct options for (a) and (b) are (iii) and (i) respectively.**

**316.** $ab \times bx = y0x$.

$\therefore$ either $b = 1$ or $x = 5$ and b is odd.

($\because$ the last digit of $y0x$ is $x$)

Case I: $b = 1$.

$\because$ $ab + bx = xy$

$\therefore$ $b + x = y$ or $10 + y$

$\Rightarrow$ $x = y - 1$ or $9 + y$ (rejected)

$\because\ ab \times bx = y0x$
$\therefore\ (xy - bx) \times bx = y0x$
$\Rightarrow\ (xy - 1x) \times 1x = y0x$
$\Rightarrow\ (10x - 9) \times (10 + x) = 101x + 100$ (using $x = y - 1$)
$\Rightarrow\ 10x^2 + 91x - 90 = 101x + 100$
$\Rightarrow\ x^2 - x = 19$
$\Rightarrow\ (x - 1/2)^2 = 77/4 \quad \Rightarrow$ Rejected

Case II: $x = 5$ and $b$ is odd
$\because\ ab + bx = xy$
$\therefore\ y = b + 5$ or $b + 5 - 10$ i.e. $b - 5$
Now $\underbrace{(5y - b5)}_{\text{For this to be positive, } b = y - 5} \times b5 = y05$ ($\because\ ab \times bx = y0x$)
$\therefore\ \{50 + y - (y - 5)\cdot 10 - 5\} \times \{10(y - 5) + 5\} = 100\,y + 5$
$\Rightarrow\ (95 - 9y)\cdot(10y - 45) = 100y + 5$
$\because\ y > 5$ and on inspection, $y = 8$ satisfies it
$\therefore\ b = 3$ and $a = 2$ ($\because\ a3 + 35 = 58$)

**So the correct options for (a), (b) (c) and (d) are (ii), (ii), (iii) and (iii) respectively.**

**317.** Note that $37 \times 3 = 111$

$$\therefore\quad 111\overline{)\,A\,B\,C\,C\,C\ldots}\ \text{quotient } A;\quad \begin{array}{l} A\,B\,C\,C\,C\ldots \\ \underline{A\,A\,A} \\ \quad A\,B\,C\ldots \end{array}$$

($\because$ it leaves the constant remainder)

$\therefore\ B - A = A$ and $C - A = B$
$\Rightarrow\ B = 2A$ and $C = 3A$
$\because\ C < 6 \quad \therefore\ A = 1$ and $B = 2$
and the remainder is $AB$ i.e. 12.

**So the correct options for (a), (b) and (c) are (i), (ii) and (i) respectively.**

**318.** $13 \times xy = 8ya = 800 + ya$

$$\Rightarrow\ xy = 61 + \frac{7 + ya}{13}$$

For $a = 8$, $y = 5$ and $xy = 61 + \frac{65}{13} = 66$,

not possible as $y = 5$.

For $a = 7$, $y = 9$ and $xy = 61 + \frac{104}{13} = 69$.

**So the correct options for (a) and (b) are (iii) and (ii) respectively.**

**319.** Let $A, B, C$ be three integers and $A', B', C'$ be them with their digits reversed. Let

$A + B + C' = 147$

$A + B' + C = 156$

$A' + B + C = 165$

$A + B + C = x$

Then $x - 165 = A - A' = \pm 9\, n$, say, where $1 \leq n \leq 9$

Also $(147 + 156 + 165 - x)$ i.e. $(143 + 154 + 165 + 6 - x)$ must be divisible by 11. $\therefore$ let $x - 6 = 11m$.

Then $11m + 6 - 165 = \pm 9n$

$\Rightarrow 11(m - 15) = 3\,(\pm 3n - 2)$

For $\pm 3n - 2$ to be divisible by 11,

$n = 8$ or 3 according as + or − sign is taken.

But for $n = 8$, $x = 237$. But $x < 200$ (as given)

$\therefore$ this case is rejected and consequently,

$n = 3$ and $x = 138$.

Now, note that

$A' - A = 3$, $B' - B = 2$ and $C' - C = 1$.

$\therefore$ $A, B, C$ may be assumed as $p(p + 3)$, $q(q + 2)$ and $r\,(r + 2)$ respectively. $\therefore$ their sum will be

$11(p + q + r) + 6 = 138 \Rightarrow p + q + r = 12$.

**So the correct options for (a), (b) and (c) are (ii), (ii) and (iii) respectively.**

**320.** Let the numbers be $x, y$ and $z$. Then

$xy + yz + zx = 406$ and

$x + y + z = 35$

$\Rightarrow x^2 + y^2 + z^2 + 2(xy + yz + zx) = 35^2 = 1225$

$\Rightarrow x^2 + y^2 + z^2 - (xy + yz + zx) = 1225 - 3 \cdot 406 = 7$

$\Rightarrow (x - y)^2 + (y - z)^2 + (z - x)^2 = 14$

Note that $10 + 12 + 13 = 35$ and

$(13 - 10)^2 + (13 - 12)^2 + (12 - 10)^2 = 14$

∴ the least number is 10 and greatest number is 13.

**So the correct options for (a) and (b) are (i).**

**321.** Note that $(a + 1 + 3 + 5)$ must be divisible by 3.

∴ $a = 0, 3, 6$ or 9.

When $a = 0$, then the integer, say $x$, can be equal to

$$\frac{960}{2} \text{ or } \frac{906}{2} \text{ or } \frac{690}{2} \text{ i.e. } 480 \text{ or } 453 \text{ or } 345$$

and $3x = 1440$ or 1359 or 1035

Now $3x = 1035$ i.e. $x = 345$ satisfies the given conditions.

Also $345 = 23 \times 15$.

**So the correct options for (a) and (b) are (iv) and (iii) respectively.**

**322.** Let the products be $2(abc)$, $2(bca)$ and $2(cab)$.

Note that the product having digits $x$, 3 and 9 will be even.

∴ $x$ has to be an even number. Let

$2(abc) = 93x$

$$\Rightarrow abc = 46\left(\frac{10+x}{2}\right)$$

$$\text{and } \quad 2(bca) = 2\left(6\frac{10+x}{2}4\right) = 13x8$$

$$\text{and } \quad 2(cab) = 2\left(\frac{10+x}{2}46\right) = 1x92$$

∴ although $x$ cannot be determined, $y = 8$.

**So the correct options for (a) and (b) are (iv) and (iii) respectively.**

**323.** Note that sum of digits of $x$ and $y$ are 22.

∴ $(x - 4)$ and $(y - 4)$ will be divisible by 9 as their sum of digits will be 18 which is divisible by 9.

Now $z - 8 = (x - 4) + (y - 4)$

∴ $z - 8$ will also be divisible by 9 as R.H.S is divisible by it. ∴ $a + 6$ will be divisible by 9, i.e. $a + 6 = 9$ or 18.

But as $a$ is a single digit integer

$\therefore \quad a = 3$

Now let us make last digit table for $z$ where each entry denotes the last digit of sum of numbers of each row (digits of $x$) and each column (digits of $y$).

| y \ x | 3 | 4 | 7 | 8 |
|---|---|---|---|---|
| 2 | 5 | 6 | 9 | 0 |
| 5 | 8 | 9 | 2 | 3 |
| 6 | 9 | 0 | 3 | 4 |
| 9 | 2 | 3 | 6 | 7 |

Now only those numbers are retained which are themselves or their predecessor are in ($a$, 3, 5, 6)

$\therefore$ in the table the valid entries are

| y \ x | 3 | 4 | 7 | 8 |
|---|---|---|---|---|
| 2 | 5 | 6 | X | X |
| 5 | X | X | 2 | 3 |
| 6 | X | X | 3 | 4 |
| 9 | 2 | 3 | X | X |

Now each row and each column should give one combination [The following just denotes the digits of $x$ and the corresponding digits of $y$ and they may not be in order]:

$$\left.\begin{matrix} x & = & 3 & 4 & 7 & 8 \\ y & = & 2 & 9 & 5 & 6 \end{matrix}\right] \rightarrow \text{Retained}$$

$$\left.\begin{matrix} x & = & 3 & 4 & 7 & 8 \\ y & = & 2 & 9 & 6 & 5 \end{matrix}\right] \rightarrow \text{Rejected}$$

$$\left.\begin{matrix} x & = & 3 & 4 & 7 & 8 \\ y & = & 9 & 2 & 5 & 6 \end{matrix}\right] \rightarrow \text{Rejected}$$

$$\left.\begin{matrix} x & = & 3 & 7 & 8 & 4 \\ y & = & 2 & 5 & 6 & 9 \end{matrix}\right] \rightarrow \text{Rejected}$$

where only first combination gave the sum having all the digits of $z$, i.e. a, 3, 5, 6.

Now it is obvious that (3 + 2) will be at the thousands place to account for 6 in $z$. $\therefore$ the numbers can be

$$\left.\begin{matrix} x=3874 \\ y=2659 \\ z=6533 \end{matrix}\right\} \quad \text{or} \quad \left.\begin{matrix} x=3784 \\ y=2569 \\ z=6353 \end{matrix}\right\}$$

**So the correct options for (a), (b), (c) and (d) are (ii), (i), (i) and (iv) respectively.**

**324.** Let the four digit number be $ABCD$ which is divisible by 7. Now $ACBD$ is divisible by 11 and $DBCA$ is divisible by 7. Note that $DBCA$ will also be divisible by 11 (as $ACBD$ is divisible by 11). Now

$ABCD + DBCA = 1001\ (A + D) + 2 \cdot BC0$

$= 11 \times 13 \times 7 \cdot (A + D) + 2 \cdot BC0$

As $ABCD$ and $DBCA$ are divisible by 7

$\therefore$ $BC0$ will be divisible by 7.

$\because$ $ABCD$, i.e. $A00D + BC0$ is divisible by 7

$\therefore$ $A00D$ will be divisible by 7

i.e. $A00A + D - A$ i.e. $(1001)\ A + D - A$

i.e. $11 \times 13 \times 7\ A + (D - A)$ is divisible by 7

$\therefore$ $D - A = \pm 7$

Now, as $ACBD$ is divisible by 11

$\therefore$ $B + A = C + D$ or $C + D \pm 11$

$\because$ $D - A = \pm 7$

$\therefore$ $B = C \pm 7$ or $C \pm 4$ (only valid options considered)

Now $BC0$ is divisible by 7 and $(B - C) = 4$ or 7

$\therefore$ the valid options for $BC$ are 84 and 70 and if $D = 0$, then $BC = 84$ as all the digits are different.

**So the correct options for (a), (b) and (c) are (iii), (iv) and (iv) respectively.**

**325.** $ABCD = 1000A + 100B + 10C + D$

$= 1000A + 100B + 10\ (10 - B) + A + B - 9$

($\because$ $C = 10 - B$ and $D = A + B - 9$)

$$= 1001A + 91B + 91$$
$$= 91\ (11A + B + 1)$$
$$= 13 \times 7\ (11A + B + 1)$$

$\therefore$ the number will be divisible by 7 and 13.

**So the correct options for (a) and (b) are (iii) and (i) respectively.**

**326.** Let $(abc)^2 = 12xy49$.

As $300^2 <$ R.H.S. $< 400^2$

$\therefore \quad a = 3$

Now $(bc)^2$ will end in 49 only if

$\quad 20b \cdot c + c^2$ ends in 49

which is possible only if $c = 7$ (c = 3 is not valid)

and $b = 5$

$\therefore \quad (357)^2 = 12xy49$

$\Rightarrow \quad 127449 = 12xy49$

$\therefore \quad x = 7$ and $y = 4$

**So the correct options for (a) and (b) are (iv) and (ii) respectively.**

**327.** Let $\quad a = 1\,2\,3\,4\,5\,6\,7\,8\,9$

$$= 10^8 + 2 \cdot 10^7 + 3 \cdot 10^6 + \ldots\ 9 \cdot 1$$

$$\Rightarrow \quad 10\,a = 10^9 + 2 \cdot 10^8 + 3 \cdot 10^7 + \ldots\ 9 \cdot 10$$

$$10\,a - a = 10^9 + 10^8 + \ldots + 10 - 9$$

$$\Rightarrow \quad 9\,(a + 1) = 1111111110 \quad \text{(nine 1)}$$

$$\Rightarrow 81\,(a^2 + 2a + 1) = 1\,2\,3\,4\,5\,6\,7\,8\,9\,7\,6\,5\,4\,3\,2\,1\,0\,0$$

On division of R.H.S. by 81, we get

$a^2 + 2a + 1 = 1\,5\,2\,4\,1\,5\,7\ \ldots$

[81) 1 2 3 4 5 6 7 8 9 ... (1 5 2 4 1 5 7 ...
    8 1
  × 4 2 4
    4 0 5
  × 1 9 5
    1 6 2
  × 3 3 6
    3 2 4
  × 1 2 7 ]

$$\begin{array}{r} 8\ 1 \\ \hline \times\ 4\ 6\ 8 \\ 4\ 0\ 5 \\ \hline \times\ 6\ 3\ 9 \end{array}$$

$\Rightarrow$ $a^2 = 1\ 5\ 2\ 4\ 1\ 5\ 7$ ... upto 16 digits

– ($a$ 9 digit integer)

$\therefore$ $u\ v\ w\ x\ y\ z = 1\ 5\ 2\ 4\ 1\ 5$

**So the correct options for (a), (b) and (c) are (ii), (i) and (iv) respectively.**

**328.**

$$\begin{array}{cccc} & A & B & C \\ + & 4 & C & D \\ \hline & D & A & B \end{array}$$

Note that

| | | | or | | |
|---|---|---|---|---|---|
| $C + D =$ | $B$ | | or | $10 + B$ | |
| $B + C =$ | $A$ | $10 + A$ | | $A - 1$ | $9 + A$ |
| $A + 4 =$ | $D$ | $D - 1$ | | $D$ | $D - 1$ |

$\therefore$ we can have two cases:

Case I: $C + D = B$, $B + C = A + (10)$, $A + 4 = D - (1)$

(where the bracket means that the number inside it may or may not be there)

$$\Rightarrow \begin{cases} B + C = D - 4 - (1) + 10 \\ C + D = B \end{cases}$$

Adding, we get

$2C = 10 - 4 \Rightarrow C = 3.$

Now $3 + D = B$, $A + 4 = D$, $B = A + 7$

$\therefore$ $A = 1$ or $2$, $B = 8$ or $9$, $D = 5$ or $6$

Case II: $C + D = B + 10$, $B + C = A - 1 + (10)$, $A + 4 = D - (1)$

$$\Rightarrow \begin{cases} B + C = D - 5 + (10) - (1) \\ C + D = B + 10 \end{cases}$$

Adding, we get,

$2C = 5 + (10) - (1)$

The possibilities are

$2C = 4$ or $14 \Rightarrow C = 2$ or $7$

For $C = 2$, $D = B + 8$, $B = A - 3$, $A = D - 5$

$\therefore B = 1$, $A = 4$, $D = 9$

For $C = 7$, $D = B + 3$, $B = A + 2$, $A = D - 5$

$\Rightarrow D = 6, 8$ or $9$

$A = 1, 3$ or $4$

$B = 3, 5$ or $6$

$\therefore$ there can be 5 possibilities for $A$ (viz. 1, 2, 4, 6, 3)
6 possibilities for $B$ (viz. 8, 9, 1, 3, 5, 6)
3 possibilities for $C$ (viz. 3, 2, 7)
4 possibilities for $D$ (viz. 5, 6, 9, 8)

**So the correct options for (a), (b), (c) and (d) are (iv), (iv), (ii) and (iii) respectively.**

**329.**

$$\begin{array}{cccc} & A & B & C \\ + & 2 & C & 8 \\ + & D & E & B \\ \hline 1 & A & 1 & E \end{array}$$

Note that $C + 8 + B = 10 + E$ or $20 + E$

$\Rightarrow C + B - E = 2$ or $12$

and $(1, 2) + B + C + E = 11$ or $21$

$\Rightarrow B + C + E = 10$ or $20$

($\because$ if $B + C + E = 9$ or $19$, then compounded with $C + B - E = 2$ or $12$, E will not be an integer)

Also $(1, 2) + A + 2 + D = 10 + A$

$\Rightarrow (1, 2) + D = 8$

Now if $B + C + E = 10$, then

$C + B - E = 2$ and consequently,

$E = 4$ and $D = 7$

If $B + C + E = 20$, then

$C + B - E = 2$ (12 not possible as it would have made $B + C + E = 9$ or $19$)

and $D = 6$.

$\therefore B + C - E = 2$ and $E + 5D = 39$ for both of the above cases.

**So the correct options for (a) and (b) are (i) and (iii) respectively.**

**330.**

$$\begin{array}{cccc} & A & 1 & B \\ + & 3 & C & D \\ + & E & F & 2 \\ \hline 1 & 6 & 6 & 5 \end{array}$$

We have B + D = 13

$\therefore$ (B, D) ≡ (4, 9) or (5, 8) or (6, 7)

Now C + F ≠ 4 $\therefore$ C + F = 14 and A + E = 12.

i.e. (C, F) ≡ (5, 9) or (6, 8) and (A, E) ≡ (4, 8) or (5, 7).

$\therefore$ We have

(B, D); (C, F) and (A, E) ≡ (4, 9); (6, 8) and (5, 7) or (6, 7); (5, 9) and (4, 8)

**So the correct options for (a) and (b) are (ii) and (i) respectively.**

**331.**

$$\begin{array}{ccccc} & A & B & C & D \\ + & B & C & D & A \\ + & C & D & A & B \\ \hline 1 & ? & D & C & A \end{array}$$

Note that $D + B = 10$

$D + A = 9$

$B + C = 9$

Now $? =$ last digit of $(1 + A + B + C)$, i.e. $(10 + A)$ which will be $A$

$\therefore$ $? = A$

Also $9 - C + 9 - A = 10$ $(\because B + C = 10)$

$\Rightarrow A + C = 8.$

**So the correct options for (a) and (b) are (i) and (iv) respectively.**

**332.** $ab \times bc \times ca = (10a + b) \times (10b + c) \times (10c + a)$

$= 1000\, a \cdot b \cdot c + 100\,(a^2 b + b^2 c + c^2 a)$

$+ 10\,(a^2 c + b^2 a + c^2 b) + a \cdot b \cdot c$

Note that $a \cdot b \cdot c$ must be less than and near 98.
Also it must end in 2.

$\therefore$ checking for $a, b, c \equiv 9, 2, 4 \rightarrow$ Not possible
$\equiv 9, 8, 1 \rightarrow$ Not possible
$\equiv 6, 4, 3 \rightarrow$ Possible

and $34 \times 46 \times 63 = 98532$

i.e. $a = 3$, $b = 4$, $c = 6$ and $d = 5$.

**So the correct options for (a), (b), (c) and (d) are (i), (i), (iii) and (ii) respectively.**

**333.**

$$\begin{array}{cccc} & a & b & c \\ & \times & d & 7 \\ \hline c & b & d & a \end{array}$$

Note that from part (c),
$c = 3, 4, 7$ or 9
We can have four cases:

| | | | | | |
|---|---|---|---|---|---|
| $c$ | = | 3 | 4 | 7 | 9 |
| $a$ | = | 1 | 8 | 9 | 3 |
| $d$ | = | 2 | N.P | N.P | 2 or 3 (3, not possible as $a$, $d$ are distinct) |

(N. P. $\rightarrow$ Not possible)
($d$ is estimated mainly with the help of $c$ in the product)
$\therefore$ we have

$$\begin{array}{cccc} & 1 & b & 3 \\ & \times & 2 & 7 \\ \hline 3 & b & 2 & 1 \end{array} \quad \text{or} \quad \begin{array}{cccc} & 3 & b & 9 \\ & \times & 2 & 7 \\ \hline 9 & b & 2 & 3 \end{array}$$

For the product to be divisible by 27, the sum of digits of the product must be divisible by 9. $\therefore$ $b = 3$ or 4 respectively. For first of the above cases, $b = 3$ is rejected as $b$, $c$ are distinct. $\therefore$ from second case $(a, b, c, d) \equiv (3, 4, 9, 2)$

**So the correct options for (a), (b), (c) and (d) are (ii), (ii), (iv) and (ii) respectively.**

**334.**

$$\begin{array}{rrrrrrr} & A & B & C & 9 & 4 & 7 \\ & & & & & \times & B \\ \hline D & B & D & 3 & B & C & A \end{array}$$

Note that from options,
$A = 1, 2, 6, 8$ correspond to $B = 3, 6, 8$ and 4.
Checking for $B$, we have

$$\begin{array}{rrrr} & 9 & 4 & 7 \\ & & \times & 3 \\ \hline 2 & 8 & 4 & 1 \end{array} \qquad \begin{array}{rrrr} & 9 & 4 & 7 \\ & & \times & 6 \\ \hline 5 & 6 & 8 & 2 \end{array}$$

$\therefore B = 6$, i.e. $A = 2$ is found to be valid.
$\therefore C = 8$ and

$$\begin{array}{rrrrrrr} & 2 & 6 & 8 & 9 & 4 & 7 \\ & & & & & \times & 6 \\ \hline - & - & - & 1 & 3 & 6 & 8 \end{array} \qquad \therefore D = 1$$

**So the correct options for (a), (b) and (c) are (ii), (iv) and (i) respectively.**

**335.**

$$\begin{array}{rrrrr} & & C & A & B \\ & & \times & B & A \\ \hline B & 2 & D & 4 & O \end{array}$$

The product is

$$\begin{aligned}(100 + AB) \times BA &= 100 \cdot C \cdot (BA) + AB \times BA \\ &= 100 \cdot C \cdot (BA) + (10A + B) \times (10B + A) \\ &= 100 \cdot C \cdot (BA) + 100\, A \cdot B + 10\,(A^2 + B^2) + A \cdot B\end{aligned}$$

Now one of $A$, $B$ must be 5.
For the last two digits of the product to be 40, the other one must be 6.
Now $B2D = C \cdot (BA) + 30 + 6$
and $BA = 56$ or 65.

Case I: $B = 5$, $A = 6$. Then
$52D = (56) \cdot C + 36$
No value of $C$, $D$ are possible.

Case II: $B = 6, A = 5$. Then

$62D = (65)\cdot C + 36$

$C = 9$ satisfies it and $D = A$

**So the correct options for (a), (b), (c) and (d) are (ii), (iii) (iv) and (i) respectively.**

**336.**

$$\begin{array}{cccc} & A & B & C \\ & \times & A & B \\ \hline B & D & D & B \end{array}$$

There can be three different cases, viz.

$C = 1$ or $C \to$ odd and $B$ or $C = 6$, $B = 8$

Case I: Let $C$ be 1. Then $A$ cannot be double figure as the product is a four digit number.

$\therefore$ $A = 2$ or 3 and correspondingly

$B = (5, 6, 7, 8)$ or 9

Checking for $A = 2$,

$$\begin{array}{cccc} & 2 & B & 1 \\ & & 2 & B \\ \hline B & D & D & B \end{array}$$, no value of $B$ is found to be valid.

Similarly, checking for $A = 3$, the case is not found to be possible.

Case II: Let $C \to$ odd and $B = 5$

$\therefore$ $A = 2$ and checking for

$$\begin{array}{cccc} & 2 & 5 & C \\ & \times & 2 & 5 \\ \hline 5 & D & D & 5 \end{array},$$

no values of $C$ (viz. 1, 3, 7, 9) are found to be valid.

Case III: Let $C = 6$, $B = 8$

$\therefore$ $A = 2$ and

$$\begin{array}{cccc} & 2 & 8 & 6 \\ & \times & 2 & 8 \\ \hline 8 & 0 & 0 & 8 \end{array}$$ is found to be valid.

**So the correct options for (a), (b), (c) and (d) are (ii), (iii), (iii) and (i) respectively.**

**337.**

$$\begin{array}{r} A\ B\ C \\ \times\ D\ 6 \\ \hline 9\ 9\ B\ C \end{array}$$

Note that $(A00 + BC) \times D6 = 9900 + BC$

$\Rightarrow A \times D6 \times 100 + BC \times (D5 + 1) = 9900 + BC$

$\Rightarrow A \times D6 \times 100 + BC \times D5 = 9900$

Now $BC \times D5$ must be a multiple of 100

which is only possible if $BC$ is an even multiple of 5 or $D5$ is a multiple of 25.

$\because C \neq 0$ from options, $\therefore D$ is a multiple of 25

and $D = 2$ or 7. From options, $D = 2$.

Now $A$ can be equal to 3 only

$\because \quad BC \times 25 < 2500$ and

$4 \times 26 \times 100 > 10000$

$\therefore \quad 3 \times 26 \times 100 + BC \times 25 = 9900$

$\Rightarrow \quad 12 \times 26 + BC = 99 \times 4$

$\Rightarrow \quad BC = (33 - 26) \times 12$

$= 7 \times 12 \quad = 84$

**So the correct options for (a), (b), (c) and (d) are (iii), (iv), (ii) and (ii) respectively.**

**338.**

$$\begin{array}{r} A\ 6\ B \\ \times\ 4\ C \\ \hline 1\ B\ C\ 8\ A \end{array}$$

$\because$ the product is a five digit number

$\therefore A$ can be equal to 2, 3 or 4.

If $A = 2$, then $B$, $C$ can be equal to (4, 8) or (8, 9)

But $A64$ or $A68$ is divisible by 4 while the product ending in 82 is not divisible by 4.

$\therefore A = 2$ is not possible.

Checking for $A = 3$, $B$, $C$ can be equal to (7, 9) or (9, 7). Now

$$\begin{array}{r} 3\ 6\ 9 \\ \times\ 4\ 7 \\ \hline 3 \end{array}$$

↳ this is not 8
∴ rejected

$$\begin{array}{r} 3\ 6\ 7 \\ \times\ 4\ 9 \\ \hline 1\ 7\ 9\ 8\ 3 \end{array}$$

Found to be valid
∴ A = 3, B = 7 and C = 9

**So the correct options for (a), (b) and (c) are (iii), (ii) and (iv) respectively.**

**339.**

$$\begin{array}{r} 1\ a\ b \\ \times\ c\ 7 \\ \hline 6\ a\ 0\ a \end{array}$$

It is prudent to ascertain the value of a and c first.
From options,

| | | | | |
|---|---|---|---|---|
| *c* can be | 3 | 4 | 5 | 6 |
| *a* can be | >5 | 3 | 1 or 2 | 1 |
| | | Rejected | Rejected | Rejected |

(as $a > 6$, from options)

$\therefore c = 3$
Now, the remainder when $6a0a$ is divided by 37 is $6 + 27a$

$$\left(\because \frac{6000 + 101a}{37} \text{ gives the remainder as } 6 + 27a\right)$$

For $6 + 27a$ to be divisible by 37,
$6 - 10a$ must be divisible by 37 which is possible for $a = 8$.
$\therefore a = 8$ and consequently $b = 4$.

**So the correct options for (a), (b) and (c) are (iii), (ii) and (i) respectively.**

**340.**

$$\begin{array}{r} a\ b\ 6 \\ \times\ 7\ a \\ \hline 2\ b\ 9\ c\ c \end{array}$$

Note that $a$ can be 3 or 4 only since the first digit of the product is 2.
If $a = 3$, then $c = 8$, $b = 5$ and

$$\begin{array}{r} 3\ 5\ 6 \\ \times\ 7\ 3 \\ \hline 2\ 5\ 9\ 8\ 8 \end{array}$$

$\therefore$ $a = 3$, $b = 5$ and $c = 8$ are verified.

**So the correct options for (a) and (b) are (iii) and (iv) respectively.**

**341.**

$$\begin{array}{r} 5\ a\ 6 \\ \times\ 2\ b \\ \hline c\ b\ 2\ d\ e \end{array}$$

Note that $a, b, c, d, e \equiv \{0, 1, 3, 4, 7, 8, 9\}$
Obviously $c = 1$ as first digit of product has to be 1.
Now $5b$ cannot be more than 20 as $b$ cannot be equal to 5, 6 or 7, 8, 9 (the first two digits of product, i.e. $1b$ cannot be possible).
If $b = 0$ or 4, $e$ will also become 0 or 4 respectively
$\therefore$ $b = 3$ is the only possibility and consequently $e = 8$.
Now $a = 0, 4, 7$ or 9
If $a = 0$, then $d = 2$, not possible
If $a = 4$, then $d = 5$, not possible
If $a = 7$, then $d = 4$
If $a = 9$, then $d = 0$
$\therefore$ there can be two cases:

$$\begin{array}{r} 5\ 7\ 6 \\ \times\ 2\ 3 \\ \hline 1\ 3\ 2\ 4\ 8 \end{array} \quad \text{or} \quad \begin{array}{r} 5\ 9\ 6 \\ \times\ 2\ 3 \\ \hline 1\ 3\ 7\ 0\ 8 \end{array}$$

**So the correct options for (a), (b) and (c) are (iii), (iv) and (iv) respectively.**

**342.** Let $ABC$ be one of the numbers. Adding all the permutations, we get the sum as

$$2 \times 111 \times (A + B + C) = 827 + 980 + 1079 \text{ (given)}$$
$$= 2886$$

$\Rightarrow A + B + C = 13$

Now from last digits of the sum, let

$A + B = 10$, $B + C = 7$ or 17 and $C + A = 9$

If $B + C = 17$, then $A = 1$, $B = 9$, $C = 8$, not possible one of the sum is 827.

If $B + C = 7$, then $A = 6$, B = 4, $C = 3$

$\therefore$ $827 = 364 + 463$

$980 = 346 + 634$

$1079 = 436 + 643$

**So the correct options for (a), (b) and (c) are (iv).**

**343.** Let $x = ab$ and $y = cde$.

Now difference of two pairs of given numbers will be of the form : $(cde) - (edc) = 99\ (c - e)$

Now from given sums,

$911 - 713 = 198$. Assuming $e < c$,

$c - e = 2$ and $ab + edc = 713$

$ab + cde = 911$

$ba + edc = 731$

Also $9(b - a) = 731 - 713 = 18 \Rightarrow b - a = 2$.

$\therefore$ $10a + (2 + a) + 100e + 10d + (e + 2) = 713$

$\Rightarrow 11a + 10d = 709 - 101e$

Note that $e$ can be equal to 6 only and consequently,

$11a + 10d = 103$

$\Rightarrow a = 103 - 10\ (a + d)$

$\because$ $a$ is single digit positive integer

$\therefore$ $a + d = 10$ and $a = 3$ which gives $d = 7$.

**So the correct options for (a), (b) and (c) are (iii), (i) and (iii) respectively.**

**344.** Note that $y \times (.8072) \simeq x$

$\Rightarrow .8y + .0072 \times y \simeq x$

$\Rightarrow 4y + .036 \times y \simeq 5x$ (one multiplication by 5)

$\Rightarrow 5x - 4y \simeq .036 \times y$

Now R.H.S. can be 1, 2 or 3 only

We will have three cases:

Case I: $.036 \times y \simeq 1 \Rightarrow y \simeq \frac{1}{.036} \simeq 27.7$

Also precisely $y \leq 27.7$

$\therefore$ $y = 27$

Case II: $.036 \times y \simeq 2 \Rightarrow y \simeq \dfrac{2}{.036} \simeq 55.5$

$\therefore y = 55$

Case III: $.036 \times y = 3 \Rightarrow y \simeq \dfrac{3}{.036} \simeq 83.3$

$\therefore y = 83$

Now $5x - 4\ (27, 55, 83) = 1, 2, 3$ respectively

$5x = (108, 220, 332) + 1, 2, 3$ respectively

only $y = 83$ and consequently $x = 67$ is found to be valid.

**So the correct options for (a), (b), (c) and (d) are (iv), (iii), (i) and (iv) respectively.**

**345. A.** Let the numbers be $a$ and $b$. Then

$$ab = 216500 + xy$$
$$\Rightarrow 4ab = 86000 + 4xy$$
$$\Rightarrow (a + b)^2 - (a - b)^2 = 866000 + 4xy$$
$$\Rightarrow 1000000 - (a - b)^2 = 866000 - 4xy$$
$$\Rightarrow |a - b| = \sqrt{134000 - 4xy}$$

Now 13400 is slightly less than 366 and $4xy$ cannot be more than 364

$$\therefore \sqrt{134000 - 4xy} = 366$$
$$\Rightarrow 134000 - 4xy = 366^2 = 133956$$
$$\Rightarrow 4xy = 44$$
$$\Rightarrow xy = 11$$

**So the correct options for (a) and (b) are (i).**

**B.** Let the number be $100 + x$ and $300 + y$

$$\therefore (100 + x)(300 + y) = 31411$$
$$\Rightarrow (3x + y)\,100 + xy = 1411$$
$$\Rightarrow xy = 1411 - (3x + y)\,100$$

Now $3x + y \le 14$

$\because x \cdot y$ cannot be greater than 100

$\therefore 3x + y = 14$ and $x \cdot y = 11$

$x = 1$ and $y = 11$

**So the correct options for (a) and (b) are (ii).**

**346.** Given $x \times 90 + 1 = y \times 90 + 1{\cdot}1y$

$\Rightarrow (x - y) \times 90 + 1 = 11y$

$\Rightarrow 88\ (x - y) + 2\ (x - y) + 1 = 11y$

$$\Rightarrow 8\ (x - y) + \frac{2(x-y)+1}{11} = y$$

| Value of $(x - y)$ possible: | 5 | 16 | 27 | 38 |
|---|---|---|---|---|
| | $\downarrow$ | $y = 131$ | $y = 221$ | $y = 311$ |
| | Rejected as $x$, $y$ are three digits integers | $x = 147$ | $x = 248$ | $x = 349$ |

**So the correct options for (a) and (b) are (ii) and (iv) respectively.**

**347.** Note that in sum, there has to be one carry for sum of digits of every place and it has to be 1 and cannot be equal to 2. Now the equivalent of digits on subtracting 5 from each digit will be (0, 1, 3, 4) and (1, 2, 3, 4).

Now the digits of the sum are 1, 2, 5, 6 and 8.

To account for 8, we must have (4, 4) in unit digit place or (4, 3) in other places.

To account for 6, we must have (4, 2) in unit digit place or (4, 1), (3, 2) in other places.

To account for 5, we must have (3, 2), (4, 1) in unit digit place or (4, 0), (3, 1) in other places.

To account for 2, we must have (0, 2), (1, 1) in unit digit place or (0, 1) in other places.

Note that 1 will be the first digit of the sum.

Case I: $\overline{(4,4)}$ in unit digit place, then other digits place will have (3, 2), (3, 1), (0, 1) which is valid as the two groups of numbers can have (0, 1, 3, 4) and (1, 2, 3, 4).

Case II: (4, 3) in other places, then such pairs can be $\overline{(4,2)}$, (3, 1), (0, 1) ; (4, 1), $\overline{(3,2)}$, (0, 1); (4, 1), (3, 1), $\overline{(0,2)}$; (3, 2), $\overline{(4,1)}$, (0, 1) or (3, 2), (4, 0), $\overline{(1,1)}$

(The bars above numbers indicate that they are at unit digit place)

**So the correct options for (a), (b), (c), (d) and (e) are (iv), (iii), (i), (ii) and (i) respectively.**

**348.** Note that $ab \times bc \times ca > a0 \times b0 \times c0$

$\Rightarrow 11xxy4 > (a \cdot b \cdot c) \cdot 1000$

$\therefore$ the product $a \cdot b \cdot c$ must be less than 4.

Checking the options for $y$, we find that y is odd.

$\therefore$ the product is divisible by 2 but not by 4.

Consequently two of $(a, b, c)$ must be odd and third even.

$\therefore$ the viable options for $(a, b, c)$ are

(3, 7, 4) or (3, 9, 2)

Now $37 \times 74 \times 43 = 117734$

$34 \times 47 \times 73 = 116654$

We need not check (3, 9, 2) as the options contain only two numbers which have already been found.

**So the correct options for (a), (b), (c) and (d) are (ii), (i), (ii) and (iv) respectively.**

**349.** Given $7 \times (5, 6, 8, 9) = (2, 6, 8, 9, 9)$

Note that the last digit of product can be 3, 6, 2 or 5 only.

Also first digit of the product can be 3, 4, 5 or 6 only.

$\therefore 7 \times \_\,\_\,\_\,6 = 6\,\_\,\_\,\_\,2$

Also third digit (ten's place) of number can be only 5 as

$7 \times 5\ (= 35) + 4\ \text{(carry)} = 39$

$$\left.\begin{array}{lll} 7 \times 8 & +4 & = 60 \\ 7 \times 9 & +4 & = 67 \end{array}\right\} \text{Rejected}$$

Now second digit of number can be only 8 as

$7 \times 8 + 3$ (carry) $= 59$

$7 \times 9 + 3 = 66$; rejected.

$\therefore 7 \times 9856 = 68992$

**So the correct options for (a) and (b) are (iii) and (iv) respectively.**

**350. (a) The correct option is (iv). EXPLANATION:**

Let $x = 123...9 = 10^8 + 2.10^7 + ... + 9$

On multiplication by 10, we get

$10x = 10^9 + 2.10^8 + ...9.10$

Subtraction gives

$9x = 10^9 + 10^8 + ...\ 10 + 1 - 10$

$$= \frac{10^{10}-1}{9} - 10$$

$\Rightarrow 81x = 10^{10} - 91$

$\therefore$ sum of digits of $(81x)$ will be

$9 + 0 + 8 \times 9 = 81$

**(b) The correct option is (iii). EXPLANATION:**

Note that $12345678987654321 = (111111111)^2$

$\therefore$ the given product is $81 \times (111111111)^2$

$= (999999999)^2$

$= (10^{10} - 1)^2$

$= 10^{20} - 2\cdot10^{10} + 1$

$\therefore$ sum of digits will be $1 + 8 + 9 \times 9 = 90$

**351.** The given number is

$10^{12}x + 10^6y + 20 + z$

$= (10^{12} - 2\cdot10^6 + 1)\, x + (2x + y)\, 10^6 + 20 + z - x$

$= (10^6 - 1)^2\, x + (2x + y)\,(10^6 - 2\cdot10^3 + 1) + 2\cdot10^3\,(2x + y)$

$+ 20 + z - 3x - y$

The first two terms are divisible by 81.

Also $2\cdot10^3 = 81 \times 25 - 25$

$\therefore$ for the given number to be divisible by 81,

$-25\,(2x + y) + 20 + z - 3x - y$ must be divisible by 81.

i.e. $-27\,(2x + y) + x + y + 20 + z$ must be divisible by 81.

i.e. $2x + y = 4$ or 7 or 10 or 13 and

$x + y + z = 7$

Now we can have four cases:

Case I: $2x + y = 4 \Rightarrow x = 1, y = 2, z = 4$

Case II: $2x + y = 7 = x + y + z \Rightarrow x = z$ which cannot be possible as $x, y, z$ are distinct.

Case III: $2x + y = 10 \Rightarrow x = 4, y = 2, z = 1$

Case IV: $2x + y = 13 \Rightarrow x - z = 6$, rejected as $x \le 6$

**So the correct options for (a), (b) and (c) are (iv), (ii) and (iv) respectively.**

**352.** Consider the following table:

| Product | Sum of digits |
|---|---|
| $7 \times 2$ | 5 |
| $7 \times 3$ | 3 |
| $7 \times 4$ | 10 |
| $7 \times 5$ | 8 |
| $7 \times 6$ | 6 |
| $7 \times 7$ | 13 |
| $7 \times 8$ | 11 |
| $7 \times 9$ | 9 |

Now let S(X) denotes sum of digits of $7 \times x$. Then

S(A) + S(B) = 14 or 24
S(B) + S(C) = 9 or 19
S(C) + S(A) = 11 or 21

Now if S = S(A) + S(B) + S(C), then S can be equal to 17, 22, 27 or 32.

For S = 17,
S(A) = 8, S(B) = 6, S(C) = 3 i.e. A, B, C ≡ 5, 6, 3 respectively.

For S = 22,
S(A) + S(B) ≠ 24 and S(C) + S(A) ≠ 21
∴ S(B) + S(C) = 19
Consequently, S(A) = 3, S(B) = 11 and S(C) = 8
⇒ A, B, C ≡ 3, 8, 5 respectively.

For S = 27,
S(B) + S(C) ≠ 9 and S(C) + S(A) ≠ 11.
∴ S(A) = 8, S(B) = 6 and S(C) = 13.
⇒ A, B, C ≡ 5, 6, 7 respectively.

For S = 32,
S(A) = 13, S(B) = 11 and S(C) = 8
⇒ A, B, C ≡ 7, 8, 5 respectively.

**So the correct options for (a), (b) and (c) are (iii), (iii) and (ii) respectively.**

**353.** Let *a*, *b*, *c* be the sum of digits of *A*, *B* and *C* respectively. Note that in any sum

$$\begin{array}{cc} x & y \\ +\ p & q \\ \hline (x+p) & (y+q) \end{array},$$

the sum of digit is $(x + p + y + q)$ or
$x + p + y + q - 10 + 1$ or $x + p + y + q - 20 + 2$.

Similarly in any subtraction,

$$\begin{array}{rcc} & x & y \\ - & p & q \\ \hline & (x-p) & (y-q) \end{array}$$

the sum of digits is $(x + y - p - q)$ or $(x - 1 - p) + (10 - y - q)$

Now $\quad a + b - c = 6$ or 15 (From subtraction explanation)

$b + c - a = 11$ or 2 (not possible)

$a + c - b = 13$ or 4 (not possible)

Now again $a + b - c = 6$ is also not possible as it makes

$2a = 6 + 13 = 19$

$\therefore a + b - c = 15$. Together with

$b + c - a = 11$ and $a + c - b = 13$, we get

$$a = \frac{15+13}{2} = 14,\ b = 13 \text{ and } c = 12$$

Now sum of digits of $(A + B + C)$ can be equal to

$$\left.\begin{array}{l} 14 + 13 + 12 = 39 \\ 39 - 10 + 1 = 28 \\ 39 - 20 + 2 = 21 \end{array}\right\} \begin{array}{l} \text{not possible as } A + B + C \text{ may} \\ \text{be 3 digit number} \le 300 \\ \text{but its maximum value} < 21 \end{array}$$

$$39 - 30 + 3 = 12$$

**So the correct options for (a), (b) and (c) are (iv), (iii), (ii) and (i) respectively.**

**354.** Note that the four digit number is not divisible by 3 (as the sum of digit of the numbers is not divisible by 3) but the product which digits are (0, 1, 4, 7, 9) is divisible by 3 or 6. We can have two cases:

Case I: $3 \times (3, 5, 8, 9) \equiv (0, 1, 4, 7, 9)$

The product of 3 and the digits of the number will be 9, 15, 24, 27 and the carries can be 1 or 2.

$\therefore$ 8 will be the last digit of the number. And 9 cannot be the first digit of the number $\therefore$ 27 will be added to one of the carries (1 or 2) and $\because$ there is no 8 in the product $\therefore$ the carry will be 2. So the number will be __ __ 98.

Now second digit has to be 5 to account for 7 in the product. ∴ the number will be 3598 and

$3 \times 3598 = 10794 \rightarrow x = 3$

$4 \times 3598 = 14392 \rightarrow$ Rejected

$5 \times 3598 = 17990 \rightarrow y = 5$,

$6 \times 3598$, not possible

$7 \times 3598 = 25168 \rightarrow z = 7$.

Case II: $6 \times (3, 5, 8, 9) = 0, 1, 4, 7, 9$

This case need not be checked as all the options can be answered by the first case only.

**So the correct options for (a), (b), (c), (d) and (e) are (i), (ii), (iii), (iv) and (iii) respectively.**

**355.** Consider the product which digits are (1, 3, 4, 9).

Note that the product can be either odd or may be divisible by 2 (but not by 4). Also it will not be divisible by 3. ∴ from options of part (a), $x = 2$.

Now the number can be $\frac{1394}{2}$ or $\frac{1934}{2}$ i.e. 697 or 967

Also note that for other products, the sum of digits is 12

∴ $y = 3$ or 6.

Now on checking, we get

$\frac{2091}{3} = 697$ and $\frac{2901}{3} = 967$.

∴ the number can be 697 or 967 while $y = 3$.

**So the correct options for (a), (b) and (c) are (i).**

**356.** Note that the sum of digits of $w, x, y, z$ are 16, 17, 14, 22 respectively, i.e. $w, x, y, z$ are of the form $9n + 7$, $9n + 8$, $9n + 5$, $9n + 4$ respectively. Now the sum of two of them will be equal to that of other two only if

$w + y = x + z$ [both of form: $9n + 12$]

$\Rightarrow (2, 5, 9) + (1, 6, 7) = (4, 6, 7) + (5, 8, 9)$

From R. H. S, the sum will have at least two carries (+1).

From the condition given in the problem (1 and 2 occupy same digit place in numbers of L.H.S) the sum (in L.H.S) will have two carries (+1)

Now if (1, 2) occupy the unit digit place or hundred digit place, then the digits at other places of the numbers can be switched, and correspondingly the digits of R.H.S. can also be switched, the new sum of both sides will still remain same.

Now if (1, 2) occupy the middle position, then they can similarly switch their positions with hundred digit place and with the corresponding change of digits of numbers of R.H.S, the new sum of both sides will still remain same.

**So the correct options for (a), (b), (c), (d) and (e) are (ii), (iv), (iv), (iv) and (iv) respectively.**

**357.** Let the product be *abcde*. Now when 13 divides 100, 1000 and 10000, the remainders are 9, 12 and 3 respectively.

$\therefore$ the product will be divisible by 13 only if

$$3a + 12b + 9c + 10d + e$$

i.e. $3(a - d) + (e - b) - 4c$ is divisible by 13.

Now $a + b + c + d + e = 2 + 4 + 5 + 7 + 9 = 27$

$\therefore$ $3(a - d) + (e - b) - 4(26 + 1 - a - b - d - e)$

must be divisible by 13.

Now the remainder $7a$, $d$, $5e$, $3b$ will leave $a$, when divided by 13, can be tabulated as:

| | | | | | | |
|---|---|---|---|---|---|---|
| $a, d, e, b$ | $\rightarrow$ | 2 | 4 | 5 | 7 | 9 |
| $7a$ | $\rightarrow$ | 1 | 2 | –4 | –3 | –2 |
| $d$ | $\rightarrow$ | 2 | 4 | 5 | –6 | –4 |
| $5e$ | $\rightarrow$ | –3 | –6 | –1 | –4 | 6 |
| $3b$ | $\rightarrow$ | 6 | –1 | 2 | –5 | 1 |

When a number from each row and distinct column is chosen, then their sum minus 4 must be divisible by 13. From inspection of above table, this sum must be

–9, –4 or 17.The possible cases can be for

$-9 \rightarrow (a, d, e, b) \equiv$ (2, 7, 4, 5); (2, 9, 5, 7) or (7, 9, 5, 4)

$-4 \rightarrow (a, d, e, b) \equiv$ (4, 7, 5, 9); (4, 9, 7, 5); (9, 2, 4, 5) or (9, 4, 5, 7)

$17 \rightarrow (a, d, e, b) \equiv$ Not possible

**So the correct options for (a), (b), (c), (d) and (e) are (iv), (ii), (ii), (i) and (ii) respectively.**

**358.** Note that $x + y = 909$ or $990$;
$y + z = 578, 587, 758, 785, 857$ or $875$;
$z + x = 247, 274, 427, 472, 724$ or $742$.

Note that $(x + y + z)$ will be divisible by 3 as the sum of sum of digits of $x + y$, $y + z$ and $z + x$ is divisible by 3.

Case I: Let 0 be at the unit digit place of $(x + y + z)$

$$\text{Then } \left.\begin{array}{lcl} x+y & = & 909 \\ y+z & = & 578 \text{ or } 758 \\ z+x & = & 274 \text{ or } 724 \end{array}\right\} \text{ or } \left.\begin{array}{ccc} & 990 & \\ 785 & \text{or} & 875 \\ 247 & \text{or} & 427 \end{array}\right\}$$

Add we have
$(909 + 587 + 724)/2 = 1110$ and
$(990 + 758 + 472)/2 = 1110$
$\therefore$ $(x, y, z) \equiv (523, 386, 201)$ and $(352, 638, 120)$

Case II: Let 1 be at the unit digit place of $(x + y + z)$

$$\text{Then } \left.\begin{array}{lcl} x+y & = & 909 \\ y+z & = & 578 \text{ or } 758 \\ z+x & = & 274 \text{ or } 724 \end{array}\right\} \text{ or } \left.\begin{array}{ccc} & 990 & \\ 785 & \text{or} & 875 \\ 247 & \text{or} & 427 \end{array}\right\}$$

And we have
$(990 + 758 + 274)/2 = 1011$ ] Not possible as
$(990 + 785 + 247)/2 = 1011$ ] $z$ is $a$ 3-digit integer
$(990 + 785 + 427)/2 = 1011$
$\therefore$ $(x, y, z) \equiv (316, 674, 111)$

**So the correct options for (a), (b), (c), (d) and (e) are (i), (iii), (iv), (iii) and (ii) respectively.**

**359.** Given : $A + 3678 = 2, 5, 6, x$ and
$A + 4321 = 1, 6, 7, y$

Taking difference, we get
$(1, 6, 7, y) - (2, 5, 6, x) = 643$
Note that the form of $(1, 6, 7, y)$ is $9n + 5 + y$
that of $(2, 5, 6, x)$ is $9n + 4 + x$ and
that of 643 is $9n + 4$

$\because$ the form of numbers on both sides of equality must be same $\therefore 1 + y - x = 4$ or $- 9 + 4$

$\Rightarrow y - x = 3$ or $- 6$

We can have two cases:

Case I: $y - x = 3$. Then

$(1, 6, 7, x + 3) - (2, 5, 6, x) = 0643$

Note that the difference of no two of the groups (1, 6, 7) and (2, 5, 6) is 3. $\therefore$ at least one of $x$ or $x + 3$ will be at the unit digit place in their respective numbers. We can have three subcases:

Subcase I: Both $x$ and $x + 3$ are at unit digit place. Then

$(1, 6, 7) - (2, 5, 6) = 064$

the only possibility is

$$\begin{array}{ccc} 7 & 1 & 6 \\ 6 & 5 & 2 \\ \hline 0 & 6 & 4 \end{array}$$

$\therefore A + 3678 = 652x$

$$\Rightarrow A = \begin{array}{cccc} 6 & 5 & 2 & x \\ 3 & 6 & 7 & 8 \\ \hline 2 & 8 & 4 & - \end{array} \quad \text{(Note that } x < 8\text{)}$$

Note that all the parts can be done with the use of above informations. So we need not check subcases II, III or Case II.

**So the correct options for (a), (b), (c) and (d) are (ii), (ii), (iv) and (ii) respectively.**

**360.** Note that the form of numbers which digits are

| | | |
|---|---|---|
| (3, 5, 7) | is | $9n + 6$ |
| (4, 6, 8) | is | $9n + 0$ |
| (1, 7, 9) | is | $9n + 8$ |
| (1, 2, 3, 8) | is | $9n + 5$ (or 14) |
| (1, 1, 5, 8) | is | $9n + 6$ |
| (1, 3, 4, 9) | is | $9n + 8$. |

$\because$ the forms also add up

$\therefore$ (3, 5, 7) + (4, 6, 8) = (1, 1, 5, 8) ...(i)

(3, 5, 7) + (1, 7, 9) = (1, 2, 3, 8) ...(ii)

(4, 6, 8) + (1, 7, 9) = (1, 3, 4, 9) ...(iii)

From equation (i), 8 cannot be first, second or fourth digit of the number (1, 1, 5, 8) $\therefore$ it will be the third digit. $\therefore$ (1, 1, 5, 8) will be 1185 or 1581.

For 1185, the numbers in L.H.S of equation (i) will be 537 and 648.

For 1581, the numbers in L.H.S of equation (i) will be 735 and 846.

For 537, the second number in equation (ii) will be 791 and for 735, the second number is not possible.

$\therefore$ the three numbers are 537, 648 and 791 and S = 1976.

**So the correct options for (a), (b), (c) and (d) are (iv), (iii), (iii) and (iv) respectively.**

## Reader's Notes

# Reader's Notes

## Reader's Notes

## Reader's Notes

# Reader's Notes

# Reader's Notes